PHARMACOGENOMICS
A Primer for Clinicians

PHARMACOGENOMICS
A Primer for Clinicians

EDITORS

Jerika T. Lam, PharmD, APh, AAHIVP
Associate Professor, Department of Pharmacy Practice
School of Pharmacy
Chapman University
Irvine, California

Mary A. Gutierrez, PharmD
Professor, Department of Pharmacy Practice (Psychiatry)
School of Pharmacy
Chapman University
Irvine, California

Samit Shah, PhD, RPh, MBA
Dean, School of Pharmacy
Rueckert-Hartman College for Health Professions
Regis University
Denver, Colorado

New York   Chicago   San Francisco   Athens   London   Madrid   Mexico City
Milan   New Delhi   Singapore   Sydney   Toronto

1 2 3 4 5 6 7 8 9   LOV   26 25 24 23 22 21

ISBN 978-1-260-45710-0
MHID 1-260-45710-9

This book was set in Adobe Jenson Pro by MPS Limited.
The editors were Michael Weitz and Peter J. Boyle.
The production supervisor was Richard Ruzycka.
The text was designed by Mary McKeon.
The cover designer was W2 Design.
Project management was provided by Jyoti Shaw, MPS Limited.

This book is printed on acid-free paper.

Library of Congress Control Number: 2021930910

I dedicate this textbook to my parents and siblings for their unwavering love and guidance. My parents' determination and strength in overcoming their struggles and challenges have taught me that anything is possible through education, perseverance, and resourcefulness. They have inspired me to go the extra distance in life, as well as kept me grounded.

—Jerika Lam

CONTENTS

CONTRIBUTORS

Lucas A. Berenbrok, PharmD, MS, BCACP, TTS
Assistant Professor
Department of Pharmacy and Therapeutics
University of Pittsburgh School of Pharmacy
Pittsburgh, Pennsylvania
Chapter 1

Christine L. Cadiz, PharmD, MA, BCPS
Health Sciences Assistant Clinical Professor
Department of Clinical Pharmacy Practice
UCI School of Pharmacy and Pharmaceutical Sciences
Susan and Henry Samueli College of Health Sciences
Irvine, California
Chapter 9

Kelly E. Caudle, PharmD, PhD, BCPS
Co-PI and Director, CPIC
Department of Pharmaceutical Sciences
St. Jude Children's Research Hospital
Memphis, Tennessee
Chapter 4

Emily J. Cicali, PharmD, BCPS
Clinical Assistant Professor
Department of Pharmacotherapy and Translational
Research
College of Pharmacy, University of Florida
Gainesville, Florida
Chapter 2

Rachel Daut, PhD
Medical Science Liaison
Myriad Neuroscience
Mason, Ohio
Chapter 8

Julio D. Duarte, PharmD, PhD
Assistant Professor
Center for Pharmacogenomics and Precision Medicine
Department of Pharmacotherapy and Translational

Research
College of Pharmacy, University of Florida
Gainesville, Florida
Chapter 2

Roseann S. Gammal, PharmD, BCPS
Assistant Professor
Department of Pharmacy Practice
MCPHS University School of Pharmacy
Boston, Massachusetts
Chapter 4

Mary A. Gutierrez, PharmD, BCPP
Professor, Department of Pharmacy Practice (Psychiatry)
School of Pharmacy
Chapman University
Irvine, California
Chapter 8

David R. Ha, PharmD, BCIDP
Infectious Diseases Pharmacist
Stanford Antimicrobial Safety and Sustainability Program
Stanford Healthcare
Palo Alto, California
Chapter 9

Kim Hamann, MS CGC
Medical Science Liaison
Myriad Neuroscience
Mason, Ohio
Chapter 8

Daniel L. Hertz, PharmD, PhD
Assistant Professor
Department of Clinical Pharmacy
University of Michigan College of Pharmacy
Ann Arbor, Michigan
Chapter 7

Jerika T. Lam, PharmD, AAHIVP
Associate Professor, Department of Pharmacy Practice
School of Pharmacy
Chapman University
Irvine, California
Chapter 6

Whitney D. Maxwell, PharmD, MBA, BCPS
Clinical Associate Professor
Department of Clinical Pharmacy and Outcomes Sciences
University of South Carolina College of Pharmacy
Columbia, South Carolina
Chapter 5

Lisa S. Parker, PhD
Dickie, McCamey, and Chilcote Professor of Bioethics
Center for Bioethics and Health Law
University of Pittsburgh
Pittsburgh, Pennsylvania
Chapter 3

Amy L. Pasternak, PharmD, BCPS
Clinical Assistant Professor
Department of Clinical Pharmacy
University of Michigan College of Pharmacy
Ann Arbor, Michigan
Chapter 7

Natasha J. Petry, PharmD, BCACP
Associate Professor, Department of Pharmacy Practice
School of Pharmacy, North Dakota State University
Fargo, North Dakota
Pharmacogenetics Clinical Pharmacist, Sanford Health
Imagenetics
Sioux Falls, South Dakota
Chapter 2

Moom R. Roosan, PharmD, PhD
Assistant Professor, Department of Pharmacy Practice
School of Pharmacy, Chapman University
Irvine, California
Chapter 2

James M. Stevenson, PharmD, MS, BCPP
Assistant Professor
Division of Clinical Pharmacology, Department of Medicine
School of Medicine, Johns Hopkins University
Baltimore, Maryland
Chapter 1

PREFACE

Since the completion of the Human Genome Project in 2003, there has been a plethora of scientific research in genetics and the molecular characterization of various diseases, such as cancer. President Obama's announcement and endorsement of precision medicine in the 2015 State of the Union address further mobilized many federal and private institutions to promote, collaborate on, and intensify efforts to use the human genome information to optimize patient care and outcomes. The main goal of the Precision Medicine Initiative was to support research in pharmacogenomics, the delivery of targeted therapeutics, and the sharing of genetic data in electronic health records.

The Food and Drug Administration (FDA) has since developed a website with labeling changes for over 130 medications and includes its recommendations or requirements for pharmacogenetics testing prior to prescribing the medications. The labeling information contains clinical evidence for genotype-guided treatments based on pharmacogenomic information that affects drug exposure and clinical response variability, risk for adverse events, and polymorphic drug target and disposition genes. Similarly, two well-known resources that offer pharmacogenomics information include the Clinical Pharmacogenetics Implementation Consortium (CPIC) and Pharmacogenomics Knowledge Base (PharmGKB). They disseminate actionable recommendations and guidelines to clinicians for genotype-guided therapy for specific drug–gene pairs.

There is also growing evidence that pharmacogenomics and precision medicine are influencing the future of professional health education and clinical practice. We have observed the incorporation of pharmacogenomics in the curricula of medical and pharmacy schools. The national professional entities that recognize the significant role of pharmacogenomics and its impact in the future of health care and how it could lead to improved patient health outcomes include the American Medical Association (AMA), American Society of Health-System Pharmacists (ASHP), and American Association of Colleges of Pharmacy (AACP).

In clinical practice, we have noticed patients who experience subtherapeutic efficacy in spite of receiving maximum daily dosages of their medications, as well as patients who experience severe adverse events from the standard recommended medication dosages. Many pharmacological treatments are complex for the myriad of conditions and diseases that a patient has, not including their genetic variability. As a result, this textbook is created for clinicians who are interested in practicing precision medicine by using the science of pharmacogenomics and making actionable, genotype-guided recommendations to optimize treatments for their patients. Furthermore, this textbook contains updated information about pharmacogenomics resources and the ethical and legal considerations to assist clinicians who are interested in implementing pharmacogenomics in practice settings.

This textbook also includes the fundamentals of pharmacogenomics and therapeutics topics that have the most significant and evidence-based recommendations from scientific and clinical studies. The therapeutics chapters are laid out in a clear and concise format that includes the mechanism of drug–gene interaction, consequences of drug–gene interaction, and genotype-guided treatment recommendations to help clinicians make evidence-based decisions and recommendations. Additionally, the textbook contains tables, figures, and case scenarios in each chapter to stimulate critical thinking and reinforce the main concepts. Each chapter also has a clinical pearls section to highlight and summarize the key takeaways.

Recognizing that research in pharmacogenomics is rapidly increasing, I hope the readers will find the textbook useful in helping them implement and apply pharmacogenomics in their clinical practice. More importantly, I hope the textbook will serve as an essential resource for clinicians who desire to practice precision medicine in order to optimize treatments based on their patients' genetic variability and promote patient safety.

Jerika T. Lam
December 2020

CHAPTER 1

INTRODUCTION AND FUNDAMENTALS OF PHARMACOGENOMICS

James M. Stevenson and Lucas A. Berenbrok

LEARNING OBJECTIVES

1. Summarize scientific advances that have furthered the field of pharmacogenomics.

2. Apply the principles of "personalized" or "precision" medicine to drug therapy.

3. Define common terms and nomenclature used in pharmacogenomics.

OVERVIEW AND HISTORY

Historical Perspective of Precision Medicine

In 2015, President Barack Obama announced the launch of the Precision Medicine Initiative in his State of the Union address to the nation. The mission of the initiative is "to enable a new era of medicine through research, technology, and policies that empower patients, researchers, and providers to work together toward development of individualized care."[1] The term "personalized medicine" has also been used to describe this individualized care; however, the term "precision medicine" is favored so as not to presume that the care that patients will receive will differ from each other.[1]

In this new era of precision medicine, treatment and prevention of disease are tailored to the individual. Such individualization contrasts with traditional approaches to care, which have largely relied on "one-size-fits-all" models. Individualized care considers unique characteristics

of individuals, including past medical history, family history, lifestyle, diet, microbiome, and genome sequence. Pharmacogenomics uses the individual's genomic sequence to predict drug response and is essential to achieving the mission of precision medicine. However, the science and art of prescribing pharmacotherapy are not perfect.

As mentioned, the selection of drug therapy has largely relied on the "one-size-fits-all" approach due to the homogeneity commonly seen in clinical trials leading to the approval of new drugs by the U.S. Food and Drug Administration (FDA). Furthermore, diverse responses to drug therapy are often not observed until postmarketing use, which can characterize and stratify drug response to the uniqueness of individuals rather than strict inclusion and exclusion criteria of the randomized, placebo-controlled clinical trial. Many individuals will fail pharmacotherapy at first, and some individuals will trial two or more unique drugs before finding effectiveness with minimal adverse effects. Pharmacogenomics enters here with the promise of predicting drug response for better clinical outcomes and less adverse events. As the data supporting specific gene–drug pairs grow, we can expect that pharmacogenomics will lead to more actionable changes to prescribing that meet the mission of the Precision Medicine Initiative.

Advances in Technology Leading to the Present State of Precision Medicine

In 1990, the Human Genome Project, an international research endeavor coordinated by the U.S. National Institutes of Health and the U.S. Department of Energy, set out to sequence a complete and accurate sequence of the human genome and to locate the exact location of an estimated 20,000 to 25,000 human genes. Fourteen years later, the sequencing of the first entire human genome was completed, including more than 3 billion DNA base pairs, and made publicly available for others to build upon the work.[2] This complete sequence of the human genome made available the first ever blueprint for human beings, a peek into the most fundamental building blocks of what makes us human. The process of mapping the human genome has since been significantly reduced to a few weeks. Such advances have opened the door for researchers and clinicians to use DNA to study, create new knowledge, and implement this knowledge into modern medicine, including pharmacotherapy. In more recent history, laboratory companies have created avenues for pharmacogenomic testing that can return results in as little as 4 to 6 weeks, which can provide clinicians and patients with preemptive or reactive testing avenues. The former refers to when pharmacogenomic testing is performed in anticipation of a possible future clinical need for the drug, and the latter refers to when testing is performed after the clinical need for the drug is determined.

The term pharmacogenetics originated in the late 1950s and has since been used to define how DNA, or individual genes, may affect drug response.[3] More specifically, pharmacogenetics refers to the effects of a specific gene, and pharmacogenomics refers broadly to genomic differences. Regardless of this nuance, the terms are often used interchangeably. For the purposes of this chapter, the term pharmacogenomics will be used throughout.

As the science of identifying individual genes predicted to affect drug response grows, so does the clinical use of drugs in terms of both safety and effectiveness of use. Over 250 drugs have pharmacogenomic biomarkers in their labeling. A current and comprehensive list of drugs with pharmacogenomic biomarkers in their labeling can be found on the FDA's website.[4] Standard drug labeling accompanies all drugs approved by the FDA. These sections of the FDA prescribing information where pharmacogenomic information appears include adverse reactions, black-boxed warning, clinical pharmacology, clinical studies, contraindications, dosage and administration, drug interactions, indications and usage, overdosage, use in specific populations, and warnings and precautions. To sample the array of FDA-approved drugs with biomarkers related to pharmacogenomics, the following therapeutic areas are represented: anesthesiology, cardiology, dental, dermatology, endocrinology, gastroenterology, gynecology, hematology, inborn errors of metabolism, infectious diseases, neurology, oncology, psychiatry, pulmonology, rheumatology, toxicology, transplantation, and urology. For further perspective, it has been estimated that nearly 50% of the U.S. population enrolled in Medicare and Medicaid received at least one drug with an available pharmacogenomic guideline.[5]

GENETICS 101

DNA Structure

DNA, or deoxyribonucleic acid, is the blueprint for life. Made up of the nucleic acids adenosine, cytosine, guanine, and thymidine (ACGT), DNA codes for every component and process of our living body. The human genome consists of approximately 3 billion base pairs intricately organized to code life. The human genome consists of 23 chromosome pairs, 22 of which are autosomal and 1 of which defines sex (Figure 1-1). One set of chromosomes is inherited from the father and the other from the mother. In each chromosome, the DNA helix is intricately woven around proteins, or histones, to form compact structures which can fit inside the nucleus of a cell. These strands are made of a helical pairing of base pairs A, C, G, and T (Figure 1-2). Understanding how this code is formed and replicated in the process of transcription and translation is necessary to understand how variants in this code can affect an individual's response to drug therapy.

Transcription/Translation

Of the estimated 20,000 to 25,000 genes that make up the human genome, approximately 1% of DNA codes for proteins. The other 99% of DNA is known as noncoding DNA. Proteins are important because they carry out the functions needed for cellular activity and ultimately for life. The process in which a gene is used to

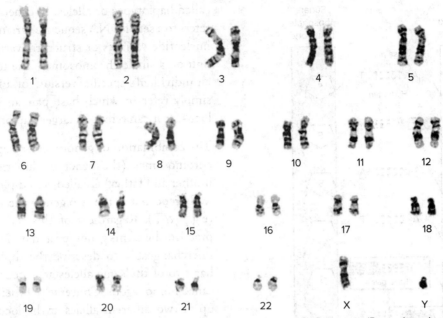

FIGURE 1-1 • The human genome: 22 pairs of autosomes and one pair of sex chromosomes. (Reproduced, with permission, from McCarthy JJ, Mendelsohn BA. *Precision Medicine: A Guide to Genomics in Clinical Practice.* New York, NY: McGraw Hill; 2017.)

direct the synthesis of proteins is called gene expression. This process begins in the nucleus of the cell with transcription. Transcription is the first step in the process of gene expression. Transcription copies information from the DNA code, found in the nucleus, into messenger RNA (mRNA). mRNA is a single strand of code, complementary to DNA, that transfers information from DNA to the cytoplasm of the cell for protein synthesis. Transcription is initiated when the enzyme ribonucleic acid (RNA) polymerase binds to a region of the DNA called the promoter region, with other proteins called transcription factors (Figure 1-3). Once transcription begins, a complementary strand of mRNA is created from the DNA template by the RNA polymerase and transcription factor complex. Ultimately, this newly created strand of mRNA will exit the nucleus of eukaryotic cells to serve as the archetype for protein synthesis, a process called translation.

Translation is the second step in the process of gene expression. Translation, or the process of protein synthesis, occurs in the cytoplasm of eukaryotic cells. Like transcription, two tools are needed for translation. These tools are called ribosomes and transfer RNA (tRNA). Ribosomes are proteins that assemble polypeptides by reading the mRNA and matching tRNA to appropriate codons. tRNA transfers amino acids, the building blocks of proteins, to the ribosome for assembly (Figure 1-4). Translation is terminated by a stop codon in the mRNA sequence. Once translation

ends, the protein may require further processing to assume the correct shape before it can be fully functional. When errors in transcription or translation occur, proteins may lose their structure and/or function.

DNA Replication

DNA replication is the process of creating two identical copies of DNA molecules from one original molecule. Each strand of the original DNA molecule, or parent strand, acts as the blueprint for the resulting identical copies or daughter strands. The process of DNA replication is necessary for cell division. DNA replication occurs in the nucleus of a eukaryotic cell in three steps. First, the double-helical structure of the DNA must be opened and separated. Second, the DNA parent strands, which serve as the templates, must be prepared for replication. Last, new DNA strands are created by the enzyme DNA polymerase. DNA replication occurs with high fidelity, and errors are estimated to be at only one incorrect base pair per 10^9 to 10^{10} nucleotides assembled.

NOMENCLATURE/TERMINOLOGY: FROM GENOTYPE TO PHENOTYPE

A specific position along a chromosome (or put in another way, location in the genome) is called a locus. A locus (plural: loci) can refer to a single base pair or a larger region such as an entire gene. An individual's DNA sequence at

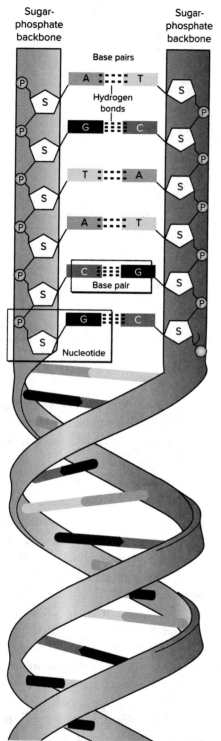

FIGURE 1-2 • The double helix structure of DNA. (Reprinted from National Human Genome Research Institute, NIH, Washington, DC. Phosphate Backbone. https://www.genome.gov/genetics-glossary/Phosphate-Backbone. Accessed August 18, 2020.)

a locus on one of their chromosomes (the chromosome inherited from *either* the mother or the father) is called a genotype. Genetic loci near one another on a single chromosome tend to be inherited together. As a result, DNA on a given chromosome tends to be inherited in "blocks"

called haplotypes or alleles. In other words, a haplotype refers to a set of DNA sequence variants, including single-nucleotide variants or structural variants, inherited as a unit on a single chromosome.[6] The term "allele" refers to an individual's specific "version" of a locus. An allele can simply refer to which base pair an individual has at a locus, or it can refer to a larger haplotype block.

The combination of genotypes or haplotypes from both chromosomes (the genotype inherited from *both* the mother and father) is called as a diplotype, which is typically reported as the two genotypes separated by a slash (e.g., A/T). Regardless of this technical difference, in practice, the terms genotype and diplotype are often used interchangeably to describe the diplotype. If a person has two of the same alleles at a locus, their diplotype is called homozygous. Conversely, if their diplotype is made up of two different alleles at the locus, the diplotype is termed heterozygous. The diplotype is translated into a predicted phenotype or metabolizer status (i.e., poor metabolizer, intermediate metabolizer, normal metabolizer, rapid metabolizer, and ultrarapid metabolizer), which clinicians use for prescribing drugs.[6]

In many well-characterized genes relevant to pharmacogenomics, a standardized nomenclature has been developed to promote research generalizability and clinical translation of research. The star (*) allele system is used to describe the versions of a gene the individual carries without requiring the investigator to describe the entire genetic sequence of the gene.[7] A regularly updated database called PharmVar documents observed star alleles and their effect on gene function (for more information, see Chapter 4).[8] Generally, the *1 allele represents the gene's "normal" version that encodes a functional enzyme.

Phenotype refers to the observable consequence of genetic variation. Classic examples of phenotypes include eye color and blood type. How the genotype determines the phenotype depends on the genetic model of the phenotype. Recessive phenotypes only occur in individuals homozygous for the causative allele. Dominant phenotypes only require one copy of the causative allele. When there is incomplete dominance, the phenotype for heterozygotes is distinct from and usually in between the phenotype of either homozygote. In addition, some phenotypes are determined by many genes, while others are determined by a single gene. Phenotypes in pharmacogenomics are related to medications or medication-related processes. For example, an individual may metabolize paroxetine poorly (slowly) because of his or her genotype in a gene

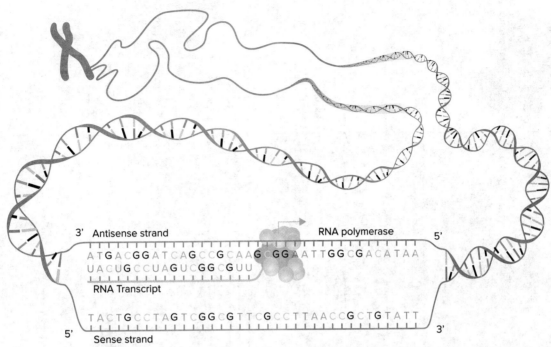

FIGURE 1-3 · Transcription—the process of creating RNA from DNA. (Reprinted from National Human Genome Research Institute, NIH, Washington, DC. Antisense. https://www.genome.gov/genetics-glossary/antisense. Accessed August 18, 2020.)

encoding a relevant drug-metabolizing enzyme. Often in clinical pharmacogenomics, we refer to the individual's "predicted phenotypes" or "metabolizer status."

An individual predicted to be an ultrarapid metabolizer for a given enzyme is expected, based on his or her genetics, to metabolize substrates of that enzyme at a faster-than-average rate. But this genetically predicted phenotype does not always match the observed phenotype. For example, an individual predicted to be an ultrarapid metabolizer based on genetics may, in actuality, metabolize enzyme substrates *slower* than average if they are concurrently treated with a strong inhibitor of the said enzyme. This mismatch between genetically predicted phenotype and observed phenotype because of environmental or clinical factors is termed phenoconversion.

GENETIC VARIATION WITHIN HUMAN POPULATIONS

Humans are roughly 99.9% identical in DNA sequence, but due to the size of the genome, this translates to 4 to 5 million base-pair differences between any two individuals.[9] Genes that encode proteins involved in essential physiologic processes are largely conserved (nearly identical) between individuals because aberrant protein function in these pathways is not compatible with life. Other genes can be highly polymorphic (varying greatly from one individual

to the next), with some individuals' genes encoding nonfunctional proteins or excessive amounts of protein.

Generally speaking, every cell in an individual's body has the same DNA sequence. Cells continually divide into two new identical cells for the purpose of growth and replacement of dead cells. During this process, DNA must be replicated so that the new cells have an identical DNA sequence to the original cell. On occasion, there are errors in this process, such as an incorrect nucleotide. Usually, cellular repair processes identify and correct these errors, but when the repair processes also fail, a new mutation is introduced into the genome of these new cells.

The spontaneous generation of mutations is not the only, or most common, source of DNA variation between individual humans. If a genetic variant confers an advantageous trait for a population—that is, one that increases the chance of producing offspring—over many generations of reproduction, that variant will become more common in that environment due to natural selection. Note that whether a trait is advantageous depends on the environment, which results in differences in variant frequency across populations. A classic example is the sickle-cell anemia trait, which causes an illness that one would assume is disadvantageous. However, the sickle-cell trait also reduces susceptibility to malaria, and having malaria reduces the probability

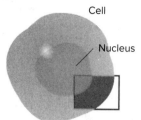

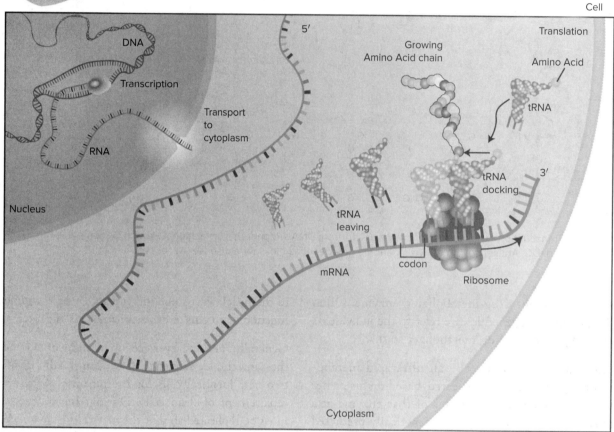

FIGURE 1-4 • Translation—the process of using RNA to create a polypeptide/protein. (Reprinted from National Human Genome Research Institute, NIH, Washington, DC. https://www.genome.gov/sites/default/files/tg/en/illustration/translation.jpg. Accessed August 18, 2020.)

of producing offspring. As a result, the genetic variants causing sickle-cell anemia are relatively more common in populations derived from areas with high malaria prevalence compared to areas where the antimalarial advantage is irrelevant.

Sexual reproduction itself produces genetic variation, as the offspring inherits its genome approximately equally from the mother and father. The offspring may be heterozygous at loci in which each parent was homozygous. In addition, there is a process called recombination, or "crossing over," in which paired chromosomes from the mother and father combine. This "shuffles" DNA on the chromosome, resulting in new alleles in the offspring that were not observed in the mother's or father's DNA (Figure 1-5).

Many genetic differences have no known biological consequence. Other variants can cause increased expression, decreased expression, or a functionally different protein. The concept of genomic differences between two individuals can reflect small differences (a single base-pair difference) or very large (absence or extra copies of a chromosome). Differences in the number of chromosomes between individuals can result in profound developmental disorders but are not directly applicable to pharmacogenomics. More subtle variations, such as insertion/deletion of genomic regions, copy number variation (CNV), and single-nucleotide variants/polymorphisms, are more relevant to the field of pharmacogenomics. In general, the more subtle mechanisms of genetic variation are more common, with individuals typically carrying

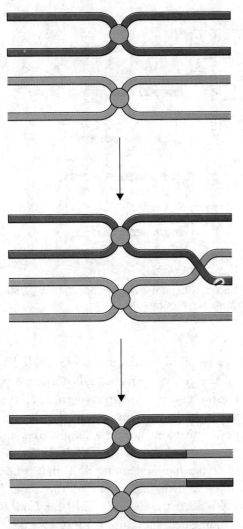

FIGURE 1-5 • Crossing over creates new combinations of al-leles. (Reproduced, with permission, from Rodwell VW, Bender DA, Botham KM, Kennelly PJ, Weil PA. *Harper's Illustrated Biochemistry.* 31st ed. New York, NY: McGraw Hill; 2018.)

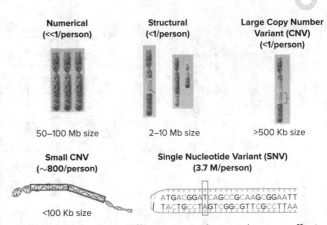

FIGURE 1-6 • Genomic differences can be very large or affect only a single nucleotide. More radical types of variation are rarer. (Reproduced, with permission, from McCarthy JJ, Mendelsohn BA. *Precision Medicine: A Guide to Genomics in Clinical Practice.* New York, NY: McGraw Hill; 2017.)

more than 3 million single-nucleotide variants compared to a reference genome (Figure 1-6).

When an individual's genotype at a given locus matches the most common "normal" genotype in a population, we refer to the genotype as "wild type." Wild type can also refer to the most common "normal" phenotype in a population. The less common genotype, or allele, at the locus is called the minor allele. Population geneticists often refer to the minor allele frequency, which describes what percentage of alleles in a population are the minor version. The terms "single-nucleotide variant" (SNV) and "single-nucleotide polymorphism" (SNP) refer to situations in which a single base pair of a sequence is altered. The term SNP is typically used instead of SNV when the polymorphism is relatively common (minor allele

frequency >1%). Because most clinically used pharmacogenomic associations deal with common genetic variants, we will use the term SNP throughout the chapter instead of SNV, though most of the principles will apply to SNVs as well.

Copy Number Variations and Deletions in Pharmacogenomics

Some genes relevant to pharmacogenomics are known to vary in copy number between individuals. Entire genes can be deleted or duplicated in some individuals. Clearly, if a genomic region is outright deleted, the protein products of deleted genes will not be produced. Duplications of genes can result in excess protein products. For practical examples of these concepts in pharmacogenomics, refer to sections focusing on the drug-metabolizing enzyme CYP2D6 in this chapter and throughout the text. Differences in copy number do not only apply to entire genes but can also be observed in smaller sections of the genome. The serotonin transporter gene *SLC6A4* contains regions in which genomic units <25 base pairs in length are tandemly repeated to different extents between individuals.

SNPs in Coding and Noncoding Regions

Though we consider SNPs a more "subtle" form of genetic variation, SNPs can have profound effects on the protein target through multiple mechanisms. Variation in regulatory regions can affect binding of transcription factors and ultimately gene expression. SNPs in splice sites can create abnormal transcripts. Single-nucleotide changes

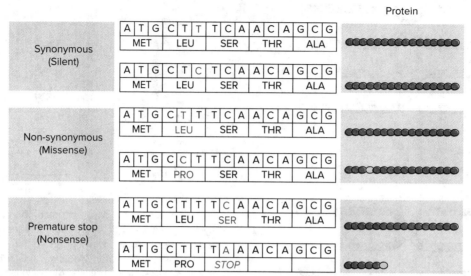

FIGURE 1-7 • The functional consequence of SNPs in coding regions. (Reproduced, with permission, from McCarthy JJ, Mendelsohn BA. *Precision Medicine: A Guide to Genomics in Clinical Practice.* New York, NY: McGraw Hill; 2017.)

to the coding region of genes can be inconsequential or can have large effects on protein function. Coding synonymous variants do not change the amino acid sequence of the protein and typically do not affect protein function. Nonsynonymous (also called missense) variants cause a substitution of one amino acid, which may or may not affect protein function. Similarly, SNPs can result in the creation of a stop codon, which halts transcription resulting in a truncated version of the protein product. Figure 1-7 provides a visual representation of these SNP consequences.

Describing Genetic Variation

Various types of nomenclature are used to describe genetic variants in research and clinical literature. SNPs are sometimes described in a format that describes the gene name, location of the polymorphism, the wild-type nucleotide, and the variant nucleotide. For example, "CYP2C19 c.681G>A" refers to a polymorphism in the gene *CYP2C19*. The "c.681" portion refers to where in the *CYP2C19* gene the polymorphism occurs. The "G>A" portion of this nomenclature tells us that G is the wild-type nucleotide that is changed to the variant nucleotide version A.

This same SNP can be described by its reference SNP ID number, often simply referred to as its rsID or rs#. The National Center for Biotechnology Information (NCBI) assigns these numbers, and its databases can be queried using this nomenclature. In this case, rs4244285 describes the exact same SNP as CYP2C19 c.681 G>A.

Sometimes we need to describe not a single SNP, but a block of the genetic sequence called a haplotype. For many important genes in pharmacogenomics, the aforementioned star allele system was developed to describe haplotypes. This nomenclature simply uses the gene name and the star allele (e.g., CYP2C19*2). Many of these haplotypes have a defining SNP that is not found in the other known haplotypes of the gene. In this case, rs4244285 is the defining SNP for CYP2C19*2. Thus, in biomedical literature CYP2C19 c.681 G>A, rs4244285, and CYP2C19*2 are essentially describing the same polymorphism.

GENETIC ASSAY TECHNOLOGY

Unsurprisingly, there have been great technological advances in the methods used to determine genetic variation. Different types of variations in genes (e.g., SNPs vs. CNVs) often require different types of assays to properly characterize the variation. For some genes that are known to have multiple forms of a genetic variation, samples may need to be tested on multiple platforms in order to provide an accurate and comprehensive genotype.

Most assays currently used in clinical pharmacogenomics applications are considered targeted genotyping. These technologies only interrogate a small and relevant subset of genes within the human genome and do not assay genes outside the areas of interest. Consequently, these technologies are not ideal for discovering new genetic associations with disease or drug outcomes, since only known variants in a small subset of genes are assayed.

This approach will most likely fail to detect a rare variant in a gene of interest that influences drug response or an important variant in a gene not covered by the targeted assay. To the contrary, these technologies are often acceptable for clinical pharmacogenomics applications, given their relatively low cost, quick turnaround time, and the fact that most pharmacogenomics associations considered "actionable" are well-defined and detectable on commercial pharmacogenomics platforms. Targeted genotyping can be deployed to detect only a single base-pair locus (assay just one SNP) or can assay thousands of predefined SNPs in a single run. These multiplexed assays, called SNP microarrays, or sometimes simply arrays, are commonly used in clinical pharmacogenomics. Arrays can also cover SNPs across the entire genome and be used in research studies to identify novel genetic associations (for more detail, see Discovery/Research Approaches later).

Sequencing is a strategy that differs from targeted SNP genotyping or arrays in that it directly assays each and every base pair in an area of interest. Sequencing techniques can be targeted toward a particular gene or locus of interest, or it can be applied across the entire exome or genome. Exome refers to the portion of the genome consisting of exons—the part of the DNA that provides coding information for peptides/proteins. Whole-genome or -exome sequencing generates large data files that can be used for genomic medicine applications beyond pharmacogenomics. The downsides to whole-genome or -exome sequencing are longer turnaround time, computational/labor demands for interpretation, data storage concerns when performed at scale, and financial cost.

The purpose of this textbook is to cover germline pharmacogenomics. In the broader precision medicine context, tumor sequencing, identification of driver mutations, and mutation-specific treatments have been well-studied and implemented clinically in oncology. However, these topics are outside the scope of the present context. Likewise, epigenetics is a rapidly growing area of study that is beyond the scope of this text. Epigenetics refers to mechanisms of gene regulation that are not dependent on differences in DNA sequence.

Can Test Results for an Individual "Change"?

With few exceptions, an individual's DNA sequence does not change throughout the lifetime. This is one reason the promise of pharmacogenomics is so appealing—pharmacogenomics testing can be performed once and will provide clinical value throughout the patient's entire life. But while the patient's DNA sequence will not change throughout one's lifetime, it is likely that testing methodology and genotype/predicted phenotype relationships will change.

In many clinical contexts today, arrays are used that do not directly interrogate each base pair of the genome. If we discover in the future that there are important genetic loci that were not covered on the arrays of today, retesting of patients may be necessary. This scenario is far from hypothetical, as new star alleles for important drug-metabolizing enzymes are described each year. Likewise, our understanding of the functional consequences of known genetic variants evolves over time. A genotype that today is predicted to produce a normal metabolizer of a particular drug-metabolizing enzyme may be reclassified to predict a rapid metabolizer phenotype in the future as research evidence accumulates. In short, DNA sequences will not change over a lifetime, but the ways that we test and interpret results are likely to.

RATIONALE FOR GENETIC INFLUENCE ON DRUG RESPONSE

Pharmacokinetic Basis for Genetic Influence on Drug Response

Drug-Metabolizing Enzymes

The human genome contains more than 50 presumably functional cytochrome P450 (CYP) genes that are responsible for the metabolism of many endogenous compounds, medications, and xenobiotics.[10] Many of the relevant drug-metabolizing enzymes are primarily expressed in the liver, but many of these enzymes are found in other tissues such as the gut and brain. There is considerable interpatient variability in CYP enzyme activity, which in some cases can be explained by genetic variation in the gene encoding a given CYP enzyme.

In addition to genetic factors, variation in enzyme function can be due to fixed (i.e., sex) or dynamic factors that change over a lifetime. Some of the most common dynamic factors that can affect enzyme function are age, drug exposure, and illness. Behavioral factors, such as medication nonadherence, also represent a source of pharmacokinetic variability.

CYP2D6. CYP2D6 is responsible for the metabolism or bioactivation of approximately 25% of all marketed drugs, spanning a wide range of indications and drug classes.[11] These drugs include several antidepressants, antipsychotics, analgesics, and anticancer agents, among others. Interpatient variability in the metabolism of CYP2D6 substrates was first described in the 1970s, with specific genetic variants first associated with metabolizing phenotype in the 1980s.[12–14]

CYP2D6 is one of the most polymorphic human genes, and the gene can be deleted outright or duplicated in some individuals. More than 130 different alleles have been documented, leading to null, decreased, normal, or increased enzyme activity.[15] For this reason, thought leaders in CYP2D6 research are constantly receiving reports of new alleles and attempting to assign a predicted function to each.

The CYP2D6 activity score (AS) is a commonly used mechanism for translating genotype to predicted phenotype. Experts assign a value to each known allele: 0 for no function, 0.25 or 0.5 for decreased function, or 1 for normal function.[16] If an allele is duplicated, the value is multiplied by the number of copies. An individual's AS is the sum of the values from their two alleles. For example, an individual with the CYP2D6 *1/*4 diplotype has one normal-function allele and one no-function allele, and thus would have an AS of $1 + 0 = 1$. An individual with the CYP2D6 $*1 \times 2/*4$ diplotype, in which the *1 allele is duplicated, has an AS of $1 \times 2 + 0 = 2$. Individuals are functionally classified as poor, intermediate, normal, or ultrarapid metabolizers (PM, IM, NM, and UM, respectively) based on their CYP2D6 AS. Current standards for converting AS to phenotype are shown in Table 1-1.

The CYP2C9 Family. The clinically important enzymes CYP2C19 and CYP2C9 are encoded by genes located in what is called the CYP2C cluster on chromosome 10, which is composed of CYP2C8, CYP2C9, CYP2C19, and CYP2C18 in that order. CYP2C19 metabolizes a wide variety of currently used drugs, including antiplatelet agents, antidepressants, proton pump inhibitors, and antifungals. Notably, the prodrug antiplatelet agent clopidogrel is primarily dependent on CYP2C19 for its activation. Several nonfunctional alleles have been described for CYP2C19, as well as the *17 allele, which confers increased expression. Individuals are often characterized by the number of functional and increased expression alleles into one of five functional groups: PM, IM, NM, rapid metabolizer (RM), or UM (Table 1-2). Population frequencies of the phenotype groups vary greatly by ethnicity. Approximately 2% to 5% of white European individuals and African Americans are

TABLE 1-1. CYP2D6 Activity Score Translated to Metabolizer Phenotype Group

Activity Score (AS)	Predicted CYP2D6 Phenotype
0	PM
$0 < x \leq 1$	IM
$1 < x \leq 2.25$	NM
>2.25	UM

TABLE 1-2. CYP2C19 Functional Metabolizer Status Definitions

Metabolizer Status	Definition	Example CYP2C19 Diplotype
PM	Two no-function alleles	*2/*2
IM	One no-function allele and one normal- or increased-function allele	*2/*17
NM	Two normal-function alleles	*1/*1
RM	One normal-function allele and one increased-function allele	*1/*17
UM	Two increased-function alleles	*17/*17

PM: Poor metabolizer, IM: intermediate metabolizer, NM: normal metabolizer, RM: rapid metabolizer, UM: ultra-rapid metabolizer

Source: Data from Caudle KE, Dunnenberger HM, Freimuth RR, et al. Standardizing terms for clinical pharmacogenetic test results: consensus terms from the Clinical Pharmacogenetics Implementation Consortium (CPIC). Genet Med. 2017;19(2):215–223.

PMs of CYP2C19, compared to 15% of individuals with Asian ancestry.[17]

CYP2C9 is primarily expressed in the liver and metabolizes endogenous compounds, as well as xenobiotics. Notable CYP2C9 medication substrates include warfarin, phenytoin, several nonsteroidal anti-inflammatory drugs, and sulfonylureas. The CYP2C9 gene has several known alleles that produce decreased-function or nonfunctional enzymes. The *2 and *3 allele account for the vast majority of the known pharmacogenomic variation in individuals of European and Asian ancestry, but *5, *6, *8, and *11 are collectively more common than *2 and *3 in individuals of African ancestry.[18] For this reason, clinicians and researchers must be mindful of whether the appropriate CYP2C9 alleles for their patient population are being tested for by their assay/testing platform.

Other CYP Enzymes

CYP1A2. CYP1A2 is responsible for the metabolism of select endogenous substrates, xenobiotics, and medications.[19] In addition to CYP1A2 induction from medications, tobacco smoking, dietary cruciferous vegetables, and polyamine hydrocarbons from grilled meats are also known to induce CYP1A2.[20] Compared to CYP2D6 or CYP3A, fewer commonly used medications are CYP1A2 dependent. Perhaps due to the relatively low number of clinically used substrates and/or the nongenetic influences on enzyme activity, current understanding of the clinical utility of CYP1A2 pharmacogenomics is underdeveloped. However, clozapine and caffeine (used therapeutically for apnea of prematurity) are narrow therapeutic index drugs and are CYP1A2 substrates that may represent opportunity for clinically oriented research.

CYP2B6. CYP2B6 makes up approximately 2% to 10% of total hepatic CYP content and is also expressed in brain tissue.[21,22] High interpatient variability in CYP2B6 expression has been described; however, polymorphisms of the CYP2B6 gene likely only explain a small fraction. CYP2B6 is highly inducible by medications and other xenobiotics and is regulated by nuclear receptors. Thus, environmental factors and genomic regulation via other genes may account for the majority of the variation in CYP2B6 activity. CYP2B6 pharmacogenomics may be clinically relevant for human immunodeficiency (HIV) antiretrovirals (e.g., efavirenz and nevirapine), antidepressants (e.g., bupropion), and chemotherapeutic agents (e.g., cyclophosphamide).

CYP3A. CYP3A enzymes are responsible for the metabolism of a wide range of endogenous substrates and drugs, including 37% of the most frequently prescribed drugs in the United States.[23] *CYP3A4* and *CYP3A5* are thought to be the most clinically relevant in human adults. The *CYP3A4* and *CYP3A5* genes share many similarities in sequence and, unsurprisingly, there is significant overlap in the substrates that their enzyme products metabolize. Individuals with two nonfunctional copies of *CYP3A4* (poor metabolizers) are rare, but *CYP3A5* poor metabolizers are more common, especially in certain ethnic groups. In fact, the majority of individuals with white European ancestry have no functional CYP3A5 alleles, while most African Americans have one or two functional alleles.[24,25]

Non-CYP Drug-Metabolizing Enzymes

TPMT. Clinically relevant pharmacogenomic associations have been demonstrated for drug-metabolizing enzymes outside of the CYP system. The gene *TPMT* encodes thiopurine S-methyltransferase, which is involved in an important metabolic pathway for the thiopurine drugs thioguanine, 6-mercaptopurine, and azathioprine. Patients homozygous for no-function TPMT variants are at increased risk for life-threatening myelosuppression when treated at conventional doses. There are known ethnic differences in allele frequencies of TPMT variants, with the *3A variant most common in European ancestry patients, and the *3C variant most common in African and East Asian populations. Thiopurine pharmacogenomics will be covered in greater detail in Chapter 7.

DPYD. The gene *DPYD* encodes dihydropyrimidine dehydrogenase, which is the rate-limiting step for metabolism of the fluoropyrimidine drugs 5-fluorouracil and capecitabine. These are narrow therapeutic index drugs used to treat solid tumors and concentration-related toxicities. Alleles conferring no function and decreased function have been described. Decreased-function alleles are carried by 3% to 7% of European and African ancestry populations.[26] More information regarding *DPYD* and fluoropyrimidine therapy can be found in Chapter 7.

UGT1A1. UGT1A1 is an enzyme in the uridine diphosphate glucuronosyltransferase family that is responsible for the glucuronidation of bilirubin from its toxic form (unconjugated bilirubin) to its nontoxic form (conjugated bilirubin), allowing for its excretion from the body. The enzyme is also involved in the glucuronidation of drugs and xenobiotics, making them water soluble for biliary or renal elimination. Atazanavir is an antiretroviral protease inhibitor used in conjunction with ritonavir or cobicistat, which are pharmacokinetic enhancers, to treat HIV infection. Atazanavir inhibits UGT1A1, which can result in increased plasma unconjugated (indirect) bilirubin concentrations, presenting as jaundice in some patients. Studies have shown that patients who are homozygous for decreased-function *UGT1A1* alleles are more likely to discontinue atazanavir/ritonavir treatment for bilirubin-related reasons[27] or for any cause,[28] though this finding was not consistent across all studies and ethnic groups.[29]

The chemotherapeutic agent irinotecan is a prodrug with an active moiety, SN-38, that is cleared by UGT1A1. The FDA-approved prescribing information for irinotecan indicates that prescribers should consider reduced doses in individuals homozygous for the decreased function *28 allele.[30] This topic is covered in greater detail in Chapter 7.

Drug Transporters

SLCO1B1. Variation in genes encoding drug transporters can also affect medication pharmacokinetics. *SLCO1B1* encodes an organic anion-transporting polypeptide that facilitates the hepatic uptake of HMG CoA-reductase inhibitors. Statin-related muscle toxicity is the most common adverse drug reaction of this drug class (incidence 1% to 5%) and is concentration-dependent. Evidence clearly shows that the *SLCO1B1* genotype affects simvastatin pharmacokinetics and myopathy risk, with less clear evidence for other statins. *SLCO1B1* is polymorphic, since 12% to 45% of patients carry at least one decreased-function allele, and published guidelines provide recommendations for altering statin therapy based on the *SLCO1B1* genotype.[31] This topic is covered in greater detail in Chapter 5.

P-glycoprotein. The drug efflux pump p-glycoprotein is encoded by the gene *ABCB1*. P-glycoprotein is expressed in the epithelial cells of the intestines, liver, proximal tubules of the kidney, and blood–brain barrier, among other sites. Across disease states, investigations of *ABCB1* variants to drug response outcomes have yielded inconsistent results, and at the time of publication, no consensus guidelines exist for altering therapy based upon the *ABCB1* genotype.

Pharmacodynamic Basis for Genetic Influence on Drug Response

Drug Targets

SLC6A4. The most obvious way in which genetic variation may influence drug pharmacodynamics is through differences in the genes encoding drug targets. The serotonin transporter is an example of a drug target in which genetic variation may influence drug response. Drugs that inhibit the reuptake of serotonin from the synapse—namely selective serotonin reuptake inhibitors (SSRIs) and tricyclic antidepressants (TCAs)—antagonize the serotonin transporter. Variation in the serotonin transporter gene *SLC6A4* has been studied for decades as a potential risk factor for affective disorders and as a pharmacogenomic marker of antidepressant response. The most widely studied variation in *SLC6A4*, called the serotonin transporter polymorphic length region (5-HTTLPR), is thought to modulate the expression of the transporter. Pharmacogenomic studies suggest it may be modestly predictive of SSRI response and tolerability, but at this time, *SLC6A4* genetics are not routinely used in clinical care. *SLC6A4* pharmacogenomics will be expanded upon in Chapter 8.

VKORC1. Another established example of drug target pharmacogenomics is *VKORC1*, which encodes vitamin K epoxide reductase, the target of the anticoagulant warfarin. Vitamin K reductase converts vitamin K epoxide to its active, reduced form. The active vitamin K then acts as a cofactor for coagulation factors II, VII, IX, and X. *VKORC1* has a well-described missense SNP rs9923231, also known as c.-1639 G>A, that has been repeatedly associated with warfarin dosage requirements. The alanine residue results in a less active vitamin K reductase enzyme, and thus, individuals with this SNP have lower warfarin dose requirements to sufficiently inhibit the enzyme. Interestingly, the frequency of the c.-1639 G>A SNP varies greatly by ancestry, with the G allele most common in African ancestry individuals, the A allele most common in Asian ancestry individuals, and Caucasians are often heterozygous. In fact, c.-1639 G>A polymorphism is a major driver of the differing average warfarin dose requirements between Black and White Americans that had been observed for decades, although it does not fully explain the dose variation. The pharmacogenomics of warfarin dosing are complex and polygenic and will be covered to a greater degree in Chapter 5.

Downstream Proteins

A second mechanism by which genetic variation can influence drug pharmacodynamics is through variation in "downstream" proteins—that is, proteins that are involved in the same physiologic pathway but are not directly targeted by medications. Recall our previous discussion of antidepressants and the serotonin transporter earlier in this chapter. While many antidepressants directly antagonize the serotonin transporter, their antidepressant effects are thought to be dependent on the increased synaptic serotonin interacting with serotonin receptors. The serotonin-2A receptor, encoded by *HTR2A*, is one such example. Although SSRIs do not directly act on this receptor, genetic variation of *HTR2A* is thought to influence the risk of side effects of SSRIs, particularly sexual dysfunction.

For another example, we return to warfarin pharmacogenomics. Although warfarin's direct drug target is vitamin K reductase, which converts vitamin K into its active form, other enzymes in the vitamin K pathway influence warfarin dose requirements. CYP4F2 does not metabolize warfarin, nor is it the drug target of warfarin;

however, it metabolizes the active vitamin K compound back into its oxidized, inactive form. Functional genetic variation is known in the *CYPF2* gene, and indeed, this variation influences warfarin dose requirements, albeit to a lesser degree than *VKORC1*.

Pharmacogenomics and Hypersensitivity Reactions

The cluster of genes called the human major histocompatibility complex (MHC) encodes cell surface proteins that present intracellular antigens to the immune system. Human leukocyte antigen (HLA) genes within the MHC are implicated in some severe drug-related hypersensitivity reactions. These genes are extremely polymorphic, with thousands of alleles described for both the *HLA-A* and *HLA-B* genes. HLA genes influence the risk of hypersensitivity reactions to medications, including carbamazepine and related compounds, such as oxcarbazepine, abacavir, allopurinol, and phenytoin, among others. The clinical manifestation of these hypersensitivity reactions can differ by drug and include severe cutaneous reactions such as Stevens-Johnson syndrome, blood dyscrasias, or generalized yet progressive flulike symptoms. For some medications with well-established evidence linking HLA genotype to hypersensitivity (i.e., abacavir), genetic testing is required before initiating antiretroviral therapy in treatment-naïve HIV-positive patients because of the severity of these adverse drug reactions. For other compounds, such as carbamazepine, the FDA-approved package insert recommends HLA testing prior to initiation only in patients that report ancestry to populations in which risk alleles are common (e.g., Thai ancestry).[32] Further research is being conducted in an attempt to associate other seemingly immunologic-mediated adverse drug reactions (e.g., heparin-induced thrombocytopenia, clozapine-related agranulocytosis) with genetic risk factors.

Summary: Genetic Influence on Drug Response

Clinical response and tolerability to medications can be influenced by genes related to pharmacokinetics, pharmacodynamics, and immunologic reactions. A key point to keep in mind is that, generally speaking, pharmacogenomic results are *predictive*, not *deterministic*. That is, pharmacogenomic variants affect the likelihood of a given treatment outcome, but do not guarantee that an outcome will certainly happen. A CYP2C19 poor metabolizer will have increased risk of stent thrombosis if treated with clopidogrel, but this outcome will not happen in every

CYP2C19 poor metabolizer. This is because genetic and nongenetic factors also affect the treatment outcome. There may be alternative metabolic pathways that can metabolize the drug when the primary pathway is compromised. Drug–drug interactions or organ dysfunction may "mask" or wash out genetic effects. And, of course, a patient who does not adhere to the treatment regimen may have a different outcome than the pharmacogenomic results predict.

Even within the scope of precision medicine, patient-specific biological mechanisms affect drug response that are not captured by traditional germline genotyping. Somatic variations—those that occur spontaneously after birth and can be tissue-specific—can have profound effects on treatment outcomes and are of particular interest in cancer treatment. Epigenetics, defined as differences in gene function *not* related to differences in genetic sequence, can alter the expression of drug-metabolizing enzymes or targets. These changes can be tissue-specific and change over the lifespan. Outside of genetic mechanisms, it is becoming apparent that individual differences in the human gut microbiome—the microorganisms within the body—can affect human health and potentially medication outcomes. While important, these mechanisms are generally outside of the scope of this text, which focuses on germline genetic sequence variation.

DISCOVERY/RESEARCH APPROACHES

The hypothesis that differences in the metabolism of xenobiotics may drive unusual response to food or drugs was speculated in the early twentieth century. Patterns of adverse drug reactions associated with certain ethnic groups and patterns of response in family studies were noted in the academic literature in the middle of the century. As the methodology for quantifying the pharmacokinetics of medications advanced, so did the ability to measure inherited or familial patterns of abnormal pharmacokinetics.[33]

As methods to phenotype (e.g., measuring relative concentration of a parent drug and its metabolite) and directly genotype individuals advanced, so did pharmacogenomics research. This led to an era that largely leaned on what is called the "candidate gene" approach. In brief, this term refers to studies in which investigators focus on genes known or thought to be mechanistically related to the drug's pharmacokinetics and pharmacodynamics. Many important pharmacogenomic associations, such as

CYP2D6 genotype affecting codeine outcomes, were first demonstrated in candidate gene studies.

New approaches became possible as genotyping microarray technology advanced in terms of breadth, reliability, and reduced cost. One popular approach made possible from advances in microarray technology is the genome-wide association study (GWAS). As the term implies, this approach typically utilizes microarrays that genotype roughly 1 million SNPs across the entire genome—from chromosome 1 to X/Y. Note that the human genome is much larger than 1 million base pairs (it is closer to 4 billion), and thus, these arrays do not provide direct information on each and every base pair of the genome. However, the SNPs on genome-wide arrays are intentionally spaced out in a fashion that allows researchers to identify *regions* of the genome that are associated with the phenotype, even if the causal SNP is not directly interrogated. By "causal SNP" we are referring to an SNP that directly leads to an altered-function protein or changes in expression. But even if the causal SNP is not genotyped on a given microarray, if there are genotyped SNPs nearby in linkage disequilibrium, they will show association with the phenotype and guide researchers to more closely interrogate the region in future studies. Results from a GWAS are typically presented in the form of a Manhattan plot, named as such because the figure resembles a skyline. The "skyscrapers" are regions of association (Figure 1-8).

An important feature of GWAS is that they are called "hypothesis-agnostic" approaches, by which the researchers humbly acknowledge that they do not know the full set of candidate genes that may affect the phenotype of the study. Thus, researchers have less incentive and/or ability to manipulate results to support an *a priori* hypothesis. This feature is useful in that it can uncover previously unknown molecular mechanisms and/or pathways affecting the phenotype.

Another important consideration in GWAS is that 1 million or more SNPs are being tested for association with the phenotype. Advanced statistical techniques and corrections are required to prevent false-positive (type I) errors. If 1 million SNPs were tested for association with a phenotype that has no genetic basis, there would be tens of thousands of false-positive associations at the standard alpha = 0.05 threshold. Thus, alpha is usually set to a much more conservative threshold ($p < 5 \times 10^{-7}$, for example) or other techniques are used to prevent type I errors.

Through genome-wide approaches, researchers have found variation in surprising genomic regions that have been associated with drug response phenotypes. And indeed, genetic variants in one region can affect the expression of genes in a fairly distant region of the genome—even on different chromosomes! GWAS can even uncover genomic regions that are associated with phenotypes in which the mechanism driving the association is poorly understood. Unsurprisingly, GWAS has uncovered important pharmacogenomic associations, such as *CYP2C19* variation and antiplatelet response to clopidogrel.

The tests of genetic association most commonly used in pharmacogenomic studies quantify the association between a single genetic marker and the odds or risk

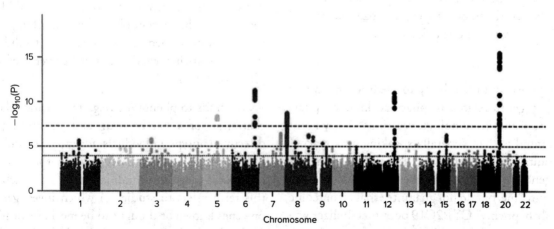

FIGURE 1-8 • A Manhattan plot depicting the results of a genome-wide association study. The x-axis depicts the location of the SNP in the genome, and the y-axis is a negative-log transformation of the p-value from the genetic association test. Higher points on the y-axis indicate more significant associations. (Reproduced, with permission, from McCarthy JJ, Mendelsohn BA. *Precision Medicine: A Guide to Genomics in Clinical Practice.* New York, NY: McGraw Hill; 2017.)

of the phenotype (often drug response). Phenotypes, including drug response phenotypes, differ in their genetic complexity. Sometimes the genotype–phenotype relationship is very simple: an individual with non-functional variants for a drug-metabolizing enzyme that is solely responsible for a given drug's metabolism will have higher parent drug compounds. But some phenotypes—schizophrenia, for example—are thought to have a strong genetic component, yet no one variant explains the majority of disease risk. How can this be? One scenario is if the phenotype is influenced by multiple genetic variants, with each variant only influencing risk of the phenotype by a small degree. To predict an individual's risk under such conditions, researchers developed a tool commonly called a polygenic score or polygenic risk score. In brief, this risk score is a sum of an individual's risk alleles across his or her genome, weighted by how much each risk allele is estimated to affect risk of the phenotype. Polygenic risk scores for many human diseases have been established, and while they are not used routinely in clinical settings at present, their clinical utility is being examined. Polygenic risk for a given disease is sometimes examined as a potential predictor for treatment response/resistance (e.g., does a high polygenic score for schizophrenia affect the likelihood of treatment resistance?). As genome-wide or sequencing data become more affordable and readily available in daily practice, it is likely that polygenic risk scores will be used in primary disease prevention strategies and determining disease treatment.

CONCLUSION

Although humans are largely the same at the genomic level, genetic differences can have large effects on medication pharmacokinetics and pharmacodynamics. While pharmacogenomics can help to predict adverse drug reactions and the probability of drug response, nongenetic factors act in concert to determine medication outcomes. Pharmacogenomics is an aspect of precision medicine that today is being implemented into routine clinical care, with pharmacogenomics information increasingly appearing in treatment guidelines and drug labeling. This text will provide dedicated chapters to resources for pharmacogenomics information (Chapter 4), clinical implementation strategies (Chapter 2), and ethical considerations (Chapter 3) for current and future leaders in pharmacogenomics.

CASE SCENARIOS

Pharmacokinetic Basis for Genetic Influence on Drug Response

Case 1

Patient Presentation

"I saw an advertisement last week about genetic testing. Can my DNA really explain what medications I should or should not take?"

Question : How can you, the clinician, best explain to the patient the limitations of pharmacogenomic testing in patient-friendly terms?

Answer: Genetic testing can tell us lots about a person's health. For some, it can confirm a genetic disease or condition. In others, it can rule it out. Genetic testing can also tell us about a person's risk of developing a genetic condition or passing one along to their children. However, pharmacogenomic testing is different. Pharmacogenomic testing looks for variation in the smallest pieces of a person's DNA, and only in specific locations, not the entire human code made up of over 3 billion base pairs. Because of this, pharmacogenomic testing will not tell you about your ancestry, character traits, diagnose you with a medical condition, or predict risk for disease. Instead, pharmacogenomic testing will help your physician and pharmacist form a more complete picture about how your body may respond to certain medications. For some, pharmacogenomics may help predict when a drug will not work. In others, pharmacogenomics may help predict when a drug is more likely to cause side effects. Pharmacogenomics results should always be interpreted by a health care clinician and with other considerations in mind.

Takeaways

- The human genome is a code made up of over 3 billion base pairs. Base pairs make up approximately 20,000 genes, which are responsible for our individual human characteristics and traits.

- Pharmacogenomics, a branch of precision medicine, is the study of how DNA, or individual genes, may affect drug response. Pharmacogenomics is not the only factor one should consider when selecting a medication.

Case 2

Clinician Inquiry

"Will pharmacogenomic testing help me select the right medication for my patients?"

Question: How can you, the clinician, best explain the benefits and the limitations of pharmacogenomic testing to a clinician colleague?

Answer : Pharmacogenomic testing can be helpful in selecting and tailoring pharmacotherapy in individual patients. When pharmacogenomic tests are performed prior to a clinical need, results should be stored for future interpretation and clinical use. When pharmacogenomic testing is performed after a clinical need arises, results should be used to tailor drug therapy reactively. When pharmacogenomic test results are in hand, the results can be best applied when considered in tandem with other subjective and objective patient data. Pharmacogenomic results can predict, but cannot determine, the ultimate outcome related to drug safety and effectiveness. Clinicians should choose to test patients for pharmacogenomic biomarkers after considering both the benefits and limitations of testing.

Takeaways

- Pharmacogenomic testing can be performed prior to clinical need for the drug (preemptive testing) or after the clinical need for the drug with polymorphic gene association (reactive testing).

- Pharmacogenomic results are predictive, not deterministic. That is, pharmacogenomic variants affect the likelihood of a given treatment outcome but do not guarantee that an outcome will certainly happen.

PHARMACOGENOMICS FUNDAMENTAL PEARLS

- Pharmacogenomics is a component of precision medicine that is being implemented into drug labeling, clinical guidelines, and routine clinical care.
- Although only a small percentage of the genome differs between individuals, these differences can cause profound changes to phenotypes, including drug response.
- Genetic variation, related to the pharmacokinetics and pharmacodynamics of drugs, can affect drug response. Types of variation include single-nucleotide polymorphisms, insertions, deletions, and copy number variation.
- Typically, pharmacogenomic variants affect the probability of drug response or adverse drug reactions. Usually, they do not solely or always determine which individuals will respond to a drug or experience adverse drug reactions.

KEY TERMS[34,35]

Allele: One of two or more DNA sequences occurring at a particular gene locus.

Autosomal: Refers to any of the chromosomes numbered 1 to 22 or the genes on chromosomes 1 to 22.

Candidate gene: A gene whose chromosomal location is associated with a particular disease or other phenotype.

Chromosome: A chromosome is an organized package of DNA found in the nucleus of the cell. Different organisms have different numbers of chromosomes. Humans have 23 pairs of chromosomes: 22 pairs of numbered chromosomes, called autosomes, and 1 pair of sex chromosomes, X and Y. Each parent contributes one chromosome to each pair so that offspring get half of their chromosomes from their mother and half from their father.

CNV: Copy number variant refers to the genetic trait involving the number of copies of a particular gene present in the genome of an individual. Genetic variants, including insertions, deletions, and duplications of segments of DNA, are also collectively referred to as CNVs. CNVs account for a significant proportion of the genetic variation between individuals.

Codon: A codon is a trinucleotide sequence of DNA or RNA that corresponds to a specific amino acid. The genetic code describes the relationship between the sequence of DNA bases (A, C, G, and T) in a gene and the corresponding protein sequence that it encodes. The cell reads the sequence of the gene in groups of three bases. There are 64 different codons: 61 specify amino acids, while the remaining 3 are used as stop signals.

Cytogenetics: The study of the structure, function, and abnormalities of human chromosomes.

Diplotype: The two alleles an individual has inherited at a genetic locus.

Genetic variant: An alteration in the most common DNA nucleotide sequence. The term variant can be used to describe an alteration that may be benign, pathogenic, or of unknown significance.

Genome: An organism's complete set of DNA, including all of its genes.

Genotype: The allele(s) an individual has inherited at a genetic locus. Sometimes used as a synonym for diplotype.

Germline: The cells from which eggs or sperm are derived.

GWAS: A genome-wide association study is a way for scientists to identify inherited genetic variants associated with the risk of disease or a particular trait. This method surveys the entire genome for genetic polymorphisms, typically single-nucleotide polymorphisms (SNPs), that occur more frequently in cases than in controls.

Haplotype: A set of closely linked genetic markers present on one chromosome that tend to be inherited together.

Microarray technology: Microarray technology is used to study the expression of many genes at once. It involves placing thousands of gene sequences in known locations on a glass slide called a gene chip. A sample containing DNA or RNA is placed in contact with the gene chip. Complementary base pairing between the sample and the gene sequences on the chip produces light that is measured. Areas on the chip producing light identify genes that are expressed in the sample.

Missense mutation: A missense mutation is when the change of a single base pair causes the substitution of a different amino acid in the resulting protein. This amino acid substitution may have no effect, or it may render the protein nonfunctional.

Multiple-gene panel test: Genetic tests that use next-generation sequencing to test multiple genes simultaneously.

Mutation: A mutation is a change in a DNA sequence. Mutations can result from DNA-copying mistakes made during cell division, exposure to ionizing radiation, exposure to chemicals called mutagens, or infection by viruses. Germline

mutations occur in the eggs and sperm and can be passed on to offspring, while somatic mutations occur in body cells and are not passed on.

Nucleotide: A nucleotide is the basic building block of nucleic acids. RNA and DNA are polymers made of long chains of nucleotides. A nucleotide consists of a sugar molecule (either ribose in RNA or deoxyribose in DNA) attached to a phosphate group and a nitrogen-containing base. The bases used in DNA are adenine (A), cytosine (C), guanine (G), and thymine (T). In RNA, the base uracil (U) takes the place of thymine.

Personalized medicine: An emerging practice of medicine that uses an individual's genetic profile to guide decisions made in regard to the prevention, diagnosis, and treatment of disease.

Pharmacogenomics: A branch of pharmacology concerned with using DNA and amino acid sequence data to inform drug development and testing. An important application of pharmacogenomics is correlating individual genetic variation with drug responses.

Phenotype: The observable characteristics in an individual resulting from the expression of genes; the clinical presentation of an individual with a particular genotype.

Polymorphism: Polymorphism involves one of two or more variants of a particular DNA sequence. The most common type of polymorphism involves variation at a single base pair. Polymorphisms can also be much larger in size and involve long stretches of DNA.

Precision medicine: An emerging approach for disease treatment and prevention that considers individual variability in genes, environment, and lifestyle for each person.

SNP: Single-nucleotide polymorphism is a DNA sequence variation that occurs when a single nucleotide (adenine, thymine, cytosine, guanine) in the genome sequence is altered; usually present in at least 1% of the population.

Somatic variant: An alteration in DNA that occurs after conception and is not present within the germline. Somatic variants can occur in any of the cells of the body except the germ cells (sperm and egg) and therefore are not passed on to children.

Wild-type gene: A term used to describe a gene when it is found in its natural, nonmutated (unchanged) form.

REFERENCES

1. The White House. President Barack Obama. The Precision Medicine Initiative. Available at https://obamawhitehouse.archives.gov/precision-medicine. Accessed February 27, 2020.

2. National Human Genome Research Institute. What Is the Human Genome Project? Available at https://www.genome.gov/human-genome-project/What. Accessed February 27, 2020.

3. Kalow W. Pharmacogenetics and pharmacogenomics: origin, status, and the hope for personalized medicine. *Pharmacogenomics J.* 2006;6(3):162–165.

4. U.S. Food & Drug Administration. Table of Pharmacogenomic Biomarkers in Drug Labeling. Available at https://www.fda.gov/drugs/science-and-research-drugs/table-pharmacogenomic-biomarkers-drug-labeling. Accessed November 4, 2019.

5. Samwald M, Xu H, Blagec K, et al. Incidence of exposure of patients in the United States to multiple drugs for which pharmacogenomic guidelines are available. *PLoS One.* 2016;11(10):e0164972.

6. Pratt VM, Del Tredici AL, Hachad H, et al. Recommendations for CYP2C19 genotyping allele selection: a report of the Association for Molecular Pathology. *J Mol Diagn.* 2018;20(3):269–276.

7. Ingelman-Sundberg M, Daly AK, Oscarson M, Nebert DW. Human cytochrome P450 (CYP) genes: recommendations for the nomenclature of alleles. *Pharmacogenetics.* 2000;10(1):91–93.

8. PharmVar. Pharmacogene Variation Consortium. The PharmVar Consortium. Available at https://www.pharmvar.org/about. Accessed February 27, 2020.

9. 1000 Genomes Project Consortium, Auton A, Brooks LD, et al. A global reference for human genetic variation. *Nature.* 2015;526(7571):68–74.

10. Zanger UM, Klein K, Thomas M, et al. Genetics, epigenetics, and regulation of drug-metabolizing cytochrome p450 enzymes. *Clin Pharmacol Ther.* 2014;95(3):258–261.

11. Ingelman-Sundberg M, Sim SC, Gomez A, Rodriguez-Antona C. Influence of cytochrome P450 polymorphisms on drug therapies: pharmacogenetic, pharmacoepigenetic and clinical aspects. *Pharmacol Ther.* 2007;116(3):496–526.

12. Mahgoub A, Idle JR, Dring LG, Lancaster R, Smith RL. Polymorphic hydroxylation of Debrisoquine in man. *Lancet.* 1977;2(8038):584–586.

13. Eichelbaum M, Spannbrucker N, Steincke B, Dengler HJ. Defective N-oxidation of sparteine in man: a new pharmacogenetic defect. *Eur J Clin Pharmacol.* 1979;16(3):183–187.

14. Skoda RC, Gonzalez FJ, Demierre A, Meyer UA. Two mutant alleles of the human cytochrome P-450db1 gene (P450C2D1) associated with genetically deficient metabolism of debrisoquine and other drugs. *Proc Natl Acad Sci U S A.* 1988;85(14):5240–5243.

15. Gaedigk A, Ingelman-Sundberg M, Miller NA, et al. The Pharmacogene Variation (PharmVar) Consortium: incorporation of the human cytochrome P450 (CYP) allele nomenclature database. *Clin Pharmacol Ther.* 2018;103(3):399–401.

16. PharmGKB. Gene-Specific Information Tables for CYP2D6. Available at https://www.pharmgkb.org/page/cyp2d6RefMaterials. Accessed February 27, 2020.

17. Scott SA, Sangkuhl K, Stein CM, et al. Clinical Pharmacogenetics Implementation Consortium guidelines for CYP2C19 genotype and clopidogrel therapy: 2013 update. *Clin Pharmacol Ther.* 2013;94(3):317–323.

18. Pratt VM, Cavallari LH, Del Tredici AL, et al. Recommendations for clinical CYP2C9 genotyping allele selection: a joint recommendation of the Association for Molecular Pathology and College of American Pathologists. *J Mol Diagn.* 2019;21(5):746–755.

19. Zhou SF, Yang LP, Zhou ZW, et al. Insights into the substrate specificity, inhibitors, regulation, and polymorphisms and the clinical impact of human cytochrome P450 1A2. *AAPS J.* 2009;11(3):481–494.

20. Gunes A, Dahl ML. Variation in CYP1A2 activity and its clinical implications: influence of environmental factors and genetic polymorphisms. *Pharmacogenomics.* 2008;9(5):625–637.

21. Miksys S, Tyndale RF. The unique regulation of brain cytochrome P450 2 (CYP2) family enzymes by drugs and genetics. *Drug Metab Rev.* 2004;36(2):313–333.

22. Wang H, Tompkins LM. CYP2B6: new insights into a historically overlooked cytochrome P450 isozyme. *Curr Drug Metab.* 2008;9(7):598–610.

23. Zanger UM, Turpeinen M, Klein K, Schwab M. Functional pharmacogenetics/genomics of human cytochromes P450 involved in drug biotransformation. *Anal Bioanal Chem.* 2008;392(6):1093–1108.

24. van Schaik RH, van der Heiden IP, van den Anker JN, Lindemans J. CYP3A5 variant allele frequencies in Dutch Caucasians. *Clin Chem.* 2002;48(10):1668–1671.

25. Xie HG, Wood AJ, Kim RB, et al. Genetic variability in CYP3A5 and its possible consequences. *Pharmacogenomics.* 2004;5(3):243–272.

26. Amstutz U, Henricks LM, Offer SM, et al. Clinical Pharmacogenetics Implementation Consortium (CPIC) guideline for dihydropyrimidine dehydrogenase genotype and fluoropyrimidine dosing: 2017 update. *Clin Pharmacol Ther.* 2018;103(2):210–216.

27. Vardhanabhuti S, Ribaudo HJ, Landovitz RJ, et al. Screening for UGT1A1 genotype in study A5257 would have markedly reduced premature discontinuation of atazanavir for hyperbilirubinemia. *Open Forum Infect Dis.* 2015;2(3):ofv085.

28. Lubomirov R, Colombo S, di Iulio J, et al. Association of pharmacogenetic markers with premature discontinuation of first-line anti-HIV therapy: an observational cohort study. *J Infect Dis.* 2011;203(2):246–257.

29. Ribaudo HJ, Daar ES, Tierney C, et al. Impact of UGT1A1 Gilbert variant on discontinuation of ritonavir-boosted atazanavir in AIDS Clinical Trials Group Study A5202. *J Infect Dis.* 2013;207(3):420–425.

30. Camptosar [package insert]. New York, NY: Pfizer; 2020.

31. Ramsey LB, Johnson SG, Caudle KE, et al. The Clinical Pharmacogenetics Implementation Consortium guideline for SLCO1B1 and simvastatin-induced myopathy: 2014 update. *Clin Pharmacol Ther.* 2014;96(4):423–428.

32. Tegretol [package insert]. East Hanover, NJ: Novartis; 2009.

33. Roden DM, McLeod HL, Relling MV, et al. Pharmacogenomics. *Lancet.* 2019;394(10197):521–532.

34. National Human Genome Research Institute. Talking Glossary of Genetic Terms. Available at https://www.genome.gov/genetics-glossary. Accessed February 27, 2020.

35. National Cancer Institute. NCI Dictionary of Genetics Terms. Available at https://www.cancer.gov/publications/dictionaries/genetics-dictionary. Accessed February 27, 2020.

CHAPTER 2

Implementation: A Guide to Implementing Pharmacogenomics Services

Natasha J. Petry, Moom R. Roosan, Emily J. Cicali, and Julio D. Duarte

LEARNING OBJECTIVES

1. Describe the resources necessary to implement pharmacogenomics services into your practice successfully.

2. Identify the key personnel needed for implementation of a pharmacogenomics service.

3. Identify the technology needed for successful pharmacogenomics implementation and maintenance.

4. Discuss the value of educational activities to support pharmacogenomics implementation efforts.

5. Recognize potential challenges to implementation and summarize possible approaches to overcome them.

INTRODUCTION

Creating and implementing a pharmacogenomics (PGx) program requires many considerations. Usually, a health system's main goal is to use PGx information to help improve drug efficacy and/or to reduce side effects in their patient population. However, the motivation of health systems to implement PGx testing may stem from varied priorities. Because of this, the process of implementation will not be uniform across institutions. A framework for implementation is presented in this chapter (Figure 2-1), but each implementing institution will need to decide the order of processes that make sense and work for them. This chapter aims to (1) describe resources needed for those interested in implementing PGx services, (2) suggest key personnel likely needed for

PGx implementation, (3) discuss the broad technology and informatics structure involved in PGx implementation, (4) discuss the value of educational activities for successful implementation, and (5) address challenges faced and strategies to overcome. This chapter expands upon the key concepts related to implementing PGx. Examples in various practice settings are highlighted throughout to provide important real-world considerations for the prospective implementers.

DESIGNING A SERVICE

While planning the details of a program, there are many factors to consider. Logistical factors include consideration of testing strategies, what testing platform will be utilized, where and how testing will be performed, and

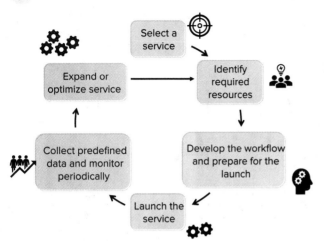

FIGURE 2-1 • A potential pharmacogenomics service implementation process. Stakeholders and the implementation team select a service to implement and identify the required resources. The implementation team will work with stakeholders to develop the workflow and prepare for launch. The team will launch the service and periodically collect and monitor the quality of the service to further optimize it.

selection of drug–gene pairs that will benefit your patient population and have strong supporting evidence. Each of these factors will be discussed in detail throughout the chapter, but it is important to realize that each institution's program may appear very different and the level of support desired around testing is a major factor that will shape the program. For example, does the institution wish to simply make it feasible for providers to order PGx tests, or are interpretation and/or consultation notes desired, or are face-to-face PGx results interpretation visits with the patient desired? The answers to these questions will help determine the workflow and personnel required for the PGx program to be successful.

Testing Approach

Deciding if a preemptive or reactive genotyping strategy will be used is a key first step when determining the testing approach. Preemptive PGx testing is typically done before the results are needed to guide pharmacotherapy decisions, while reactive testing is ordered once the results are desired for a specific pharmacotherapy decision. Table 2-1 lists key differences between reactive and preemptive testing approaches to consider for defining the workflow.

Preemptive testing allows PGx information to be available at the time of initial therapeutic decision-making because the test was previously ordered and the results are readily available. This eliminates the need to order a test and wait for the result. Preemptive testing often involves ordering a panel of multiple tests to cover the many potential therapeutic situations surrounding multiple drugs. However,

preemptive panels are not generally yet covered by insurance, in part due to lack of randomized controlled trials showing cost or efficacy benefits.[1] While it may be tempting to order PGx testing for all patients, until further research is done, it might be more cost-effective to target high-risk patients, those likely to be prescribed a medication with an actionable variant.[2]

Reactive testing is ordered in response to a medication event where PGx data may inform decision-making. For reactive testing, PGx tests may be ordered in response to a side effect from a medication or lack of efficacy of a medication where there is PGx evidence (Figure 2-2). Providers may also order a PGx test using the reactive approach if contemplating use of a new medication. Reactive PGx testing may be for one gene or multiple genes depending on the medication of interest.

Both preemptive and reactive testing approaches can be done as either a single gene test or a panel-based test, and deciding which one to use is another key component of the testing approach. Some institutions may start with one drug–gene pair with strong levels of evidence and continue to add single genes as the program grows. Other institutions may begin with a panel test and only validate certain genes to be released into the medical record, starting with interpretation for the validated gene(s) before validating and providing interpretations for subsequent genes as the program grows. Others may choose to start with a panel that covers drug–gene pairs with high levels of evidence and provide interpretation for all genes on the panel. Many institutions choose drug–gene pairs based off of evidence from Clinical Pharmacogenetics Implementation Consortium (CPIC) guidelines.[3] Utilizing CYP2C19 genotype results to guide antiplatelet therapy following percutaneous coronary intervention (PCI) is one of the most commonly implemented drug–gene pairs and is an example of a single-gene reactive approach.[4] With significant supporting evidence established, CYP2C19 testing for clopidogrel might be a relatively established option for beginning PGx implementation and allow further expansion after initial systems and procedures are built.[5] While CYP2C19 testing for clopidogrel may work well for the inpatient setting, a panel-based preemptive testing program may be more appropriate in the context of primary care and is another common implementation approach. Often, programs with preemptive testing also offer reactive testing, and the use of each approach can be patient specific.[6-8]

Other institutions may choose to focus on specific disease states, such as depression, when implementing a

TABLE 2-1. Comparison of Reactive and Preemptive Testing Approaches

	Preemptive Testing	Reactive Testing
Availability of results	Ordered before a drug–gene pair is indicated for PGx testing. Result is already available.	Ordered at the time drug initiation/change is being considered. Result availability depends on the turnaround time.
Turnaround time	Days to weeks; but if done preemptively, information is available immediately at time of provider decision/prescribing.	Hours to days.
Gene test	Usually multiple genes in panel.	Usually single-gene test or a few genes related to a single drug.
Funding/Reimbursement	Less likely to be reimbursed by insurance; current limitations include no CPT code for billing purposes.	Potentially reimbursable when associated with certain diagnoses.
CDS alert for identifying patients for testing	All applicable patients receive a PGx test order if results are not available.	Suggestive PGx order message as interruptive alert or within an order set with specific medication order.
Pharmacotherapy decisions	Are able to be made immediately, as results are already available.	May be delayed if provider opts to wait for results.

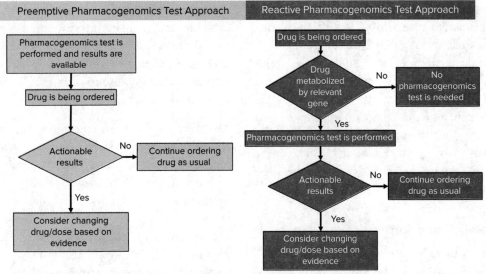

FIGURE 2-2 • A comparison of preemptive and reactive pharmacogenomics testing approaches. In the preemptive setting, PGx testing is done and results are ready to interpret in an event of a drug–gene interaction. On the other hand, PGx testing is done after a drug–gene interaction is identified in a reactive setting.

program, and this will guide their testing approach. Consider the utility of PGx testing to help predict efficacy and avoid toxicities of specific medications. Some laboratory companies market PGx panels focused on specific disease states (e.g., depression, pain, or cardiology) that can aid the test selection. However, caution should be used with these targeted panels, as these companies' evidence threshold for clinical use may differ from those of a particular health care institution. In addition, it is worth noting that the utility of a selected genetic test may have ramifications for other pharmacotherapy decisions. For example, a cardiology panel would likely include

CYP2C19, but CYP2C19 results can also guide prescribing of select antidepressants in addition to other noncardiology medications.[9] Additional factors, including many mentioned in this chapter, should also be considered (see Testing Platform) when deciding on a reactive or preemptive and single-gene versus panel approach.

Patient Population

Evaluating the target patient population is critical when designing an implementation program. Many issues must be considered when selecting a target population, including age, genetic ancestry, and medications used at the institution in question. Compared to the adult population, guidelines in the pediatric population are generally lacking for dosing recommendations. However, if an institution specializes in pediatric care, specific examples exist that lend themselves to PGx testing in pediatric patients, such as testing patients with leukemia or lymphoma for *TMPT* to help identify patients at higher risk for toxicities from thiopurines, or *CYP2D6* to aid selection of pain medications.[10–12] For example, St. Jude Children's Hospital started PGx implementation by testing patients likely to be prescribed a medication influenced by *TPMT, UGT1A,* or *CYP2D6.* Their approach eventually grew to include testing for multiple genes preemptively.[13] Pediatric implementers may need to rely on primary literature, if available, and/or extrapolate from adult recommendations.

A person's genetic ancestry is also important to consider, given the broad variation in some allele frequencies between ancestral groups. Supplemental data from CPIC guidelines report specific allele frequencies within major race/ethnic groups, and this can help guide decision-making on which specific variants to test for based on populations served by the health system.[14] For example, if the population served is largely Asian, testing for *HLA-B*15:02* and *HLA-B*58:01* should be a careful consideration due to increased frequency of those specific variants in that population.[15,16] In a health system whose population is mostly Caucasian, African American, or Latino, testing for *HLA-B*15:02* may not be a priority due to the allele largely being absent in these populations.[17]

Drug–Gene Pair Selection

The selections of which genes to test and which drug–gene pairs to implement should be rooted in strong evidence for clinical utility. Thus, a key factor to consider in the selection of drug–gene pairs is the availability of evidence to guide clinical action recommendations. The threshold for an acceptable level of evidence for actionable recommendations is determined by each institution. Chapter 4 on PGx resources describes in detail the different resources and guidelines available to help determine which drug–gene pairs to test for and the clinical recommendations that should follow from the test results.

The most prominent professional body providing clinical PGx guidelines in the United States is CPIC. One of CPIC's main goals is to assist in translating genetic test results into actionable medication recommendations.[14] However, they opt to avoid providing recommendations on whether to test a patient. CPIC provides the strength

of recommendations listed in the guidelines as strong, moderate, or optional and lets clinicians decide if testing is warranted. CPIC assigns the evidence supporting use of each drug–gene pair an evidence level from A to D. Level A drug–gene pairs have evidence for prescribing action, with high or moderate evidence supporting the action (i.e., strong or moderate strength). Level B drug–gene pairs have weak evidence for prescribing action, with at least one optional action, whereas levels C and D drug–gene pairs are not generally associated with enough evidence for prescribing actions. Many current PGx-implementing institutions follow CPIC guidelines, tending to focus on drug–gene pairs with evidence graded as Level A or B.[3]

Commercial laboratories may provide an interpretation report, which could include drug–gene pairs with varying levels of evidence. Recommendations between companies may vary, possibly because of differences in evidence thresholds used, variants tested, and phenotype definitions.[18] Each institution should decide their threshold for evidence and evaluate interpretation reports in relation to CPIC resources before deciding what recommendations to use. Factors to consider when selecting a PGx laboratory test are discussed in the Testing Platform and Laboratory Personnel sections.

The disease conditions treated within the health system should also be considered. For instance, if there is an institutional focus on psychiatry, it may be most useful to implement *CYP2D6* and *CYP2C19* testing to assist in the selection of selective serotonin reuptake inhibitors (SSRIs) and tricyclic antidepressants (TCAs). For a cardiology-related focus implementation, clopidogrel–*CYP2C19* would likely be a drug–gene pair to implement and guide antiplatelet therapy following PCI. Other cardiology-related drug–gene pairs with evidence worth considering include simvastatin–*SLCO1B1* for myopathy and rhabdomyolysis and warfarin–*CYP2C9, VKORC1,* and *CYP4F2* to guide initial warfarin dosing. Decisions such as these are important to make early in the planning process to guide the development of policies and procedures in addition to planning the service workflow (see Testing Platform).

Testing Platform

Selection of an appropriate PGx laboratory test depends on multiple factors, as summarized in Table 2-2. One way to identify genetic variants is to sequence the entire genome or exome. Although whole-genome or -exome sequencing assays are variant agnostic, they are rarely

TABLE 2-2. Factors to Consider in Selecting a Pharmacogenomic Test to be Implemented[19,20]

Target population to be tested
Drug–gene pair with significant clinical impact
Single-gene or multigene test needed
Flexibility for future plans to expand program
In-house or off-site/third-party laboratory
CAP/CLIA-licensed laboratory or FDA-cleared test
Analytical accuracy, sensitivity, and specificity
Genotyping platform used
Specific variants to be tested
Turnaround time for results
Time and labor to run the test
Cost (genotyping platform, training and education, maintenance)

used clinically for PGx due to higher cost, the need for complex bioinformatics analysis, challenges in assessing copy-number variations, and the identification of variants with unknown clinical significance that can interfere with clinical decision-making.[19] Targeted assays test for a specific list of known variants and currently are the most popular method of testing. The University of Florida (UF) Health, St. Jude Children's Hospital, Mayo Clinic, Sanford Health, and Vanderbilt University all implemented targeted assays for their PGx testing. The variants selected for testing in targeted assays are often chosen from common variants in specific ethnic populations, usually from those of European descent because of the data available. Other ancestral groups such as African and Native American populations are less studied, and some alleles frequent in these understudied populations may not be included in targeted assays. Therefore, frequencies of the known genetic variants in the target patient population should be considered in identifying the gene variants to be tested. The Association for Molecular Pathology (AMP) Pharmacogenomics Working Group recommends a minimum set of alleles (Tier 1 variants) and an extended set of alleles (Tier 2 variants) to be included in the clinical genotyping panels. So far, AMP has published recommendations for *CYP2C19* and *CYP2C9* genes, with more genes likely to follow.[21,22] Best practice would be to at least consider genotyping Tier 1 variants whenever AMP recommendations are available.

Another consideration is whether to select a test that is commercially available or customize based on the need of the health system. Commercially available off-the-shelf tests are generally not customizable and may or may not include the preferred alleles to meet the need for the target population or disease condition. The PGx implementation team may have to explore some customizable allele panels from molecular testing companies. However, these customizable tests are not approved by the Food and Drug Administration (FDA), and it is up to the users to validate the test and maintain the Clinical Laboratory Improvement Amendments (CLIA) certification of the laboratory. Therefore, it is unlikely that a health system, without a significant molecular pathology laboratory infrastructure, would likely use such customizable allele panels for clinical management of patients.

As an example, UF Health has used two different target variant PGx tests while starting up their clopidogrel–*CYP2C19* service. Since UF Health has a large population of cardiac patients and anticipated *CYP2C19* genotype usage was for more than 1000 patients per year, they implemented a preemptive *CYP2C19* genotyping approach with their College of American Pathologists (CAP)/CLIA–licensed pathology laboratories.[23] In addition to the required quality assurance and control, the laboratory used two testing platforms for clinical validation: the custom Quant Studio Open Array platform and an off-the-shelf genotyping test GenMark Dx for the first year. With the Quant Studio Open Array, the UF Health team was able to select the *CYP2C19* gene variants to be tested. This array was also scalable to their plan of expanding the service. Eventually, UF Health expanded the array to include 252 variants, and each could run 12 samples simultaneously at a cost of $42 per sample.[24] On the other hand, St. Jude Children's Hospital selected *TPMT* and *UGT1A1* for their initial implementation in 2005 as a preemptive test for their acute lymphoblastic leukemia (ALL) patients.[25] Since the hospital anticipated fewer than 100 tests per year for each test, the implementers opted for sending samples to an off-site/third-party laboratory for single-gene genotyping as more cost-effective. As the hospital expanded their PGx service over the years, they transitioned from single-gene tests to a multigene platform employing Affymetrix DMET Plus Array with a *CYP2D6* copy number detection capability.[26] This array investigated more than 1900 variants in 230 genes in a CLIA-certified third-party laboratory.

A few options are available when considering the approach to sample collection. Although whole blood yields a high-quality DNA sample, less invasive options such as saliva or buccal cell collection may be preferable for pediatric patients or institutions without on-site phlebotomy services.[27] Currently, most commercial genotyping platforms support the use of DNA from saliva, buccal cell, and blood samples. However, some platforms recommend using DNA from whole blood to avoid reprocessing of poor-quality or contaminated DNA. If drawing blood is not feasible, implementers should consider a platform that supports genotyping from saliva or buccal cells, allowing any trained personnel to collect the sample.

Regardless of the type of genotyping platform, the PGx test must be adopted from a laboratory that is CAP-accredited/CLIA-licensed in order to use the results clinically. While the FDA clears commercial tests for clinical use, the FDA has only an "enforcement discretion" for single laboratory developed tests (LDTs), which are developed and performed by a single laboratory. If an on-site CAP/CLIA-certified laboratory is used for genotyping, they will have to validate and maintain compliance status by appropriately training licensed personnel and maintaining certifications, which should be considered when deciding on an in-house or off-site/third-party laboratory. The Genetic Testing Registry (GTR), a National Center for Biotechnology Information (NCBI) initiative where companies voluntarily report information regarding genetic and PGx tests, provides many key information important in selecting appropriate tests.[28]

STAKEHOLDERS

Creating an interdisciplinary team with complementary expertise is important to the success of a PGx program. Thus, implementation will require participation from many stakeholders within the health care institution. Depending on the implementing institution, this may not all be required, but its involvement should at least be considered. Communication with the stakeholders is essential to gain their support and assure the established program runs efficiently.

Pharmacogenomics Clinical Team

At a minimum, the PGx implementation team should be led by a clinician with a background in PGx. Ideally, the clinician should have undergone residency, fellowship, or other advanced training program in PGx. Many current examples of successful PGx programs are led by physicians (such as those implemented at Vanderbilt University and the University of Maryland) or pharmacists (such as those implemented at UF and St. Jude Children's Hospital), but this is not an absolute requirement for a program's success.[25,29–31] Other members who work on the team will also need some level of training, whether that be formal training or on-the-job training.

If PGx training is an institutional priority, a resident or fellow could assist with the day-to-day clinical activities. This would also provide a pipeline for trained clinicians who can join the team after training is completed. For instance, both UF and St. Jude Children's Hospital offer advanced pharmacy residencies in PGx and precision medicine.

The day-to-day duties of the PGx clinical team will vary based on the model chosen, but they will often include interpreting test results, making clinical recommendations based on these results, and answering questions related to PGx testing and providing education to other stakeholders (see the Defining the Workflow section). While using electronic clinical decision support (CDS) tools greatly facilitates communication among the team members and with collaborating providers, regular PGx team meetings will also be needed. These meetings allow team members to assess clinical and administrative performance, as well as address workflow- or personnel-related issues and communicate any changes in procedures—which may occur frequently at first (see the Continuous Monitoring and Improvement Processes section). Initially, frequent team meetings (perhaps weekly or monthly) will likely be necessary and can be adjusted to less frequent meetings according to need.

Collaborating Providers

Having buy-in from applicable health care providers at individual institutions is imperative to the success of a PGx program. Because physicians are often the leaders of the health care team, having at least one physician champion can greatly increase the chance of program success. Physician champions can advocate for drug–gene pairs for which they feel that evidence supports implementation, particularly if the physician is made aware of key evidence (see Chapter 4). Furthermore, they can provide valuable input with regard to CDS creation, educate other physicians, and provide sponsorship in relation to administrative approval. Ideally, this physician champion should be highly regarded by his or her peers, knowledgeable, invested, and autonomous. The physician champion can also advocate for the appropriate use of PGx testing to his or her peers and to senior administration. The Mayo Clinic found success in identifying clinical champions to secure clinical acceptance of PGx and to provide guidance on drug–gene pairs.[32]

Once the PGx program is implemented, a PGx clinician should maintain open lines of communication with the collaborating medical and pharmacy teams to ensure that appropriate medication recommendations are provided based on both genotype and clinical data. A pager and/or email and phone number specific to the PGx service will allow a centralized contact point for anyone requesting consultation from the service or if any questions arise.

Institutional Leadership

Institutional leadership can include both high-level administrators and administrative supervisors of departments that may be involved with the PGx implementation efforts. Cooperation is more likely to be obtained from personnel in these departments if they are aware that their supervisors approve and, ideally, are enthusiastic about the implementation (see the Administration Approval section). Regularly scheduled meetings providing updates to leadership will increase the likelihood of their continued engagement, particularly if these updates include data showing some benefit (whether it be clinical or financial) to their department or the institution as a whole. In addition to administrative leaders, these meetings can include clinicians who are well respected and consulted often for their clinical expertise and knowledge. Physicians who meet this requirement would also make ideal physician champions for the PGx program.

Laboratory Personnel

The extent of laboratory personnel involvement on the PGx implementation team will depend upon the laboratory chosen for use. The clinical laboratory selected to conduct clinical genotyping should be accredited and licensed by CAP and CLIA, respectively, with appropriately trained and licensed personnel. If these services are not available at the institution where the PGx program is being established, an off-site/third-party laboratory can be used. In addition to the standard commercial laboratories, some academic medical centers and universities offer genotyping services to other institutions. Use of an off-site/third-party laboratory may involve a longer test turnaround time from sample collection to genotype result. This could potentially diminish the usefulness of genetic data, particularly when results are needed for urgent therapeutic decisions, so the impact of delays in receiving test results should be considered if off-site/third-party testing services are used. To illustrate this point, a recent review of 12 institutions implementing *CYP2C19* genotyping to inform antiplatelet therapy in patients undergoing PCI showed that every site conducted genotyping within their institution. This makes sense due to the timely need to dose effective antiplatelet therapy post-PCI.[4] Within this group of institutions, those conducting rapid point-of-care genotyping had a higher proportion of patients with a *CYP2C19* no-function

allele prescribed alternative antiplatelet prescriptions at discharge compared to institutions conducting standard genotyping.[4] In order to minimize post-PCI cardiovascular risk, minimizing time on less effective antiplatelet agents is clearly ideal.

The PGx implementation team, nursing staff, and/or phlebotomist must coordinate getting the patient's genetic sample to the laboratory in a timely manner. Such coordination is usually more complicated when using an off-site/third-party laboratory. If the laboratory used is within the institution, the electronic health record (EHR) system can be used to facilitate the coordination of sample collection and its transport to the laboratory. Whether using an internal or external off-site/third-party laboratory, it is helpful to have a single point of contact who is familiar with PGx testing and can provide information regarding specific sample logistics, test turnaround time, and communication of results to the clinical team. Ideally, this contact person will also be either directly or indirectly involved in performing the actual PGx testing.

Information Technology and Informatics Staff

To facilitate communication among the PGx team and ensure the sharing of timely, easily accessible, and accurate PGx information, successful clinical PGx implementation will likely require an institutional EHR system. Informatics and/or information technology (IT) expertise will be needed to create the CDS infrastructure (see **the** Integration of Pharmacogenomics Result in the EHR section) for recording and integrating PGx test results into the EHR. Including a member with this expertise on your implementation team can facilitate this development. PGx tests are most useful if they can be easily ordered by clinicians and the results can be quickly and easily found. Unlike most clinical laboratory results, a patient's genotype will almost never change, so this information remains clinically useful throughout their lifetime. Thus, storing PGx test results in a designated location within the EHR can allow access to this information over time. If a preemptive PGx panel is chosen for implementation, the storing of data becomes even more important, as some panel data may not be applicable until future changes in the patient's drug therapy. Regardless of the level of informatics implementation, it is imperative to keep in mind that building such areas within the EHR to house genotype results and creating CDS tools may take significant time to create. Thus, it is important that informatics/IT personnel are engaged early in the process of PGx program development.

Third-Party Payers

As with other clinical laboratory tests, PGx tests ordered for most patients will likely be billed to a third-party payer for payment. When developing the PGx program model, it is important to consider whether the tests implemented will be covered by major third-party payers. Thus, contacting representatives early in the planning process to assess their willingness to pay may be prudent. Any data you can provide on how your proposed PGx program will improve patient outcomes or reduce cost will greatly increase your chance of success (see the Funding section).

Patients

The most important stakeholders to be considered during the development of a PGx program are the patients. Not only should the program cater to the individual institution's patient population (see Designing a Service) but it should also consider the patient's interests and priorities. Thus, acquisition of data that provide the patient's perspective on PGx testing will be beneficial. These data will likely be of interest to many of the other stakeholders discussed earlier. One way to gather these data would be to administer questionnaires to the applicable patient population as a preliminary step to strengthen the rationale for program implementation.

Once the service is established, communication with patients serviced by the program is highly recommended. A process should be in place to disseminate genotyping results and interpretations to patients (e.g., by mail, phone, or online access) in the event that they are not present when test results are finalized. Beyond simply reporting their genotype results, patient communication should also include educational materials that explain what genotyping is and why it is performed (see the Education section).

ADMINISTRATION APPROVAL

As discussed previously, implementing PGx into clinical practice will often require participation from multiple specialties/departments. In addition, some amount of funding will be needed to get the program started. Thus, it is essential to obtain support from institutional leadership. Depending on the organizational structure of the institution, this could require engaging a medical director or even the chief executive officer. At larger institutions, the leadership structure may be such that the appropriate person to contact may not be obvious.

Support will be needed from multiple departments, including health system administration, pharmacy, medicine, laboratory, and health IT. Whether it makes sense to start at a higher administrative level and then engage department heads or discuss with department heads first before moving up will depend on the procedure and culture of your institution. Having buy-in from the leadership of each department involved will help establish legitimacy for the program, as well as increase the likelihood of a smooth start. A physician and/or administrative champion can greatly assist in this endeavor (see the Stakeholders section).[19,20,26,27]

In addition, approval from a clinical regulatory body will be required, but the exact committee may vary by institution. Often, the pharmacy and therapeutics (P&T) committee will serve this role. The P&T committee should consider including, when relevant, PGx data for the purpose of evaluating formulary medications. P&T committees may consider consulting resources to aid in decision-making regarding formulary integration. Examples of such resources include the World Health Organization's (WHO) Model List of Essential Medicines (EML), the Pharmacogenetics Knowledgebase (PharmGKB), and the International Society for Pharmacoeconomics and Outcomes Research (ISPOR). The FDA also maintains a list of medications with information regarding PGx biomarkers in the drug labeling.[33,34] Some institutions may have a sub-P&T committee for PGx, but this is not a requirement for implementation. A medical executive committee or other similar bodies may also be necessary in some settings depending on factors such as institution size, committee structure, and assigned tasks. Additional approvals from technical approval boards may also be required.

FUNDING

Establishing who will pay for the service is another critical step. Key players and stakeholders, such as philanthropists or senior administration, may be willing to contribute funding/resources toward implementation. While helpful, philanthropic monetary donations are not a necessary step for implementation. Buy-in from stakeholders often requires a cost analysis of return on investment. Multiple factors play into cost, including IT needs, workforce, overhead space, and upkeep of the program. Funding for the service can be categorized into two parts: (1) the PGx test and (2) the PGx service (e.g., interpretation and recommendation).

Funding Pharmacogenomic Testing

It is possible that institutions may have funding that can at least initially cover the test. If this is the case, it should be determined how long that funding will last and develop a plan for if it runs out. Seed funding may help to get a service off the ground but may not be a sustainable model.

Alternatively, billing for PGx testing may allow for a sustainable model, albeit reimbursement for tests is variable at the present. Direct reimbursement for PGx testing is currently only available in the United States in the outpatient setting. Tests ordered for inpatients are only reimbursable through the diagnosis-related group (DRG) billing, which lumps all payments for a particular diagnosis/procedure into one payment.[35] The laboratory may directly bill the hospital for an inpatient PGx test, and it will be up to the institution if they want to encourage the test to be a part of the DRG. The PGx implementation team will need to consider overall costs and if PGx testing reduces cost to the institution to be accepted as financially viable. For example, in the post-PCI setting, testing for *CYP2C19* could have a positive economic impact by preventing hospital readmissions.[36]

In the outpatient setting, the PGx test can be billed to the patient's medical insurance. Like any other laboratory test, the patient may have to pay a copay or be responsible for the remainder of the charge unpaid by their insurance (including the whole amount if uncovered by insurance). Whether the patients have met their deductible may influence the amount they are required to pay. Currently, reimbursement for PGx tests is variable; therefore, if the service has direct patient interaction, it may be valuable to have a discussion with the laboratory to determine the maximum out-of-pocket cost to the patient. If patients are concerned with out-of-pocket costs, they should contact their insurance company prior to testing. It will be important for the patient to have the Current Procedural Terminology (CPT) or medical billing code of the PGx test to provide to their insurance company, which can be obtained from the laboratory. Insurance coverage for PGx panel testing is currently unconventional, with a majority of coverage related to oncology indications.[37] Some insurance companies may cover single-gene tests for a specific purpose, such as *CYP2C19* to determine appropriateness of clopidogrel post-PCI, depending on evidence available for clinical utility and cost-effectiveness of the test.[38] Third-party payers may pay for specific genes when certain diagnosis codes are present. Typically, third-party payers have their policies posted online, but this information may be difficult to find. For example, Medicare will pay for *CYP2C19* (CPT 81225) with certain ICD-10 codes (e.g., I21.3 [ST elevation (STEMI) myocardial infarction of unspecified site]); however, local coverage determinations should be reviewed.[39] Additionally, some third-party payers may require a prior authorization before they will pay for the test. The clinician or patient can call to find out if a prior authorization is needed. In certain scenarios, the clinician can prepare the prior authorization before ordering the test. Laboratory personal can also help with prior authorizations or resubmitting declined bills. Having a good relationship between the laboratory and clinician can help when discussing these situations up-front.

Funding a Pharmacogenomics Service

When thinking about the funding or payment for the interpretation service, the workflow will dictate billing capabilities. If the health system appreciates the value of a PGx service and wants to offer it to patients as a part of normal clinical services, the PGx program members may be able to provide this service as part of their employment without needing additional funding for their time. This model would be similar to other clinical services, such as an infectious disease service. If the PGx clinician is seeing patients face-to-face in the outpatient setting and desires to bill third parties for the time spent with the patient, billing capabilities in the United States will depend on the medical degree and state laws. If the PGx clinician is a health care provider who is currently allowed to bill for patient visits (e.g., a physician), then PGx interpretation can be worked into other general clinical visits or as separate dedicated visits. If the implementer is a clinician who is not universally allowed to bill for their time (e.g., a pharmacist), then billing strategies will vary by state and partnering with a billing provider may be necessary. Some successful models include pharmacist-led services within research hospitals and academic medical centers, such as St. Jude Children's Hospital and UF. In one model, utilized at institutions such as Sanford Health, all PGx test results are reviewed by a pharmacist who writes a consultation note. Another model, utilized at institutions such as Northshore University Health-System, includes a multidisciplinary approach led by a pharmacy and working with a provider who is able to bill, such as a physician or nurse practitioner. Some models, such as those used at UF, Vanderbilt University, Indiana University, Sanford Health, and Mount Sinai, focus on multigene approaches, while others, like University of Maryland, take a single-gene approach to their interpretation service.[8,23,40,41]

Regardless of the billing structure, it is important to track metrics that reflect value that the service is generating (see the Continuous Monitoring and Improvement Processes section). Metrics that show value will be dictated by the institution's priorities. Some metrics to consider tracking are dollars generated (or estimates of if not billing), relative value units (RVUs) generated from billing, insurance reimbursement of a PGx test and what diagnosis codes were paid for, medication-related recommendations, acceptance of recommendations, and potential cost savings associated with PGx-informed therapeutic changes.

Financial Analysis

A common barrier to PGx implementation is a lack of studies showing cost-effectiveness for PGx testing. As more entities implement PGx testing, more data are becoming available. While not all drug–gene pairs show positive economic outcomes, there is literature to support advancements made in the cost-effectiveness of using PGx information to guide pharmacotherapy. One must use caution in analysis of the studies due to lack of what some would consider high-quality clinical evidence.[42] One of the first drug–gene pairs shown to be cost-effective was HLA B*57:01 and abacavir.[43] In addition, CYP2C19 has been shown to be cost-effective for guiding antiplatelet therapy following PCI.[44] In a study evaluating medications from the FDA Biomarker table, ten medications were examined from 44 studies. Of the 44 studies, 30% showed cost-effectiveness, while another 27% were shown to be cost-saving. As a positive point for encouraging implementation, the study concluded that if genetic testing was freely available, 25% of evaluations would be projected as cost-effective and 50% cost-saving.[45] More targeted studies examining a cost-savings model related to PGx and depression predicted large health care savings, including factors of clinical outcomes and quality of life.[46,47] With the advent of multipanel PGx tests and the possibility of lifelong use of PGx data, PGx tests are anticipated to become increasingly more cost-effective.

DEFINING THE WORKFLOW

Ordering the Test

Allowing for intuitive ordering options will assist providers in ordering PGx tests, which should be available to order in the EHR the same as any other standard laboratory test. It is worth considering having single-gene and panel tests appear as options under a common term, such as "genetic" or "pharmacogenetic," so providers are not required to remember specific gene names. Adding PGx test options to an existing order set may be worthwhile in some instances. For example, at UF Health, a CYP2C19 test is included on the cardiac catheterization lab order set to assist in antiplatelet therapy selection.[23]

Sample Collection

As discussed earlier, sample collection is usually done via blood draw or buccal swab. Buccal swabs are rubbed inside a patient's cheek. The sample may be performed in-house or sent to an off-site/third-party laboratory. In the case of off-site/third-party laboratories and buccal samples, patients sometimes might mail the sample directly to the laboratory (see the Testing Platform section).

Integration of Pharmacogenomics Results in the EHR

Active CDS that interprets genetic data and guides clinicians within the prescription process has been recognized as one of the vital ingredients for successful PGx implementation.[48] How the information is integrated will dictate how effectively CDS may be employed. In some cases, PGx results may come from an off-site/third-party lab that provides a downloadable PDF or XML version of the report, which are often the hardest to incorporate into the EHR. One significant concern of including PDF reports is that active interruptive CDS would not be feasible with such reports, as CDS depends on discrete variables. There is also a workflow challenge of who would receive the results and be responsible for incorporating this PDF file into the EHR. Although data in XML format are more computable for providing active CDS, even most modern EHRs are not equipped to use XML-formatted data directly for CDS. This is because (1) there is no standard way of reporting PGx results from outside laboratories that would be interoperable in an EHR-agnostic manner; (2) EHRs currently do not support standard CDS algorithms (e.g., drug interactions, drug-dose checking) for PGx gene–drug pairs; and (3) CDS alerts may vary significantly across health care settings for each drug–gene pair.[49]

Once results are incorporated into the EHR, how the results are stored to enable long-term access remains a challenge. St. Jude Children's Hospital created a separate PGx tab within their EHR, which prevents genotype results from being buried under other laboratory test results as time passes.[13] However, this level of integration may not be possible for all institutions. Others, such as the University of Illinois at Chicago, simply created a new patient note category within their EHR system specifically for PGx consults, and individual notes were written by a pharmacist and placed in this section to achieve a similar effect.[50] Institutions may also consider inquiring what is already offered by their EHR vendor, often at an additional cost. For example, Epic recently implemented "genomic indicators" that the institution can use in various ways to meet their needs.

Although it might be easier to streamline the integration of PGx results from an on-site laboratory, significant informatics infrastructure development is still required to automate this process.[49] Use of an on-site laboratory generally has the advantage of providing discrete laboratory results directly into the EHR. Custom CDS rules may then be more easily designed to work with those discrete results. In building such extensive IT infrastructure, the implementation team must work with a multidisciplinary informatics board, P&T committee, or similar governing body of the organization to obtain approval and ensure the resiliency and accuracy of the system performance. UF Health invested significant resources in developing a streamlined informatics workflow to order a test and receive results from their molecular pathology laboratory. Their custom CDS alerts provided test

interpretation and clinical recommendations with formulary alternatives.[23] The custom rules check if any PGx results are available for the ordered drug and only provide guidance when results are actionable. When results are available and actionable, an interruptive CDS alert with alternative formulary recommendations appears. In other instances, when PGx data are not discrete but are available, an alert may prompt the clinician to review the available PGx results. The clinician is then responsible for reviewing, identifying actionable results, and finally making the changes recommended.

CPIC guidelines recommend converting genotype information to phenotype so that the phenotype-specific guidelines may be used in the clinical setting.[51] To support clinicians at the point-of-care with active CDS, CPIC provides pre-test and post-test alert flow charts with each clinical guideline.[52] Thoughtful workflow design may also support quality monitoring and facilitate the future expansion of PGx services to other drug–gene pairs. Resources such as PheKB knowledgebase,[53] CDS knowledgebase,[54] sequence and phenotype integration,[55] and IGNITE Tool Box[56] provide many helpful examples of CDS alerts and workflows in various EHR systems. Figure 2-3 illustrates potential pre-test and post-test CDS alerts using CPIC guideline for phenytoin.[57] At the present, it is up to the

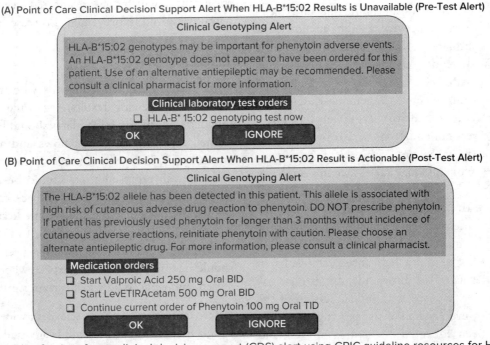

(A) Point of Care Clinical Decision Support Alert When HLA-B*15:02 Results is Unavailable (Pre-Test Alert)

Clinical Genotyping Alert

HLA-B*15:02 genotypes may be important for phenytoin adverse events. An HLA-B*15:02 genotype does not appear to have been ordered for this patient. Use of an alternative antiepileptic may be recommended. Please consult a clinical pharmacist for more information.

Clinical laboratory test orders
☐ HLA-B* 15:02 genotyping test now

[OK]   [IGNORE]

(B) Point of Care Clinical Decision Support Alert When HLA-B*15:02 Result is Actionable (Post-Test Alert)

Clinical Genotyping Alert

The HLA-B*15:02 allele has been detected in this patient. This allele is associated with high risk of cutaneous adverse drug reaction to phenytoin. DO NOT prescribe phenytoin. If patient has previously used phenytoin for longer than 3 months without incidence of cutaneous adverse reactions, reinitiate phenytoin with caution. Please choose an alternate antiepileptic drug. For more information, please consult a clinical pharmacist.

Medication orders
☐ Start Valproic Acid 250 mg Oral BID
☐ Start LevETIRAcetam 500 mg Oral BID
☐ Continue current order of Phenytoin 100 mg Oral TID

[OK]   [IGNORE]

FIGURE 2-3 • Example of point-of-care clinical decision support (CDS) alert using CPIC guideline resources for HLA-B*15:02 when a phenotype is being ordered. (A) A pre-test CDS alert notifying the clinician that an HLA-B*15:02 test may be important and allowing the clinician to order the test. (B) A post-test CDS alert on an actionable genotyping result with potential alternative recommendations.

implementers to develop their own process because there are currently no established guidelines on how to store the PGx data in the EHR.

Developing an informatics infrastructure aligned with the designed workflow will undoubtedly help facilitate consistent, timely, accessible, and accurate PGx information communication among all relevant individuals. If a third-party PGx test provider is selected, an option for EHR integration of results might include one of the following options: (1) the ordering/consulting clinician is responsible for reviewing the PGx results and manually uploading the PDF version of the results with a clinical note; (2) automatic uploading of PGx results directly from the laboratory when available and notifying the consulting clinician of the new results; and (3) automatic uploading of the PGx results directly from the laboratory, when possible with automated phenotype translation, and alerting clinicians of actionable recommendations.[49,58]

Interpretation of Results

It is important to determine who will handle and interpret the PGx results once they are returned from the laboratory. Approaches may depend on how the results are integrated into the EHR. Results may be returned to the ordering clinician, primary care physician, pharmacy team, or, in some cases, just documented in the patient chart with no active comprehensive review. Interpretation approaches include reviewing and charting on all results or reviewing all results but only charting on actionable results. Providers might acknowledge the PGx results similar to other laboratory tests. Some institutions may depend solely upon CDS. Institutions may have a process for consults/referrals to a pharmacist/pharmacy team or medical geneticist. Consults may constitute a comprehensive chart review by a pharmacist to make recommendations to a provider, while others involve actively meeting with patients to discuss the PGx results. Consults may take place in a specialty environment or within the primary care setting. Not all institutions have the means to hire a team of medical geneticists or devote a pharmacist's time completely to PGx. Certain pharmacists may be identified who have an interest in PGx and can help interpret results in addition to other assigned duties. Ideally, all pharmacists would be able to assist with interpretation of the PGx results. However, not all of the existing pharmacy workforce has been educated in the area of PGx and utilization of patient specific results (see the Education section). Nurses may also play a key role in alerting providers of actionable PGx results.

TESTING THE PROPOSED WORKFLOW

After defining the service workflow by actively collaborating with stakeholders and obtaining administrative approval, the PGx implementation team will work on developing the pilot service for testing. A pilot service may include PGx implementation at one site or for a subset of the overall targeted patient population. If the team decides to include PGx test ordering with electronic order sets, changes may be tested in the EHR testing environment. CDS may be used to check for existing orders or available PGx results to avoid duplicate ordering. Human factors engineering (HFE) should also be considered in developing a new service to ensure patient safety in the clinical setting. With regular meetings of the PGx team, an iterative designing of the new service can be developed.

An approach for identifying potential vulnerability is to apply failure mode and effect analysis. Multiple studies have shown the value of employing this system in improving patient safety and reducing errors in the process.[59–61] Evaluation of pilot sites, mock-ups, and prototypes should be considered until usability and safety goals are attained. These evaluations should help identify issues, vulnerabilities, and workarounds, allowing the team to address them. Finally, the team should plan for monitoring the effectiveness of the new services for the predefined evaluation (quality and performance) metrics to analyze the extent to which they are affected (see the Continuous Monitoring and Improvement Processes section).

EDUCATION

Once ready to launch, clinicians who will be ordering PGx tests, receiving results, reviewing results, and/or interacting with any CDS alerts should be educated and trained regarding new workflows and alerts they may encounter. Training should occur before the launch date, and clinician representation should be involved in the educational planning so that feedback can be obtained, as providers who use the affected medications on a daily basis will likely have helpful insight to aid in the integration of the workflow. All potential users of the service should be trained on what to expect, where results will be stored, and what to do when certain alerts display.

Before launching the PGx service, a wide variety of personnel may require training. It is advisable to discuss this with the health care providers involved to determine their knowledge and comfort with PGx. This could be done either formally (e.g., surveys to obtain quantitative data) or informally. Regardless of the results, education prior to the launch should be done. The inquiry will just help inform the depth of topic area(s) and quantity of education needed. It would be helpful to consider beginning PGx education during the development of the PGx service so when the service is ready to launch, training of the pertinent health care professionals on the basics of PGx is completed so new trainings can focus on the service's processes and workflows. If the health care professionals need continuing education (CE) or continuing medical education (CME), educational sessions that provide this credit might be valued. Online CMEs are less well attended, and in-person education may be preferred.[27] Offering personal genotyping to the health care providers is a method that has been shown to be beneficial in educating providers and students on PGx.[27,62] This will not only engage the clinicians but also allows the opportunity to model the type of service that will be provided to their patients (e.g., consult note) to obtain buy-in and feedback. Consistent engagement and education with health care professionals will ultimately result in a successful service. Interesting patient cases could be used and shared at the "case conferences," where lessons learned and clinical pearls could be discussed among providers. Health care professionals often prefer to learn utilizing real-life patient cases, and it will make the education more meaningful if they know that they or their colleague referred that patient into the PGx service.

Educational materials are important to develop for both providers and patients. Genomic medicine resources for clinicians, researchers, educators, and patients can be found within the IGNITE Tool Box.[56] Providers will appreciate quick reference guides (e.g., who to refer, how to refer, where to go to apply results). Patients will also appreciate visit summary handouts, but it is important to create it in patient-friendly terminology and language. The Joint Commission states that patient education materials should be written at or below a fifth-grade reading level.[63] Of note, using the word "pharmacogenomic" will significantly increase the reading level. As long as the terminology is defined, you can typically use a higher reading level and still achieve patient comprehension.

Patients should receive education prior to undergoing PGx testing (pre-test education) so they understand the purpose, risks, limitations, and anticipated outcomes. Specifically, patients should be educated about the Genetic Information Nondiscrimination Act (GINA) and what it protects and does not protect against as far as insurance coverage, as well as potential incidental findings. PGx testing is less risky as compared to whole-genome testing in terms of incidental findings; however, it could reveal that one's parents or siblings are not blood-related if multiple family members have test results. Additionally, setting realistic expectations for patients is key, as PGx is one piece of the clinical picture, and it will not solve all of the patient's medication-related problems. Some programs have used patient educational videos,[64] while others may use written or verbal education. These educational components should be considered when developing a patient consent form. The logistics of a consent form are not covered in this chapter and should be discussed with the individual institution's legal departments.

Post-PGx test education for patients should include communication of results, significance of results to current medications, impact on future medications, and familial implications. Providing PGx results to patients will vary based on the health care system—some will provide a copy of the laboratory report to the patient in the patient portal, and others may depend on the provider to communicate the results. Some laboratory reports may not be patient friendly, so you may opt to create your own format of results to hand out or mail to patients. As patients may go to another health care system where their laboratory results do not transfer, it would be up to the patient to bring their PGx results with them. Patients must be educated that PGx results are lifelong, so they are empowered to bring their results with them and be aware of potential future medications that may be affected by their results.

LAUNCH THE SERVICE

Institutions may have their own required approvals before starting, and these should all be in place before launching the PGx service. After reading through this chapter, implementers will hopefully have an idea of how to shape their PGx service. It is then advisable to create a checklist of all items that need to be in place before launching the service. Table 2-3 provides a general framework of such a checklist, and implementers can use this as a starting point in order to create their own checklist. Before the first patient undergoes testing, all items described here should be in place.

CONTINUOUS MONITORING AND IMPROVEMENT PROCESSES

Any health care service is rarely perfect at the time of the launch. Based on the key performance indicators (KPIs) and outcome indicators defined pre-launch of the PGx service, data should be collected after launching the service. This step is crucial for assuring the quality of the service provided, analyzing cost, and evaluating evidence to continue to offer the service. Implementers may have to plan for obtaining additional approval if collected data will be used beyond internal quality assurance purposes (e.g., for publication).

TABLE 2-3. Summary Checklist of Considerations Prior to Launching a PGx Service

Obtain health system support and ability to advertise new service
Develop a marketing plan and identify resources
Set up billing capabilities and create a financial plan
Establish a collaborative practice agreement (if applicable)
Work with laboratory to establish sample transportation workflow and result return
Determine need for education for health care providers, schedule, and plan appropriately
Create patient education materials (if applicable)
Determine the language for recommendations and delivery format
Create CDS tools and accompanying educational materials
Establish a plan for continuous CDS alert monitoring and updating
Establish how results will be tracked and monitored
Establish a continuous metric monitoring plan (see Continuous Monitoring and Improvement Processes)
Establish an ongoing educational plan for health care providers

Major categories of KPIs for PGx service are (1) service process, (2) service utilization, and (3) patient and provider satisfaction. Although outcome indicators may vary depending on the drug–gene pair selected, these indicators are fundamental to assess how the PGx service affects the outcome compared to historical data. These outcome indicators may also be used for cost analysis. Table 2-4 contains the list of KPIs and outcome indicators that are potentially applicable for a PGx service.

After KPI data are analyzed, consider changes to optimize the service. Often, education is a key component of improving workflow and expansion of the service. When changes are made, those affected should be notified through email, presentation, other modes of communication, or a combination of methods. Feedback on the process from both patients and providers can draw attention to issues that were not realized during the planning or previous revision processes. For example, during implementation of clopidogrel–*CYP2C19* at UF Health, the following KPI data were collected: numbers of tests ordered, results, the turnaround time, number of accepted recommendations, research consent and enrollment, pathology processes, and quality improvement. The UF Health team also encountered challenges in sample collection during their initial implementation—specifically, there was unfamiliarity with PGx tests. Through collecting KPI data and being aware of encountered

TABLE 2-4. List of Common Key Performance and Outcome Indicators Relevant for a PGx Service Implementation

Type of Indicators	Category	Variables
Key performance indicators (KPIs)	Service process	Turnaround time of genotype results, turnaround time of service communication, time from available genotyping result to service recommendation, % of service completed within a year, % of results available within a time frame or prior to a dose given, number of inappropriate orders, number of delayed genotype results
	Service utilization	Consultation number, number of genotype tests ordered and performed, number of patients who have actionable genotypes, % of accepted PGx recommendation, % of ignored PGx recommendation
	Satisfaction	Overall satisfaction of the patients and providers by a survey, overall acceptance rate by medical services
Outcome indicators	Encounters	Length of stay, number of hospitalizations, emergency department visits due to adverse drug events
	Therapeutic level	Time to a therapeutic level, average time within the therapeutic window, number of patients with therapeutic level upon hospital discharge, the proportion of supratherapeutic drug monitoring level
	Alternatives	Use of more expensive drugs, duration of patients on more expensive alternative drug

challenges, the need for educating registered nurses and phlebotomists was identified.[23] In the case of the University of Illinois Hospital and Health Sciences System's genotype-guided warfarin implementation, additional clinical data such as time to achieve a therapeutic international normalized ratio (INR), INR levels outside the therapeutic window, age, prior bleeding event, concomitant medications, and duration of low-molecular-weight heparin use were collected.[65]

In addition to optimizing the workflow, planning for expansion of the service is an important consideration. Because PGx is an emerging field and new data are constantly being generated, it is important to plan ahead and anticipate new guidelines, testing platforms, and IT updates.

CHALLENGES/BARRIERS

Ideally, utilizing the steps outlined in this chapter will mitigate the major challenges. However, each institution is different and will present its own unique challenges. Table 2-5 summarizes major challenges from the literature and provides potential solutions to overcome them[23,27,66,67] Institutions are encouraged to keep track of the challenges they encounter and disseminate how they overcome them to help other intuitions that are early in the PGx implementation stage.

CONCLUSION

PGx implementation requires collaborating with multiple stakeholders and significant research in evidence,

TABLE 2-5. A Summary of Perceived Barriers and Potential Solution to Pharmacogenomic Implementation Service[23,27,66,67]

Challenge	Potential Solution
Provider knowledge gaps	Provide case-based education before implementation and intermittently throughout
Referrals to PGx service and/or identifying who to test in context of a lack of guidelines indicating who should undergo testing	Create quick reference guides of who might benefit from testing (e.g., providing what medications are affected by the test), provide constant reminders of the service, screen for patients experiencing side effects or ineffectiveness with affected medications and flag those patients for referral by provider, get face time with providers who are referring to remind them of the PGx service
Sample collection	Have options (i.e., blood, saliva, and buccal collection)
Interpretation of results	Have a dedicated PGx specialist on the PGx implementation team or set up easy-to-use references and resources that can help interpret (e.g., automated interpretation notes)
Evolving knowledge	Periodic review of the literature and appropriate dissemination; involvement in PGx implementation groups (i.e., CPIC)
Lack of EHR integration	Work with informatics group and the EHR provider to integrate results as discrete fields
Patient perception	Provide education and give realistic expectations on how the PGx results will affect medication regimens
Timing and access to PGx results	Preemptive testing allows for the result to be acted upon by the health care provider when they are face-to-face with the patient
Time to discuss results with the patient	Implement service in a setting where time constraint is not a barrier
Reimbursement of test	Track data and contribute to literature to aid in overcoming this challenge in the future
Lack of evidence demonstrating cost-effectiveness	Track data and contribute to the literature to assist in overcoming this challenge in the future
Discrepancies between PGx guidelines of different organizations	Define process for evaluating discrepancies (i.e., scorecards and monographs) and decide on evidence thresholds for uptake
Lack of physician acceptance of PGx testing	Continuous education and provide summary of PGx outcomes literature and real-life patient cases
Lack of patient acceptance of PGx testing	Education and demonstration of the benefits of having a PGx test
Lack of expertise among prescribing clinicians to determine whether a PGx test is appropriate	Partner with a PGx specialist

feasibility, and workflow development. The implementation process may seem overwhelming at first. Throughout this chapter, there are many essential factors to consider, resources to support, case-specific scenarios to provide real-world challenges, and some approaches to address them. Note that every health care system, its patients, and clinicians are different and there is no single implementation approach that works for everyone. Therefore, every PGx implementation will need to be customized to the health care system, even with the resources and guidelines provided in this chapter. It may be useful to reach out to other institutions that have successfully implemented PGx. Also, rarely will an implementation be flawless the first time. Therefore, continuous monitoring, reevaluation of quality, communication, addressing failures, education, and maintenance are necessary.

RESOURCES

CPIC informatics https://cpicpgx.org/informatics/

PharmGKB https://www.pharmgkb.org

Genetic Testing Registry https://www.ncbi.nlm.nih.gov/gtr/

eMERGE network https://emerge.mc.vanderbilt.edu

Phenotype knowledgebase https://phekb.org

CDS knowledgebase https://cdskb.org

Sequence and phenotype integration https://www.emergesphinx.org

IGNITE SPARK TOOLBOX and implementation guide https://gmkb.org/

CASE SCENARIOS

1. While standing in line for coffee Dr. Carridy, a cardiologist, sees Dr. Pharmington also waiting in line. Dr. Pharmington is a pharmacist who Dr. Carridy knows because their daughters play on the same soccer team. While they work in the same health system, Stone Oak Health, they rarely see each other due to their varying practice specialties. Dr. Pharmington spends most of his time in psychiatry as the psychiatric pharmacy specialist, while Dr. Carridy is busy with her inpatient and outpatient cardiology practices. Dr. Carridy asks Dr. Pharmington if he thinks Stone Oak Health should look into implementing PGx into their health system. Dr. Carridy currently utilizes PGx testing occasionally within her practice but has not heard of other Stone Oak Health providers using it. Dr. Pharmington's training had a strong precision medicine focus, and he thinks PGx services would be beneficial to Stone Oak Health. While both Drs. Carridy and Pharmington have some experience in PGx, they still feel a bit overwhelmed with the idea of implementation. Dr. Pharmington agrees that he and Dr. Carridy should pursue this idea. They decide to survey a group of stakeholders and identify potential implementation team members to discuss the possibility of the health system–wide implementation of PGx.

    After reviewing some initial information, Drs. Carridy and Pharmington survey a group of stakeholders to gauge the level of support for PGx implementation. After support from stakeholders is obtained, Drs. Carridy and

    Pharmington build a PGx implementation team and suggest the team consider using the CPIC Level A guidelines to help decide which drug–gene pairs to test. This suggestion is based on the high level of evidence included in the CPIC guidelines.

    Question: Based on CPIC guidelines, and as a cardiologist, which drug–gene pair(s) might be important to Dr. Carridy's practice?

    Answer: As a cardiologist, Dr. Carridy is likely to be interested in clopidogrel–CYP2C19 and may also be interested in simvastatin–SLCO1B1 and warfarin–CYP2C9, VKORC1, CYP4F2.

    Question: Based on CPIC guidelines, and as a pharmacist specializing in psychiatry, which drug–gene pair(s) might be important to Dr. Pharmington's practice?

    Answer: As a pharmacist specializing in psychiatry, Dr. Pharmington is likely to be interested in CYP2D6 and CYP2C19 to assist in the selection of SSRIs and TCAs.

2. **Question:** How should Dr. Carridy approach which PGx test to use for her patients?

    Answer: After reviewing the PGx evidence for clopidogrel, warfarin, and simvastatin, Dr. Carridy wants to implement a PGx test for clopidogrel for all of her acute coronary syndrome (ACS) patients and patients undergoing PCI instead of just using PGx occasionally.

In her practicing hospital, a significant proportion of the patients are of European and Asian ancestry. According to the CPIC clopidogrel–CYP2C19 guideline, up to 45% and 15% of the Asian patients may exhibit intermediate and poor metabolizer phenotype, respectively (compared to 27% and 2.5% in those of European descent). Dr. Carridy asks the PGx implementation team to gather gene–allele coverage, sample source, and an approximate turnaround time for CYP2C19 genotyping assays. The team identifies AMP recommended Tier 1 variants for CYP2C19 to be *2, *3, and *17 alleles.[21] A search in the GTR resulted in 42 CLIA-certified tests with the CYP2C19 gene. However, since this team is inexperienced with PGx services and a longer turnaround time is associated with LDTs, the team leaned towards using an in-house FDA-cleared device.

3. Stone Oak Health debates launching an in-house quick clopidogrel–YP2C19 pharmacogenomics service.

Question: Why should administration approval be required before launching the clopidogrel–CYP2C19 pharmacogenomics service?

Answer: The PGx implementation team for clopidogrel and CYP2C19 in a single hospital inpatient setting may require approval from the P&T committee, cardiology team, laboratory services, informatics team, and financial administration before the implementation of the service. A formal approval process keeps everyone involved aware of the process, have a contact person for education and challenges, and understand the workflow and the vulnerabilities. Since PGx test turnaround time may vary significantly depending on the type of test used, the core team may have to coordinate the PGx service during the transition of care (from hospital to the outpatient setting). For example, the patient may be discharged from the hospital by the time the PGx test result is available if an off-site/third-party lab-provided PGx test is used. The PGx implementation team may have to coordinate the transfer of the actionable PGx results in the outpatient setting. The cardiologist may make necessary changes to clopidogrel therapy during the follow-up appointment. This coordination-of-care process may not be trivial when inpatient and outpatient EHRs are different and do not communicate with each other. In this case, additional approval from the risk management team may need to be considered. Since Dr. Carridy is using an in-house quick CYP2C19 test (e.g., Spartan RX), she will be able to intervene as appropriate, while the ACS/PCI patients are in the hospital. However, having discrete PGx results with CDS alerts in the EHR (inpatient and outpatient)

will ensure the continuity of care. If anyone wants to order clopidogrel on CYP2C19 suboptimal (poor or intermediate) metabolizers as a cost-saving measure, a CDS alert will warn the ordering clinician about the risk.

4. Dr. Carridy is busy in her practice and concerned about the increase in PGx test results that will be returned to her.

Question: What is a possible solution to ensure Dr. Carridy is not missing anything?

Answer: Dr. Carridy would like to have a pharmacist place an interpretation note in her patients' charts once the PGx results return so she does not miss any drug–drug–gene interactions. Dr. Pharmington thinks this is a great idea, and he sets out to engage pharmacists within cardiology to join their team and brainstorm how to fund the PGx interpretation service. (See Interpretation of Results.)

5. **Question:** How should Dr. Pharmington decide what PGx test to use for his patients?

Answer: Since multiple genes affect many psychiatry medications (e.g., CYP2C19, CYP2D6), Dr. Pharmington may consider a preemptive test with a multigene panel for all his patients at his practice. He may be okay with a PGx test that takes a longer turnaround time but would require a test with broader gene–allele panel (e.g., GeneSight, YouScript Psychotropic). He may consider using an off-site/third-party lab that uses whole blood for high-quality DNA for CYP2D6 copy-number variant detection. This way, he does not have to worry about having a CAP/CLIA-certified laboratory and a phlebotomist on-site. Another point for him to consider is that insurance reimbursement can be challenging with preemptive testing. His patients may have to go through a prior authorization process to avoid the high out-of-pocket cost associated with preemptive PGx testing.

6. Dr. Carridy and Dr. Pharmington's practice settings vary significantly. Dr. Carridy has her practice in the hospital, whereas Dr. Pharmington practices at the clinic.

Question: How may the PGx result integration vary for their practice settings?

Answer: CYP2C19 genotype-guided antiplatelet therapy following PCI is the top drug–gene that is clinically implemented by the early PGx adopters.[4,5] Since an in-house CYP2C19 test will be used for all of Dr. Carridy's ACS/PCI patients, the results may be automatically uploaded as discrete data in the EHR after developing a streamlined workflow. On the other hand, Dr. Pharmington is *opting for an off-site/third-party company for the test, so he will likely receive the results in PDF format. Therefore, all results for his patients may have to be manually imported and coded as discrete data into the EHR. In this case, the PGx implementation team may decide the pharmacist interpreting the pharmacogenetic results (i.e., Dr. Pharmington in most cases) would be the assigned individual for this manual process. Ideally, Stone Oak Health would use the same laboratory for PGx testing to simplify workflow and results. However, this example helps to illustrate different approaches.*

7. **Question:** *How might the clopidogrel–CYP2C19 service be set up with an informatics infrastructure?*

Answer: *Depending on the workflow of the service implementation, the informatics infrastructure may vary significantly. Dr. Carridy may want to include the PGx test (e.g., Spartan RX test for CYP2C19) within the ACS/PCI order set. Once the result is generated from the Spartan RX test, the PGx clinical team, including Dr. Carridy, may receive an automated notification to review the results. The CYP2C19 genotyping result from Spartan RX is quick and straightforward for Dr. Carridy to review and intervene if necessary. It may also be feasible to set up a CDS alert that will trigger for the ordering physician only when actionable results are generated and provide formulary alternatives based on the PGx result. For example, all post-ACS/PCI patients may start with a clopidogrel 75 mg PO daily order. If the PGx result for a patient returns as a CYP2C19 intermediate or poor metabolizer, the CDS alert may recommend Dr. Carridy change clopidogrel to ticagrelor 90 mg PO bid (or prasugrel 10 mg PO daily if it is on the formulary). If PGx results are coded in the EHR and an automated CDS alert process is set, clinicians may receive alerts when an actionable PGx result is applicable for other medications. For example, Mr. Johnson had a CYP2C19 PGx test done while he underwent PCI 3 years ago. His test result indicates he is a poor CYP2C19 metabolizer. Mr. Johnson was diagnosed with depression and was being considered for citalopram 20 mg PO daily as a starting dose by his psychiatrist. Based on CPIC guidelines for a CYP2C19 poor metabolizer, 10 mg of citalopram as a starting dose is recommended for Mr. Johnson to minimize the risk of side effects. In this case, the ordering physician may not be aware of the availability of the actionable CYP2C19 result for Mr. Johnson. However, discrete CYP2C19 genotyping results in the EHR may trigger a point-of-care CDS alert and prompt the ordering physician about the potential intervention. On the other hand, if Mr. Johnson was a CYP2C19 ultrarapid metabolizer, the CDS alert may recommend other SSRIs that are not predominantly metabolized by CYP2C19 (e.g., fluoxetine, paroxetine) on the formulary.*

PHARMACOGENOMICS IMPLEMENTATION PEARLS

- Implementation of a PGx involves many components.
- Consider patient characteristics and relevant disease states when designing a service.
- Identifying and engaging key stakeholders and implementation team members are crucial.
- Select a test considering patient population, disease condition, gene–allele coverage, turnaround time, and cost.
- Investigate pharmacogenomics resources that provide strong evidence.
- Design a workflow that works for your individual institution.
- An IT infrastructure can streamline workflow and can be leveraged for continuous improvement measures.
- Repetitive education is key.

ABBREVIATIONS AND ACRONYMS

ACS: Acute coronary syndrome

AMP: Association for Molecular Pathology Pharmacogenomics Working Group

CAP: College of American Pathologists

CDS: Clinical decision support

CLIA: Clinical Laboratory Improvement Amendments

CPIC: Clinical Pharmacogenetics Implementation Consortium

CPT: Current procedural terminology

DPWG: Dutch Pharmacogenetics Working Group

EHR: Electronic health record

GTR: Gene testing registry

KPIs: Key performance indicators

LDTs: Laboratory developed tests

PCI: Percutaneous coronary intervention

PGx: Pharmacogenomics

REFERENCES

1. Keeling NJ, Rosenthal MM, West-Strum D, Patel AS, Haidar CE, Hoffman JM. Preemptive pharmacogenetic testing: exploring the knowledge and perspectives of US payers. *Genet Med.* 2017; 21(5):1224-1232.

2. Roden DM, Van Driest SL, Mosley JD, et al. Benefit of preemptive pharmacogenetic information on clinical outcome. *Clin Pharmacol Ther.* 2018;103:787-794.

3. CPIC. CPIC Implementation. 2020. Available at https://cpicpgx. org/implementation/. Accessed June 5, 2019.

4. Empey PE, Stevenson JM, Tuteja S, et al. Multisite investigation of strategies for the implementation of CYP2C19 genotype-guided antiplatelet therapy. *Clin Pharmacol Ther.* 2018;104:664-674.

5. Cavallari LH, Lee CR, Beitelshees AL, et al. Multisite investigation of outcomes with implementation of CYP2C19 genotype-guided antiplatelet therapy after percutaneous coronary intervention. *JACC Cardiovasc Interv.* 2018;11:181-191.

6. Dawes M, Aloise MN, Ang S, et al. Introducing pharmacogenetic testing with clinical decision support into primary care: a feasibility study. *CMAJ Open.* 2016;4:E528-E534.

7. Weitzel K, Cavallari L, Lesko L. Preemptive panel-based pharmacogenetic testing: the time is now. *Pharm Res.* 2017;34:1551-1555.

8. Petry N, Baye JF, Aifaoui A, et al. Implementation of wide-scale pharmacogenetic testing in primary care. *Pharmacogenomics.* 2019;20:903-913.

9. Oberg V, Differding J, Fisher M, Hines L, Wilke R. Navigating pleiotropy in precision medicine: pharmacogenes from trauma to behavioral health. *Pharmacogenomics.* 2016;17:499-505.

10. Hoffman J. How Pharmacogenomics Can Improve Pediatric Patient Safety. 2019. Available at https://www.childrenshospitals. org/Newsroom/Childrens-Hospitals-Today/Articles/2019/03/ How-Pharmacogenomics-Can-Improve-Pediatric-Patient-Safety. Accessed February 12, 2020.

11. Maagdenberg H, Vijverberg SJH, Bierings MB, et al. Pharmacogenomics in pediatric patients: towards personalized medicine. *Paediatr Drugs.* 2016;18:251-260.

12. Van Driest S, McGregor T. Pharmacogenetics in clinical pediatrics: challenges and strategies. *Per Med.* 2013;10.

13. Hoffman JM, Haidar CE, Wilkinson MR, et al. PG4KDS: a model for the clinical implementation of pre-emptive pharmacogenetics. *Am J Med Genet C Semin Med Genet.* 2014;166C:45-55.

14. CPIC. What is CPIC? Available at https://cpicpgx.org/. Accessed 22 July, 2019.

15. Hung S, Chung W, Chen Y. Genetics of severe drug hypersensitivity reactions in Han Chinese. In: W. Pichler, ed. *Drug Hypersensitivity.* Basel, CH: Karger. 2007:105-114.

16. Nakkam N, Kongyoung P, Kanjanawart S, et al. HLA pharmacogenetic markers of drug hypersensitivity in a Thai population. *Front Genet.* 2018;9:277.

17. Dean L. Carbamazepine therapy and HLA genotype. 2015 Oct 14. In: V. M.H. Pratt, W. Rubinstein, et al. eds. *Medical Genetics Summaries.* Bethesda, MD: National Center for Biotechnology Information; 2012. Available at https://www.ncbi.nlm.nih.gov/ books/NBK321445/. Accessed July 9, 2019.

18. Bousman CA, Dunlop BW. Genotype, phenotype, and medication recommendation agreement among commercial pharmacogenetic-based decision support tools. *Pharmacogenomics J.* 2018;18:613-622.

19. Mukerjee G, Huston A, Kabakchiev B, Piquette-Miller M, van Schaik R, Dorfman R. User considerations in assessing pharmacogenomic tests and their clinical support tools. *NPJ Genom Med.* 2018;3:26.

20. Arwood MJ, Chumnumwat S, Cavallari LH, Nutescu EA, Duarte JD. Implementing pharmacogenomics at your institution: establishment and overcoming implementation challenges. *Clin Transl Sci.* 2016;9:233-245.

21. Pratt VM, Del Tredici AL, Hachad H, et al. Recommendations for clinical CYP2C19 genotyping allele selection: a report of the association for molecular pathology. *J Mol Diagn.* 2018;20:269-276.

22. Pratt VM, Cavallari LH, Del Tredici AL, et al. Recommendations for clinical CYP2C9 genotyping allele selection: a joint recommendation of the association for molecular pathology and college of American pathologists. *J Mol Diagn.* 2019;21:746-755.

23. Weitzel KW, Elsey AR, Langaee TY, et al. Clinical pharmacogenetics implementation: approaches, successes, and challenges. *Am J Med Genet C Semin Med Genet.* 2014;166C:56-67.

24. Johnson JA, Burkley BM, Langaee TY, Clare-Salzler MJ, Klein TE, Altman RB. Implementing personalized medicine: development of a cost-effective customized pharmacogenetics genotyping array. *Clin Pharmacol Ther.* 2012;92:437-439.

25. Crews KR, Cross SJ, McCormick JN, et al. Development and implementation of a pharmacist-managed clinical pharmacogenetics service. *Am J Health Syst Pharm.* 2011;68:143-50.

26. Dunnenberger HM, Crews KR, Hoffman JM, et al. Preemptive clinical pharmacogenetics implementation: current programs in five US medical centers. *Annu Rev Pharmacol Toxicol.* 2015;55:89-106.

27. Cicali EJ, Weitzel KW, Elsey AR, et al. Challenges and lessons learned from clinical pharmacogenetic implementation of multiple gene-drug pairs across ambulatory care settings. *Genet Med.* 2019;21(10):2264-2274.

28. GTR. Genetic Testing Registry. 2020. Available at https://www. ncbi.nlm.nih.gov/gtr/.

29. Cavallari LH, Weitzel KW, Elsey AR, et al. Institutional profile: University of Florida Health Personalized Medicine Program. *Pharmacogenomics.* 2017;18:421-426.

30. Pulley JM, Denny JC, Peterson JF, et al. Operational implementation of prospective genotyping for personalized medicine: the design of the Vanderbilt PREDICT project. *Clin Pharmacol Ther.* 2012;92:87-95.

31. Shuldiner AR, Palmer K, Pakyz RE, et al. Implementation of pharmacogenetics: the University of Maryland Personalized Anti-platelet Pharmacogenetics Program. *Am J Med Genet C Semin Med Genet.* 2014;166C:76-84.

32. Caraballo PJ, Hodge LS, Bielinski SZ, et al. Multidisciplinary model to implement pharmacogenomics at the point of care. *Genet Med.* 2017;19:421-429.

33. United States Food and Drug Administration. Table of Pharmacogenomic Biomarkers in Drug Labeling. Available at https://www.fda.gov/drugs/science-research-drugs/table-pharmacogenomic-biomarkers-drug-labeling. Accessed 26 March, 2019.

34. Poppe L, Roederer M. Global formulary review: how do we integrate pharmacogenomic information? *Ann of Pharmacother.* 2011;45:532-538.

35. Berndt ER, G.D., Rowe J. Economic dimensions of personalized and precision medicine. Berndt ER, Goldman DP, Rowe J, eds. Chicago, US: University of Chicago Press. 2019:300 .

36. Borse MS, Dong OM, Polasek MJ, Farley JF, Stouffer GA, Lee CR. CYP2C19-guided antiplatelet therapy: a cost-effectiveness analysis of 30-day and 1-year outcomes following percutaneous coronary intervention. *Pharmacogenomics.* 2017;18:1155-1166.

37. Park S, Thigpen J, Lee I. Accessibility and coverage of pharmacogenomic tests by private health insurance companies. *AJPE.* 82(5):71580.

38. Cohen JP, Felix AE. Personalized medicine's bottleneck: diagnostic test evidence and reimbursement. *J Pers Med.* 2014;4:163-175.

39. CMS. 2020. Available at https://cms.gov. Accessed October 10, 2019.

40. Dunnenberger HM, Biszewski M, Bell GC, et al. Implementation of a multidisciplinary pharmacogenomics clinic in a community health system. *Am J Health Syst Pharm.* 2016;73:1956-1966.

41. Cavallari LH, Beitelshees AL, Blake KV, et al. The IGNITE Pharmacogenetics Working Group: an opportunity for building evidence with pharmacogenetic implementation in a real-world setting. *Clin Transl Sci.* 2017;10:143-146.

42. Grosse SD. Is pharmacogenetic-guided treatment cost-effective? No one size fits all! In: *Genomics and Precision Health.* Atlanta, GA: CDC 2017. Available at https://blogs.cdc.gov/genomics/2017/07/24/is-pharmacogenetic-guided/Accessed July 28, 2019.

43. Hughes D, Vilar J, Ward C, Alfirevic A, Park B, Pirmohamed M. Cost-effectiveness analysis of HLA B*5701 genotyping in preventing abavavir hypersensitivity. *Pharmacogenetics.* 2004;14:335-342.

44. Okere AN, Ezendu K, Berthe A, Diaby V. An evaluation of the cost-effectiveness of comprehensive MTM integrated with point-of-care phenotypic and genetic testing for U.S. elderly patients after percutaneous coronary intervention. *J Manag Care Spec Pharm.* 2018;24:142-152.

45. Verbelen M, Weale M, Lewis C. Cost-effectiveness of pharmacogenetic-guided treatment: are we there yet? *Pharmacogenomics J* 2017;17:395-402.

46. Maciel A, Cullors A, Lukowiak A, Garces J. Estimating cost savings of pharmacogenetic testing for depression in real-world clinical settings. *Neuropsychiatr Dis Treat.* 2018;14:225-230.

47. Groessl EJ, Tally SR, Hillery N, Maciel A, Garces JA. Cost-effectiveness of a pharmacogenetic test to guide treatment for major depressive disorder. *J Manag Care Spec Pharm.* 2018;24:726-734.

48. Shuldiner AR, Relling MV, Peterson JF, et al. The Pharmacogenomics Research Network Translational Pharmacogenetics Program: overcoming challenges of real-world implementation. *Clin Pharmacol Ther.* 2013;94:207-210.

49. Gottesman O, Kuivaniemi H, Tromp G, et al. The electronic medical records and genomics (eMERGE) network: past, present, and future. *Genet Med.* 2013;15:761-771.

50. Nutescu EA, Drozda K, Bress AP, et al. Feasibility of implementing a comprehensive warfarin pharmacogenetics service. *Pharmacotherapy.* 2013;33:1156-1164.

51. Relling MV, Klein TE. CPIC: clinical pharmacogenetics implementation consortium of the pharmacogenomics research network. *Clin Pharmacol Ther.* 2011;89:464-467.

52. CPIC. CPIC Guidelines. 2020. Available at https://cpicpgx.org/guidelines/. Accessed July 9, 2019.

53. PheKB. What Is the Phenotype KnowledgeBase? 2020. Available at https://phekb.org. Accessed January 4, 2020.

54. CDSKB. CDS KnowledgeBase Is the Engine that Drives Precision Medicine. 2020. Available at https://cdskb.org. Accessed January 4, 2020.

55. Sphinx. Sequence and Phenotype Integration Exchange (SPHINX). 2020. Available at https://www.emergesphinx.org. Accessed January 4, 2020.

56. IGNITE. Genomic Medicine Knowledge Base. 2020. Available at https://gmkb.org/. Accessed January 4, 2020.

57. Caudle KE, Rettie AE, Whirl-Carrillo M, et al. Clinical pharmacogenetics implementation consortium guidelines for CYP2C9 and HLA-B genotypes and phenytoin dosing. *Clin Pharmacol Ther.* 2014;96:542-548.

58. Herr TM, Peterson JF, Rasmussen LV, Caraballo PJ, Peissig PL, Starren JB. Pharmacogenomic clinical decision support design and multi-site process outcomes analysis in the eMERGE Network. *J Am Med Inform Assoc.* 2019;26:143-148.

59. Asllani A, Lari A, Lari N. Strengthening information technology security through the failure modes and effects analysis approach. *Int J Qual Innov.* 2018;5.

60. DeRosier J, Stalhandske E, Bagian JP, Nudell T. Using health care failure mode and effect analysis: the VA National Center for Patient Safety's prospective risk analysis system. *Jt Comm J Qual Improv.* 2002;28:248-267.

61. Bonnabry P, Cingria L, Sadeghipour F, Ing H, Fonzo-Christe C, Pfister RE. Use of a systematic risk analysis method to improve safety in the production of paediatric parenteral nutrition solutions. *Qual Saf Health Care.* 2005;14:93-98.

62. Weitzel KW, McDonough CW, Elsey AR, Burkley B, Cavallari LH, Johnson JA. Effects of using personal genotype data on student learning and attitudes in a pharmacogenomics course. *Am J Pharm Educ.* 2016;80:122.

63. *Advancing Effective Communication, Cultural Competence, and Patient- and Family-Centered Care: A Roadmap for Hospitals.* Oakbrook Terrace, IL: The Joint Commission. 2010.

64. Mills R, Ensinger M, Callanan N, Haga SB. Development and initial assessment of a patient education video about pharmacogenetics. *J Pers Med.* 2017. 25;7(2):4.

65. Cavallari LH, Lee CR, Duarte JD. Implementation of inpatient models of pharmacogenetics programs. *Am J Health Syst Pharm.* 2016;73(23):1944-1954.

66. Hippman C, Nislow C. Pharmacogenomic testing: clinical evidence and implementation challenges. *J Pers Med.* 2019; 9(3):40.

67. Roden DM, McLeod HL, Relling MV, et al. Pharmacogenomics. *Lancet.* 2019;394:521-532.

ETHICAL, LEGAL, AND SOCIAL ISSUES IN PHARMACOGENOMICS

Lisa S. Parker

LEARNING OBJECTIVES

After reading this chapter, readers will be able to:

1. Explain the relevant ethical, legal, and social (ELS) considerations to patients/clients considering pharmacogenomics (PGx) testing.

2. Respond to questions from the media and public about ELS issues associated with PGx.

3. Participate in institutional or industry-level policy making about PGx in light of ELS concerns.

INTRODUCTION: NOT AS SIMPLE AS IT SEEMS

Precision medicine, the classification of "individuals into subpopulations that differ in their susceptibility to a particular disease or their response to a specific treatment" so that "preventive or therapeutic interventions can then be concentrated on those who will benefit, sparing expense and side effects for those who will not"[1] is recognized as raising multiple and difficult ethical, legal, and social issues.[2] Pharmacogenomics (PGx), the study of the relationship between genetic variation among individuals and their drug responses in order to develop new drugs and to inform prescribing practices, is sometimes considered the least ethically challenging domain of precision medicine. Who can reasonably object to precision medicine's tagline: "the right drug for the right patient at the right time"? Why shouldn't social policy embrace giving drugs only to those who may benefit, thereby minimizing the risk of adverse drug reactions (ADRs)? What negative sequelae could possibly accompany a revelation of genetic factors related to one's ability to respond to drugs? While one might worry about living in the shadow of an increased risk for cancer or Alzheimer disease, what shadow is cast by being a rapid or slow metabolizer?

Yet, the title of a 2008 article correctly suggests that PGx is "not as simple as it seems".[3] Some of the PGx-related ethical, legal, and social (ELS) issues differ from those associated with other domains of precision medicine, but some overlap. The issues also differ depending on whether the response-relevant genetic variation is an acquired variant (tissue-specific) or an inherited variant (found in an individual's genotype). Moreover, different participants in PGx face different ELS challenges as PGx matures and is implemented. These participants include patients, clinicians, pharmacists, researchers, the pharmaceutical industry, and insurers. This chapter will consider the ELS issues of PGx most salient from the different parties' perspectives.

PATIENTS AND CLINICIANS: OPPORTUNITIES AND CHALLENGES

Risks, Potential Benefits, and Limitations of PGx

Clinical decision making about any intervention, including testing to guide other interventions, is based on the intervention's risks and potential benefits, weighed in light of the patient's values and preferences.[4] The risks of PGx testing are informational risks—risks to privacy, of discrimination, and of psychosocial implications. For patients to realize the benefits of PGx testing, the information must be useful to guide their treatment. To be useful, PGx information must be accurate and available; for it to benefit the individual patient, it must be employed in the patient's interests.

Pharmacogenomic Information: Entering the Clinic, Evolving over Time

There are two main pathways that PGx information may enter the clinical context: PGx testing may be ordered by a clinician, or the patient may have had testing and brings the results to the current clinical encounter—either in hand or through the electronic health record (EHR). Someday it may become routine to order genomic sequencing or PGx testing as a part of preventive care so that the information is available in the EHR when it is needed to guide future care. However, today, if a clinician orders PGx testing, it is usually to inform a current treatment plan. The testing may be of a specific tissue, as when genetic tumor typing is conducted to determine the likelihood that a particular cancer will respond to a chemotherapeutic agent or immunotherapy. Or PGx testing may involve genotyping or genome/exome sequencing to determine whether inherited variants will affect a person's absorption, distribution, metabolism, and excretion of a drug or class of drugs. This type of testing may be ordered by a clinician or obtained from direct-to-consumer (DTC) testing companies.

If a patient brings PGx information acquired through DTC testing, clinicians may need to ascertain whether it is accurate and up-to-date. Although people's genotypes are mostly stable throughout their lifetimes, the interpretation of genes is still evolving; therefore, reinterpretation

of genomic sequencing or gene panels may be necessary.[5] Moreover, prior to 2013, when some DTC genetic testing results included some health-related information, a Government Accounting Office investigation discovered that DTC companies interpreted variants differently and produced conflicting health-risk reports.[6] Concerns about quality control and accuracy are one reason that, in 2013, the Food and Drug Administration (FDA) prohibited DTC companies from reporting health-relevant genetic test results. In 2017, the FDA once again permitted the DTC company 23andMe to report some health-related genetic information[7] and in early 2019 approved the company to report 33 variants of eight pharmacogenes related to approximately 50 drugs, as supported by the Clinical Pharmacogenetics Implementation Consortium (CPIC) guidelines.[8] It is suggested, however, that the company's report is more accurate in reporting positive results than negative ones and does not report on some common variants, including some common in African populations.[9]

Therefore, clinicians may be well-advised—for reasons of sound medical care, ethics, and legal liability—to retest using commercially available clinical genomic testing, particularly if possible false-negative results are relevant in a particular clinical context. Moreover, when patients bring DTC PGx test results or when results of clinically ordered testing are reported, it is ethically incumbent upon clinicians to explain the test's limitations and the evolving interpretation of genomic testing results. Finally, if patients were to adjust their medications without consulting their prescribers and pharmacists, neither their welfare nor their autonomy (right of self-determination) would be well-served; only acting on sound information serves those interests.

Limitations to Generalizability of PGx Results

For clinicians assessing the potential benefit of ordering PGx testing or of a particular result, it is important to be aware of the vast overrepresentation of people of European ancestry in PGx studies and in genomics studies.[10,11] The underrepresentation of people of non-European ancestry in PGx studies raises concerns about fairness and about the probability that they will benefit from clinical PGx testing.

Moreover, when enrolling research participants, PGx studies have used self-reported race as a rough approximation for the individuals' continental ancestry. The inferences being made from phenotype/self-report, to race, to continental ancestry, to variation in genotype when enrolling participants allow for substantial "slippage." Because in past

PGx research the pre-existing categories employed—races and ethnicities—are not genomically defined, "it is important to keep in mind that the ways in which individuals are grouped together determine the genetic frequencies that are attributed to such populations, not that genetic frequencies determine how to group individuals into populations."[12] Although studies show that self-reported race aligns fairly well with continental ancestry determined by genotype,[13] racial admixture complicates attribution or self-report of continental ancestry based, for example, on skin pigmentation or received views of family history and ancestral origins.[14,15] When PGx testing is employed clinically, the meaning of a variant identified will have been established. This is in part based on studies that employed race (or perhaps continental ancestry) to enroll subjects from whom the probabilities of various genotype–treatment response associations were derived. In the clinical setting, unless PGx testing is performed, clinicians may rely on self-reported or attributed (based on phenotypic characteristics) race of their patients to predict their drug response and guide prescribing and dosing decisions, based on what they read in the literature about PGx and race/ethnicity.

Clinicians at least need to be prepared to address questions about ancestry or race, in relation to PGx test results as the relevance of some variants for drug response, or for clinical outcomes that may not be adequately known for some racial/ethnic/ancestry populations. Particularly in the stressful context of needing effective medical treatment, it will be justifiably distressing for some patients to learn that the meaning of PGx test results is not clear for people of their particular racial/ethnic/ancestry background and may increase some patients' historically grounded mistrust of medicine.[16]

Finally, it is important for clinicians, patients, and the public to understand that even upon full realization of its promise, precision medicine, including PGx, will remain probabilistic and epidemiologically based, just as evidence-based nongenomic interventions have always been. A clinical drug trial yields only an average result across a given population of patients, even if that population is stratified based on genotype. Based on that trial a treatment recommendation still holds only a population-based probability of success for the individual patient.

Informational Risks of PGx Testing

As with any genetic testing, the risks of PGx testing are informational. Some could arise from the breach of privacy of a patient's medical information. Therefore, security must be maintained not only at every step of

the information pipeline (i.e., the transmitting, recording, and storing of test results) but also with regard to the storage and disposition of the samples (e.g., blood, saliva, or tissue) from which the information is generated. Genetic material within the samples is uniquely identifying, given both the requisite expertise and equipment for processing it and the means to connect the sample to personally identifying information. Therefore, samples should be stored in a deidentified manner to make connection back to an individual person more difficult even if the physical security measures of the storage facility or laboratory were breached.

It is not readily apparent that PGx information presents the same risks of discrimination and stigma, or concerns about psychosocial sequelae, that are associated with other health-related genetic/genomic information, or even that it presents the same possibility of changes in self-concept or origin stories presented by ancestry-related genetic testing.[17,18] As discussed below, however, learning PGx information is not entirely informational risk-free, particularly given pleiotropy and uncertainties regarding how insurers will incorporate PGx information about the risk of ADR and probable treatment effectiveness into their policies and practices.

Informed Consent for PGx Testing

Informed consent is both a process and a decision. As a process, it involves disclosure by a clinician of relevant information (the point of a procedure, its risks and potential benefits, and alternatives to it), understanding and deliberation about that information by a patient, and communication of the decision voluntarily made by the patient.[19] The decision and outcome of the process may be either an informed consent or an informed refusal (i.e., the informed, voluntary consent/refusal of a competent patient). A patient is considered competent to make the decision at hand when she or he is able to understand the risks and potential benefits of the proposed intervention, appreciate that those possible outcomes apply to her or him, reason and deliberate about the options (including the option of doing nothing) in light of a stable set of values, and communicate a decision.[20]

Particularly when performed to guide contemporaneous clinical care, PGx testing resembles other medical testing, including diagnostic testing, like testing for blood sugar level, cholesterol, or blood pressure. Specific informed consent is typically not obtained for such testing, unless the test itself presents risk of physical harm. The question arises in the case of PGx testing that involves a simple blood draw or noninvasive acquisition of the patient's

DNA (i.e., buccal swab, saliva sample, and tissue typing) whether testing should be preceded by informed consent or whether the patient should simply be informed that PGx testing is being done to guide treatment. At least two considerations support engaging in an informed consent process for PGx testing: the familial nature of genotype information and the possibility of PGx testing discovering incidental findings, "a finding concerning an individual … that has potential health or reproductive importance and is discovered in the course of conducting research [or clinical testing] but is beyond the aims of the study" or the clinical indication for testing.[21]

PGx and the "Duty to Warn"

Information about one's genotype, including information about drug response, may be relevant to one's family members in two senses. It may be information also true of them, and they may find it valuable to know. Thus, for both patients and clinicians the question arises of whether to share PGx information about inherited, not tissue-specific variants with the patient's family members, particularly because ordering PGx testing is not as common as ordering cholesterol testing. For example, it may be especially helpful to family members to learn that one of their relatives has a genetic variant relevant to drug absorption or metabolism. But sharing that information within one's family may be tantamount to sharing information about one's health, disease, or diagnosis, which many people would prefer to keep private.

Despite some arguments to the contrary—in ethics literature and court cases—it is generally accepted that clinicians fully discharge their responsibility to a patient's family by first, explaining to the patient that reported genetic information has implications for other family members and, if there are no strong reasons to the contrary, should be shared with them; and second, offering to provide written information that the patient may use to provide accurate information to his or her relatives. This was the court's finding in the frequently cited case, *Pate v. Threlkel*.[22] In another frequently cited case, *Safer v. Estate of Pack*, the appellate court stated that "we see no impediment, legal or otherwise, to recognizing a physician's duty to warn those known to be at risk of avoidable harm from a genetically transmissible condition," but remanded the case back to a trial court to determine whether in the particular case the clinician had a legal duty to (try to) inform a patient's relatives of pertinent genetic information; however, the case was settled before a jury ruled on that question.[23] Neither of these classic "duty to warn of genetic information" cases involved PGx information, but instead genetically based increased risk for disease.

Nor do they or any other cases clearly settle the question of legal responsibility to inform a patient's relatives of genetic information potentially relevant to their health.

From an ethical perspective, however, it is incumbent upon a clinician to inform his or her patient when information, like a PGx test result, may have relevance for genetically related family members. Further, it would be appropriate for a patient with information of potential importance to the health of his or her relatives to assume some degree of burden to inform them of the potentially relevant PGx variant.[24] On the other hand, given that PGx information is becoming increasingly relevant to the prescribing of many drugs, it may soon be the case that a relative's own indication for a drug would constitute an indication for PGx testing (i.e., without any family history of PGx-relevant genetic variations). That fact reduces the importance of intrafamilial sharing of PGx test results. Nevertheless, insofar as PGx testing may occasion an obligation to share, or at least the ethical desirability of sharing, information with family members, engaging in informed consent to PGx testing will help prepare a patient for this possibility, and even enable him or her to refuse PGx testing if that prospect is too onerous. (Whether the patient refusing such testing may or should still be prescribed a drug for which PGx testing is indicated is a question discussed later.)

Management of Incidental Findings

The possibility that PGx testing will yield incidental findings (IFs) is another reason that PGx testing warrants an informed consent process. There is strong consensus that, as a matter of "preventive ethics," clinicians should discuss the possibility that any type of genetic testing may yield IFs. Preventive ethics, modeled on preventive medicine, involves noticing patterns of recurrent problems—here ethical concerns or conflicts—and devising policies, practices, or guidelines to prevent future occurrences or mitigate their negative sequelae.[25]

Particularly given pleiotropy, it is reasonable to assume that PGx testing, like other genetic/genomic testing, may yield unwelcome information about disease risk. Indeed, over a decade ago, a third of PGx genes were found to be related to risk for disease.[26] Moreover, in 2013, the American College of Medical Genetics and Genomics (ACMG) recommended that laboratories conducting clinical sequencing should "seek and report" pathogenic variants in a set of medically actionable genes associated with serious conditions, despite the fact that "there are insufficient data on clinical utility to fully support these recommendations" and, therefore, also recommended "updating these recommendations at least annually as further data are collected."[27] Though this is not a legal requirement, it is reasonable to expect that adopting these recommendations may become the standard of care and that laboratories, clinicians, and health care institutions may face legal liability if they do not search for and offer to patients information about clinically actionable IFs, now termed "secondary findings," in recognition that they are to be specifically sought.[28] Currently there are 59 genes that the ACMG recommends searching for as a matter of opportunistic screening.[29]

The fact that new genes or variants are discovered and that variants are reinterpreted—in the case of disease risk–related genes, reclassified from "pathogenic" or "likely pathogenic" to "variant of uncertain significance," or the reverse—raises the question of the obligation of clinicians and health care institutions to inform patients of these reclassifications. The impact of such reinterpretation of variants on patients' psychological well-being, attitudes about the veracity of health information, and health-related decisions or behaviors is unknown. (Also unknown is how such changing interpretations will affect clinicians' attitudes and clinical workflow.) At the very least, if IFs are to be offered to patients, or if receiving such information is a mandated component of PGx testing, then patients need to be informed of the evolving state of the field's understanding of the information and told whether their information will be reinterpreted and whether (and how) they will be informed of revised interpretations.

It is also possible that PGx testing may suggest unwelcome information about family relationships. If, for example, a patient has an inherited pharmacogenetic variant not shared by anyone else in his or her family, this may raise questions about misattributed parentage, assisted reproduction, or adoption. Some might be prompted to question their presumed ancestry if they are discovered to have variants that are substantially more frequent in people with a particular continental ancestry they had not believed to be their own.

Finally, the possibility of PGx testing revealing genetic information that people may not want has implications for PGx testing of children for inherited variants. While it is medically and ethically appropriate to provide them the same quality of care as adults, and thus to employ PGx testing to guide their care, it would not be ethically appropriate to engage in routine PGx profiling of children just so the information would be available should they need it for future treatment.[30] It is not true that "a one-time test, given early in life, should be part of routine medical care,"[31] at least not before a person is sufficiently mature to make an autonomous decision about such testing. Because of the potential need for reinterpretation and the likelihood of new PGx variants being discovered, the concept of a "one-time test" is false. Moreover, it is generally accepted that children should have preserved, for future exercise, their right to choose whether or not to learn genetic information about themselves, information that PGx testing may reveal due to pleiotropy.[3]

May Patients Refuse Testing?

As with other recommended interventions, informed consent for PGx testing should include discussion of its risks and potential benefits and alternatives, including not having the test. Whether patients should be permitted to refuse testing and allowed to assume the risks of ADR or less effective treatment is not clear and should depend on multiple factors. These include the likelihood, likely timing, and severity of potential ADR and their treatability (and also whether the patient will be monitored in a hospital or taking the drug as an outpatient); whether treatment effectiveness (not an ADR) is the issue; what the alternative agents may be and their risk:benefit profile; and the patient's reasons for refusing PGx testing. For some drugs, for example, the risk of ADR may be so great that PGx testing is mandated by the FDA, health care institution, or health insurer. It is ethically important that patient welfare, not concern about liability or increased costs alone, drive any mandating of PGx testing, given that there are reasonable considerations that support a patient's preference not to have PGx testing and to assume the risk of less effective treatment or even an ADR. For other drugs, a traditional trial-and-error approach may be acceptable, even if PGx testing would be clinically preferable. For some patients, the risk of learning IFs may outweigh the potential benefit of PGx testing.

HEALTH CARE INSTITUTIONS: PRACTICAL AND ETHICAL CHALLENGES OF INFRASTRUCTURE

Health care institutions will need to develop policies regarding PGx testing and the issues outlined earlier, including management of IFs and reinterpretation of genomic test results. As discussed below, they will also need to implement a systematic and fair way to review appeals for exceptions to policies that generally promote patient health and safety but that may impose particular risks or burdens on some patients.

The greatest practical PGx challenge facing health care institutions is how to manage PGx information (i.e., how to store it; ensure timely access to it; and ensure that it is accurate, up-to-date, and properly used). Ideally, clinical practices and health care institutions will enable the automatic inclusion of PGx test results in the EHR, but such recording and secure storage are only part of the challenge of intrainstitutional information flow. Institutions will need to implement clinical decision support (CDS) to enable clinicians, most of whom will not have had substantial education in genetics/genomics/PGx, to employ PGx information, accurately inform patients about its meaning, and make referrals for counseling about genomic IFs.

Research suggests that patients are comfortable sharing their PGx information among their treating clinicians, and such sharing would avoid the financial costs and time delay involved in duplicate testing.[32] PGx test results could be recorded in the EHR, stored in pharmacy databases, and/or retained by patients. Storing the results so that clinicians and pharmacists need not rely on patient self-report should increase accuracy and, with appropriate CDS alerts, trigger reinterpretation of older results as new information becomes available. Self-reported results of PGx testing should be recorded in the same way that drug allergies and medications being taken are recorded in medical records and EHR.

PHARMACISTS, PHARMACIES, AND FORMULARY DECISIONS

Educating and Alerting Professionals and Patients

Education and continuing education in pharmacy are critical to expand PGx expertise and have that expertise integrated into all health care institutions and communities. Inclusion of regularly updated PGx information related to particular drugs in commercial databases (e.g., Medi-Span) and patient-focused information sources (e.g., mayoclinic.org) would also expand access to relevant information. Particularly because pharmacists are among the professionals most trusted by the public, they may play an important role in educating the public about the benefits and limitations of not only PGx testing but also about genetic testing/genomic sequencing more generally. Efforts to educate professionals and the public are supported by concern to reduce health and health care disparities and to provide equitable access to health care.

Professional Responsibility and Liability

The growing importance of PGx information may lead to changes in the relationship between pharmacists and physicians and may prompt consideration of enabling pharmacists' access to patients' EHR, perhaps even outside of hospitals for pharmacists in commercial pharmacies.[32] At the very least, a patient's PGx information could be stored in pharmacy records along with drug allergy information and medication history. If pharmacies become points of access to patient health records, or if they store genomic information, the security of pharmacies and their electronic records will become even more important because of the expanded potential for harm that a privacy breach would involve. This expanded risk would include potential harm to patients' family members because of the familial nature of genetic information, as well as the potential for PGx information to reveal associated disease-risk information.

Whether practicing within a hospital or in a stand-alone pharmacy, pharmacists have an ethical obligation to alert patients and physicians if a drug is prescribed for which PGx testing is required or recommended or to confirm that such testing was performed prior to prescribing. The development of PGx knowledge means that what was previously an unfortunate outcome of prescribing and dispensing a drug may become an ethically and legally culpable act of negligence.[33] The possibility of legal liability for a failure to inform prescribers or end users of such requirements or recommendations should also be considered.

Institutional Policies, Exceptions, and Patients' Assumption of Risk

A growing knowledge of PGx will influence health care institutions' decisions regarding inclusion of drugs on institutions' formularies and development of guidelines (or requirements) for using PGx testing to guide prescribing and administering drugs. Like other clinical guidelines, PGx-informed guidelines should seek to serve patients' health interests, not be designed primarily to protect institutional financial or reputational interests. Like all clinical guidelines, those based on PGx research will be implemented to enhance the well-being of groups of patients, not individuals; yet it is ethically important to establish a process to determine when individual patient welfare warrants an exception.[34]

In drafting PGx guidelines to direct interventions to those likely to respond positively and avoid an ADR, care must be taken not to categorically deny an intervention to an individual whose genotype indicates a relatively lower probability of positive treatment response, so long as three conditions are met. First, the intervention is otherwise available on the formulary. Second, no other intervention has been developed or is available that is (more) effective for patients with that genetic variation. Third, the risk or burden of the intervention to the individual (i.e., the probability and magnitude of an ADR) is not unduly burdensome given the possibility of benefit. It may also be argued that, following discussion of risks and potential benefits, the individual should be allowed to assume those risks and not be denied the opportunity to seek even remote benefit when no other good alternative exists. This is especially true when others with a different genotype have access to the intervention.

Particularly if the intervention or drug with remote prospect of benefit would be administered at the patient's own expense, it would seem quite reasonable to allow this assumption of risk. Most patients, however, would be unable to afford the full cost of many interventions. Moreover, it may seldom be the case that a patient could be required to assume the full cost, particularly if a serious ADR resulted. It is reasonable for institutions to consider these downstream costs when considering exceptions to clinical guidelines. Nevertheless, decisions to deny an individual, on the basis of her or his genotype, an intervention available to others cannot be made lightly or categorically, and appropriate appeal processes should be established.

INSURERS: PRIVACY, DISCRIMINATION, AND POLICY ISSUES

The Genetic Information Nondiscrimination Act of 2008 (GINA) prohibits the use of genetic information by employers in hiring, promotion, and firing decisions and by health insurers in underwriting.[35] Together with the provisions of the Health Insurance Portability and Accountability Act of 1996, GINA prohibits health insurers from requesting or requiring genetic information and/or using it for decisions regarding coverage, rates, or pre-existing conditions (Table 3-1). However, life, disability, long-term care, automobile, and other insurers are not addressed by GINA and are not thereby prohibited from using genetic information. It seems that GINA would prohibit the use of PGx test results to deny to a particular patient coverage for a specific drug or set of drugs which are part of the plan's covered package of treatments.

On the other hand, health insurance plans might argue that the particular drug(s) does not constitute medically appropriate treatment for an individual whose genotype suggests she or he is unlikely to respond or is likely to suffer from an ADR or whose acquired genetic variant in specific tissue (e.g., tumor) suggests a particular treatment is unlikely to be effective.[36] Insurance companies are permitted minimal access to genetic information,

TABLE 3-1. Legal Regulations

Genetic Information Nondiscrimination Act of 2008 (GINA)	This act seeks to prohibit discrimination on the basis of genetic information with respect to health insurance and employment.
Health Insurance Portability and Accountability Act of 1996 (HIPAA)	This act specifies how personally identifiable information maintained and transmitted by health care organizations, health plans, and health care insurance entities ("covered entities") should be protected from fraud and theft; it also addresses some limitations on health care insurance coverage.

including test results and family history information, in order to determine medical need. For example, a strong family history of breast cancer or positive *BRCA1* mutation testing may be used to establish a young woman's medical need and insurance coverage for mammography that would not otherwise be covered until age 40. Since insurers are permitted access to genetic information to make such coverage decisions, by analogy, they could presumably use PGx test results to grant or refuse coverage for particular drugs. Health care institutions should consider the same factors (described in the previous section) when evaluating possible exceptions to PGx-informed prescribing guidelines, which should be considered by insurers when considering exceptions to their PGx-informed coverage guidelines that would otherwise deny coverage to an individual patient for a particular drug(s).

Decisions to deny an individual on the basis of her or his genotype an intervention available to others should not be made categorically. Insurers must establish processes for appeal, with weight given to the possibility that the patient may benefit from a drug that PGx testing would suggest denying coverage for.

ETHICAL ISSUES IN PGX RESEARCH

For researchers, the ethical issues raised by PGx research are largely the same as for other genomic research.[37] These include informed consent, the necessity of planning for and managing IFs, reporting aggregate research results, and whether to offer return of individual research results. Of particular importance in PGx research are issues of participant recruitment. The underrepresentation of people of non-European ancestry in PGx studies results in the problems of generalizability discussed earlier and raises concern about fairness. In recruiting, it is important for researchers not to exaggerate the potential direct benefit that prospective participants may receive if they enroll in such studies, particularly if results may be less generalizable to some participants than others.

A second ethical issue particularly salient to PGx research is the use of genotype-informed recruitment (GIR). The promise of smaller, less expensive, faster clinical trials rests on the possibility of such recruitment. GIR depends on previous research recruitment that resulted in the genotyping or genomic sequencing, having obtained participants' consent to be recontacted for future studies, and then figuring out how to respect people's right not to know unwanted genomic information, while providing the information necessary for them to make an informed decision about current study participation.[38] Alternatively, researchers could employ an honest broker to search the EHR to identify a pool of potential participants with the genotype of interest. Researchers could then ask the clinicians of those identified to recruit them into the study. Or GIR could involve issuing a call for research participants who know their genotypes from either DTC testing or previous clinical testing/sequencing.[39] Any of these approaches would require suggesting to individuals already stratified into a particular population of interest based on their genotype that the current study's research question may particularly, though not certainly, pertain to them. For PGx studies, this suggestion is less likely to cause anxiety and presents a lower risk of stigmatization than would GIR to studies of disease risk. Nevertheless, these concerns about imposing risks of anxiety and stigma are not entirely negligible, and given pleiotropy, there is no fixed distinction between PGx information and genomic disease-risk information. It is also important to avoid "invitation fatigue" for those whose genotypes are highly sought for research, as well as the potential for such individuals to mistakenly and self-stigmatizingly believe that there is something fundamentally wrong with them.[39] Finally, designing trials employing GIR to maximize the chance of successful study outcomes will minimize the generalizability of study results, much as past practices of excluding women, the elderly, or pediatric patients have resulted in the development of drugs that were neither generalizable to nor approved for those populations.

THE PHARMACEUTICAL INDUSTRY

Competing Incentives and Considerations of Justice

For the pharmaceutical industry, PGx presents the opportunity to rescue drugs that have been abandoned because while they were safe and effective for many people, they had serious ADRs for a few. Shifting from the development of blockbuster drugs effective for the majority of the population needing treatment for a condition to developing and marketing drugs for those with particular PGx-relevant genotypes may allow manufacturers to abandon fewer drugs on the "cutting room floor" of research and development. Thus, PGx may reduce the cost of drugs not just through smaller, faster, GIR-based trials but by enabling cost recovery by bringing more drugs to market as specialized medications. The result—an increase in effective treatments, albeit specialized medications appropriate for a more narrowly defined patient population and the potential for lower overall costs of drug development—would promote both social welfare and social justice.

On the other hand, PGx may actually increase health and health care disparities and social injustice insofar as there would be a simultaneous incentive to develop effective medications for particular hard-to-treat genotypes. There may be a need for additional regulatory measures and incentives—beyond current orphan drug measures—to encourage development of drugs not only for rare diseases but also for rare genotypes or patients with common conditions who are "nonresponders."[40]

It is also possible that drugs would be developed to be effective in one genotype-defined population in preference to drugs for another genotype-defined population if the former genotype were more prevalent in a population with more extensive drug insurance coverage or greater purchasing power (i.e., a wealthier population).[40] This possibility is troubling in itself. It would be even more unjust if access to effective treatment for those in developing countries were thereby reduced or if race- or class-based discrimination and/or health care disparities were exacerbated within developed societies.

Finally, phenotype-wide association studies (PheWAS)—which begin with a genetic variant that known drugs target and then identify the phenotypes/conditions associated with it—may intensify some ethical concerns, as they seek to "characterize the genetic architecture of complex traits and identify novel pleiotropic relationships."[41] The reporting of the latter will require special care to avoid "hyperbole" and unduly increase anxiety in people with one of the phenotypes (e.g., reporting the apoE genotype association with lipid metabolism, Alzheimer disease, and major depression).[42] Furthermore, it remains to be seen whether the approach of beginning with known variants targeted by known drugs will build in and exacerbate biases of previous studies or instead reduce them and the disparities in PGx-informed care.

Concerns about Liability

Finally, it is possible drugs that present increased risk of an ADR for some individuals may be removed from the market to protect them but eliminate the potential benefit of the drug for others. This may occur either due to companies acting on study findings or in response to (risk of) litigation, or both. For example, a class action suit was brought against SmithKline Beecham alleging that it failed to warn that some portion (perhaps 30%) of the population has a genetic variant (HLA-DR4+) that increases the risk of developing an arthritis-related condition and/or Lyme disease upon receiving the LYMErix vaccine it had marketed to protect against Lyme disease.[31,43] Because LYMErix was not on the recommended vaccination schedule, it was not covered by the National Vaccine Injury Compensation Program. The suit was settled, and LYMErix was withdrawn from the market, though the veracity of the suit's claims was not established.[44]

While PGx testing could be used to identify individuals at increased risk of drug-specific ADR and avoid marketing or supplying the drug to them, the current stage of PGx and the fear of adverse publicity and/or litigation may lead to blanket withdrawal of drugs from the market. A review analyzing the Pharmacogenomics Knowledgebase (PharmGKB) and FDA recommendations of PGx testing found that labels directed clinicians to employ PGx testing in only 14 cases, although 12% of drugs licensed between 1998 and 2012 had PGx information included in their labels.[45]

Vaccines

The study of ELS issues of "vaccinomics" is in its infancy.[46] In a domain of public health that has traditionally depended upon population-wide vaccination and creation of a state of herd immunity, the prospect of stratifying populations to vaccinate some subpopulations and not others is a striking departure. In light of current, unfounded anti-vaccination sentiment in the wake of Andrew Wakefield's fraudulent publications falsely connecting a vaccine and autism, there is reasonable concern about promoting "personalized vaccination."[47–49] While the ability to identify those at increased risk of an ADR from a vaccine might allay fears of some "anti-vaxxers," there is a chance that anti-vaccination sentiment may only be fueled by the field of "adversomics" that seeks to "identify, characterize, and predict adverse, or maladaptive, immune responses to vaccines."[49] Does asking the question: "Does it make sense in the 21st century to give the same vaccine, dose, and at the same frequency to everyone, regardless of age, weight, gender, race, genotype, and medical condition?" primarily (or at least at the present time) lend support to those who would spare their child the presumed potential of an ADR? Considerations of public welfare make critical the need for clear communication about personal and population-wide risks, potential personal and population-level benefits, and the special needs of subpopulations (e.g., those who are immunocompromised or who have particular genotypes). Legislation—both mandating vaccination guided by PGx and providing compensation to treat ADR—would be supported by considerations of public welfare and justice.

CASE SCENARIOS

Mr. Gordon, a 55-year-old African American man, is persuaded by his wife to tell his doctor that he has been feeling depressed since his mother died three years ago. Missing her prompted him to do DTC genetic testing to search for more family connections. Receiving both ancestry and health-related results, he was disconcerted to learn he is "35% Caucasian/European," as well as that he has elevated risk for type 2 diabetes and a CYP2D6 variant related to drug metabolism. He wants to feel less sad and hopeless and to avoid premature death.

1. **How should Mr. Gordon's physician address his complicated grief and depression? What use should be made of the DTC PGx test result?**

Answer: Mr. Gordon's physician needs to use professional judgment to determine whether pharmacological intervention is warranted as an adjuvant to grief counseling and/or psychotherapy. If so, the physician needs to consider the reliability, accuracy, and relevance of the genetic test results from the DTC company. Is the laboratory reliable and certified to return these types of results? How well-established is the knowledge based upon which the interpretation of the results was made? Mr. Gordon's physician also needs to consider whether his patient's continental ancestry was taken into account in interpreting his genomic test results. In some cases when a patient brings DTC genetic test results to a clinician, the clinician may want to retest because of questions about the laboratory's standards or the accuracy and currency of the laboratory's interpretation of the results.

Finally, the physician needs to determine whether *CYP2D6* gene variants are relevant to the prescription of an antidepressant or another medication that might be prescribed to Mr. Gordon. The *CYP2D6* gene encodes for production of the CYP2D6 enzyme, which is involved in the metabolism of some drugs, including many antidepressants. If a drug is metabolized too quickly, its efficacy may be decreased; if it is metabolized too slowly, toxicity and an ADR may result.

2. What limitations of PGx testing and genetic testing might the physician explain?

Answer: The physician might explain that PGx, like genomic medicine in general, is an evolving field. Therefore, while a person's genotype may be relatively stable across the person's lifetime, the interpretation of genotype information continues to evolve. Moreover, the physician might explain that the interpretation of genetic/genomic variation is "epidemiologically based," or in other words, while the interpretation may generally be true of a population of people sharing a particular genotype, individuals and their response to a drug may vary because of differences in environment, lifestyle, or other genetic factors not accounted for by the PGx test.

Furthermore, the physician might explain that currently most genomic knowledge, including current understanding of PGx, is based on studies in which people of European descent were vastly overrepresented, while people of other continental ancestries were vastly underrepresented. Therefore, there is reason to question the generalizability of some genetic/genomic test results to individuals from groups that were underrepresented in the studies, including African Americans like Mr. Gordon.

3. How might the physician address Mr. Gordon's feelings about his ancestry results?

Answer: First, physicians need to recognize that an African American patient may or may not be surprised to learn that he or she has ancestors of European descent. Many African Americans assume that they may have genotypes reflecting both African and European ancestry because they are well aware of the history of rape of African slaves by white slave owners and slave traders. Receiving genetic test results that demonstrate this legacy, however, can be a painful and concrete personalization of that history. Clinicians should be prepared to acknowledge the fraught meaning of ancestry test results.

Within the United States, the persistence of structural racism within the health care system and existence of both health and health care disparities among groups of different ancestries may make recognizing genetic admixture more upsetting for some patients and may complicate the ability of clinicians to address adequately and sensitively the connection of genetic findings to both this historical legacy and current racism.

Moreover, anyone may experience a disrupted sense of self-identity if genetic test results challenge long-held beliefs or assumptions, for example, about place or family of origin, or about relationships. Receiving results that indicate a previously unknown adoption or misattributed parentage may be thought to be more disruptive than learning unexpected ancestry information; however, people's responses are highly individualized and vary in terms of intensity and duration. For some people, their ethnicity or ancestral cultural heritage is an important part of their identity and a source of pride or feeling of connection to the world. Disruption of that self-image may represent a substantial loss.

Second, how Mr. Gordon's physician addresses his patient's feelings about being found to be "35% Caucasian/European" may depend on the nature of their clinician–patient relationship, their degree of rapport, and the other concerns competing for attention within the clinical encounter. Nevertheless, because Mr. Gordon shared that he had sought DTC genetic testing in search of more family connections to assuage his sadness over the loss of his mother, it would seem relevant for his physician to address his disrupted sense of ancestral genetic connectedness in the context of addressing his mood. The physician may want to validate Mr. Gordon's feelings and suggest that this is a topic he might also explore with a grief counselor.

4. Based on this appointment, what information should the physician place into Mr. Gordon's EHR and what should be done about his apparently increased risk for type 2 diabetes?

Answer: What genetic test results are placed into Mr. Gordon's EHR depends partly on what his physician decides about the previously raised questions. In other words, it matters whether the results are from a reliable source and were interpreted accurately according to a current and generalizable knowledge base. The physician may decide not to record the genetic information as test results but as issues of concern to the patient. Either way, it would be important to note that the information is the product of DTC genetic testing, not testing ordered for a clinical indication.

The focus of this appointment was on Mr. Gordon's mood, not his risk for diabetes. It may not be appropriate therefore to record the self-reported genetic test result related to his diabetes risk. At least the information should not be recorded without discussion with Mr. Gordon. Moreover, despite the high prevalence of type 2 diabetes among African Americans, the genetics of type 2 diabetes is less well understood in African Americans than in Americans of European ancestry. Thus, reliance on and recording of that genetic test result should proceed, if at all, with caution.

Another reason for caution in recording the DTC genetic test results in the EHR concerns the risks of discrimination in underwriting for life, disability, and long-term care insurance. As a 55-year-old, Mr. Gordon may have reason to seek such insurance and would not want his medical record to indicate increased risk for debilitating or life-threatening conditions. Of course, Mr. Gordon would be required to answer any insurance company health questionnaire honestly, so his having received genetic risk information may already expose him to potentially higher rates or refusal of coverage. Still, information in a medical record may be regarded by the company as more veracious than self-reported information or DTC test results.

Nevertheless, especially because Mr. Gordon expressed interest in avoiding premature mortality (and, presumably, also morbidities), his physician might use the genetic indication of increased risk for diabetes to discuss steps Mr. Gordon could take to reduce his risk. The physician would need to explain that type 2 diabetes is a complex condition; in other words, a combination of genetic, environmental, and lifestyle or behavioral factors affect an individual's risk of developing type 2 diabetes. While Mr. Gordon cannot alter his genotype, he may be able to alter the other factors affecting his level of risk. The presence of genetically based increased risk could lead Mr. Gordon to be fatalistic about this health risk, especially if he is currently feeling hopeless, or it could motivate him to positively influence what he can (e.g., his diet, exercise activities, and stress levels). His physician could point out that some of these interventions may have a positive effect on his mood as well. Assuming that Mr. Gordon is currently exhibiting no signs of a diabetic or prediabetic condition, his genetic test result would not indicate pursuing any measures beyond those of a healthy lifestyle. Even in the absence of any genetic test result, the prevalence of type 2 diabetes among African Americans could be an indication to test Mr. Gordon annually for prediabetes, particularly if he has other risk factors.

5. **If Mr. Gordon shared his PGx test result with his pharmacist when picking up an antidepressant medication, what might his pharmacist discuss?**

Answer: Mr. Gordon's pharmacist should ask whether he had discussed the test result with his prescriber and could offer to call the prescriber to discuss the result. The pharmacist could also offer Mr. Gordon counseling about the meaning of the PGx information and should be prepared to discuss the issues raised earlier. The pharmacist might assume that the antidepressant was prescribed for depression and not some other, perhaps off-label use, and might assume that there is therefore relatively low risk of serious ADR. The pharmacist might be concerned, however, that an antidepressant may not be effective and that feelings of depression and hopelessness might therefore be worsened (particularly when the expectation of relief from the drug has been created by its prescription). With or without access to a PGx test result, the pharmacist might counsel Mr. Gordon to contact the prescriber if he feels that his mood is worsening or if he has any new or disconcerting symptoms, either somatic or mood related.

PHARMACOGENOMICS AND BIOETHICAL CLINICAL PEARLS

- PGx testing presents many of the same ethical concerns as other genomic testing, both because of pleiotropy and the resulting possibility that PGx testing reveals non-drug-related information (incidental findings) and because of the implications of predicting drug response. These concerns center on privacy, the rights to know and not-to-know information about one's current and future health, familial implications of genetic/genomic information and the question of whether relatives have an obligation to share information with family members to whom it might be beneficial. Risks of discrimination and stigmatization, of being prevented from accessing potentially beneficial therapies, and risks associated with either misunderstanding genetic information or relying on outdated genetic information are also of concern. These concerns suggest that it is appropriate to seek specific informed consent for PGx testing, because such testing presents risks that are not associated with other types of medical testing. In addition, clinicians and pharmacists should be prepared to advise patients about these risks—and the potential benefits—associated with their participation in PGx research.

- PGx is an evolving field. While a person's genotype may be relatively stable across the person's lifetime, the interpretation of genotype information is likely to continue to evolve for many decades. In addition, prescribers and pharmacists should be aware that patients may have obtained their PGx information through DTC testing. DTC genetic testing companies vary with regard to quality control, how they interpret genetic variants, and how well they inform customers of the implications of testing and specific test results. These factors have implications for the appropriateness of relying on genetic test results when prescribing for patients, as well as for patients' own understanding of their health, health risks, and likelihood to benefit from or be harmed by pharmacological interventions.

- PGx information and prescribing guidelines are epidemiologically based, and ethical concerns are associated with the generalizability of findings and guidelines to individual patients. A PGx test result may be generally true of the population of people sharing a particular genotype; however, an individual patient with that genotype may respond differently, and thus the prescribing guideline may not be appropriate for that patient. This fact has implications both for prescribing practices and for health insurers' decisions regarding coverage for a particular drug for a particular person. Exceptions to general guidelines may be ethically justified by concern for both justice and patient well-being.

- An important feature of the current state of PGx and all genomic knowledge is that it is based on studies that vastly overrepresent people of European descent and vastly underrepresent people of other continental ancestries. This fact both raises an additional concern about the generalizability of findings and exacerbates health care disparities and injustice in health care with regard to people of color. It also suggests that in order to promote patient well-being, prescribers and pharmacists must take special care when employing PGx information and must consider whether it is relevant to the individual patient, particularly if that patient is of mixed, unknown, or non-European continental ancestry.

- Prescribers, pharmacists, their employers, and institutions must consider whether patients should be allowed to assume the risks of taking a drug that PGx testing indicates is less likely (or unlikely) to be beneficial or more likely to cause an ADR. The availability, burdens, and cost of alternatives, as well as patient preferences, should be taken into account in order to respect patients' values, decisional autonomy, and their well-being. Policy makers and lawmakers, as well as the health care and pharmaceutical industries, need to consider how to manage issues of legal liability and the assessment of professionals' performance metrics when PGx test results are employed and when PGx-informed guidelines are overridden.

- Like all genetic information, PGx information is sensitive information. Its security must be maintained, and the privacy of individuals vis-à-vis this information must be protected. Current legal protections against discrimination based on genetic information apply only to employers' and health insurers' use of such information; other types of insurance and other social uses of genetic information (e.g., in education or law enforcement) are not addressed by laws like GINA.

KEY TERMS

Autonomy: Derived from *auto* (self-) and *nomos* "law or rule," autonomy refers to the capacity of persons to rule themselves and their right to decide for themselves.

Justice: The ethical principle of justice requires treating relevantly similar things or people similarly, particularly with regard to distributing goods, holding people responsible, or protecting people from harm.

Negligence: Negligence is the failure to use reasonable care. In law, a person may be liable for damages due to negligence when she or he breaches a duty of care (a duty to exercise the level of care that someone of ordinary prudence would have exercised under the same circumstances) and that breach results in compensable damage.

Personally identifiable information (PII): PII is information that can be used to distinguish or trace an individual's identity, either alone or when combined with other personal or identifying information that is linked or linkable to a specific individual. Some PII is publicly available (e.g., first and last name, or telephone numbers in phone books); some is not publicly available (e.g., Social Security or bank account numbers).

Welfare: Similar to "well-being," welfare refers to what is conducive to a person's or a society's good or what is in the person's or society's interest, which is objectively ascribable to the person/society and does not necessarily depend on the person's/society's particular values and preferences.

ABBREVIATIONS AND ACRONYMS

ACMG: American College of Medical Genetics and Genomics
ADR: Adverse drug reaction
BRCA: Breast cancer gene
CDS: Clinical decision support
DTC: Direct-to-consumer
EHR: Electronic health records
ELS: Ethical, legal, and social
GINA: Genetic Information Nondiscrimination Act
GIR: Genotype-informed recruitment
HIPAA: Health Insurance Portability and Accountability Act
IF: Incidental findings
PGx: Pharmacogenomics
PharmGKB: Pharmacogenomics knowledgebase

REFERENCES

1. President's Council of Advisors on Science and Technology. Priorities for Personalized Medicine. Available at https://bigdatawg.nist.gov/PCAST_Personalized_Medicine_Priorities.pdf. 2008. Accesed October 20, 2020.
2. Brothers KB, Rothstein, MA. Ethical, legal and social implications of incorporating personalized medicine into healthcare. *Personal Med.* 2015;12(1):43–51.
3. Haga SB, Burke W. Pharmacogenetic testing: Not as simple as it seems. *Genet Med.* 2008;10(6):391–395.
4. Brock DW. The ideal of shared decision making between physicians and patients. In: *Life and Death: Philosophical Essays in Biomedical Ethics.* Cambridge, UK: Cambridge University Press. 1993:55–79.
5. Shirts BH, Parker LS. Changing interpretations, stable genes: Responsibilities of patients, professionals, and policymakers in the clinical interpretation of complex genetic information. *Genet Med.* 2008;10(11):778–783.
6. Kutz G. Direct-to-consumer genetic tests: Misleading test results are further complicated by deceptive marketing & other questionable practices. Testimony before the Subcommittee on Oversight and Investigations, Committee on Energy and Commerce, House of Representatives, 2010.
7. Hayden KC. The rise, fall and rise again of 23andMe. *Nature.* 2017;550:174–177.
8. Anonymous. DTC pharmacogenomics testing under scrutiny. *Nat Biotechnol.* 2019;37:1101.
9. McCarthy J. 23andMe Is Offering Pharmacogenetic Testing, But Is It Any Good? Available at https://www.precisionmedicineadvisors.com/precisionmedicine-blog/2019/1/16/23andme-is-offering-pharmacogenetic-testing-but-is-it-any-good. Accessed January 16, 2019.
10. Bustamante CD, Burchard EG, De La Vega FM. Genomics for the World. *Nature* 2011;474:163–165.
11. Coriell Institute for Medical Research. Personal Genome Project (PGP). 2019. https://www.coriell.org/0/Sections/Collections/NIGMS/PGPs.aspx?PgId=772&coll=GMrence-Materials. Accessed October 20, 2020.
12. Foster MW, Sharp RR. Beyond race: Towards a whole-genome perspective on human populations and genetic variation. *Nat Rev Genet.* 2004;5:790–796.
13. Tang H, Quertermous T, Rodriguez B, et al. Genetic structure, self-identified race/ethnicity, and confounding in case-control association studies. *Am J Hum Genet.* 2005;76(2):268–275.
14. Murphy E, Hou L, Maher BS, et al. Race, genetic ancestry and response to antidepressant treatment for major depression. *Neuropsychopharmacology.* 2013;38:2598–2606.
15. Bamshad M. Genetic influences on health: Does race matter? *JAMA.* 2005;294(8):937–946.
16. Parker LS, Satkoske VB. Ethical dimensions of disparities in depression research and treatment in the pharmacogenomic era. *J Law Med Ethics.* 2012;40(4):886–903.
17. Hamilton R. Being young, female, and BRCA positive. *AJN.* 2012;112(10):26–31.
18. Phelan JC, Link BG, Zelner S, et al. Direct-to-consumer racial admixture tests and beliefs about essential racial differences. *Soc Psychol Q.* 2014;77(3):296–318.
19. Berg J, Appelbaum PS, Lidz CW, et al. *Informed Consent: Legal Theory and Clinical Practice.* 2nd ed. Oxford University Press; 2001.

20. Buchanan A, Brock DW. *Deciding for Others: The Ethics of Surrogate Decision Making.* Cambridge, UK: Cambridge University Press. 1990.

21. Wolf SM, Lawrenz FP, Nelson CA, Kahn JP, et al. Managing incidental findings in human subjects research: Analysis and recommendations. *J Law Med Ethics.* 2008;36(2):219–248.

22. *Pate v. Threlkel.* 661 So2d 278 (Fla 1995).

23. *Safer v. Estate of Pack.* 677 A2d 1188 (NJ Super Ct App Div 1996).

24. Buchanan A. Testing and telling?: Implications for genetic privacy, family disclosure and the law. *JHCLP.* 1998;1(2):391–420.

25. Forrow L, Arnold RM, Parker LS. Preventive ethics: Expanding the horizons of clinical ethics. *J Clin Ethic.* 1993;4:287–294.

26. Henrikson NB, Burke W, Veenstra DL. Ancillary risk information and pharmacogenetic tests: Social and policy implications. *Pharmacogenomics J.* 2008;8:85–89.

27. Green RC, Berg JS, Grody WW, et al. ACMG recommendations for reporting of incidental findings in clinical exome and genome sequencing. *Genet Med.* 2013;15(7):565–574.

28. Clayton EW, McGuire AL. The legal risks of returning results of genomic research. *Genet Med.* 2012;14(4):473–477.

29. Kalia SS, Adelman K, Bale SJ, et al. Recommendations for reporting of secondary findings in clinical exome and genome sequencing, 2016 update (ACMG SF v2.0): A policy statement of the American College of Medical Genetics and Genomics. *Genet Med.* 2017;19(2):249–255.

30. Moran C, Thornburg CD, Barfield RC. Ethical considerations for pharmacogenomic testing in pediatric clinical care and research. *Pharmacogenomics.* 2011;12(6):889–895.

31. Wertz C. Ethical, social and legal issues in pharmacogenomics. *Pharmacogenomics J.* 2003;3:194–196.

32. Haga SB, Kawamoto K, Agans R et al. Consideration of patient preferences and challenges in storage and access of pharmacogenetic test results. *Genet Med.* 2011;13(10):887–890.

33. Alcalde MG, Rothstein MA. Pharmacogenomics: Ethical concerns for research and pharmacy practice. *Am J Health-Syst Pharm.* 2002;59:2239–2240.

34. Parker LS, Brody H. Comparative effectiveness research: A threat to patient autonomy? *Health Progress.* 2011;92(5):64–71.

35. H.R. 493, the Genetic Information Nondiscrimination Act of 2008 / Public Law 110–233, 122 STAT. 881, 110th Congress.

36. Caufield T, Zarzeczny A. Defining medical necessity in an age of personalised medicine: A view from Canada. *Bioessays.* 2014;36:813–817.

37. Parker LS. Genetics and genomics research. In: MacKay D, Iltis A, eds. *Oxford Handbook of Research Ethics.* Oxford, UK: Oxford University Press; 2020.

38. Beskow LM, Fullerton SM, Namey EE, et al. Recommendations for ethical approaches to genotype-driven research recruitment. *Hum Genet.* 2012;131(9):1423–1431.

39. Budin-Ljøsne I, Soye KJ, Tasse AM, et al. Genotype-driven recruitment: A strategy whose time has come? *BMC Medical Genom.* 2013;6(19):1–7.

40. Lipton P. Pharmacogenetics: The ethical issues. *Pharmacogenomics J.* 2002;3:14–16.

41. Pendergrass SA, Brown-Gentry K, Dudek S, et al. Phenome-Wide Association Study (PheWAS) for detection of pleiotropy within the Population Architecture using Genomics and Epidemiology (PAGE) network. *PLoS Genet.* 2013;9(1):1–26.

42. DrugBaron. PheWAS—The Tool That's Revolutionizing Drug Development That You've Likely Never Heard Of. Available at http://drugbaron.com/phewas-the-tool-thats-revolutionizing-drug-development-that-youve-likely-never-heard-of/. Accessed October 20, 2020.

43. Gershon ES, Alliey-Rodriguez N, Grennan K. Ethical and public policy challenges for pharmacogenomics. *Dialogues Clin Neurosci.* 2014;16(4):567–574.

44. Abbott A. Uphill struggle. *Nature.* 2006;439:524–525.

45. Tutton R. Pharmacogenomic biomarkers in drug labels: What do they tell us? *Pharmacogenomics.* 2014;15:297–304.

46. Anonymous. NIH Names Johns Hopkins Berman Institute a Center of Excellence for Bioethics Research on Genomics and Infectious Disease. Available at http://www.bioethicsinstitute.org/media/press-release-nih-names-johns-hopkins-berman-institute-a-center-of-excellence-for-bioethics-research-on-genomics-and-infectious-disease. Accessed October 20, 2020.

47. Hopf H, Krief A, Mehta G, et al. Fake science and the knowledge crisis: Ignorance can be fatal. *R Soc Open Sci.* 2019;6:190161.

48. Opel DJ, Diekema DS, Marcuse EK. Assuring research integrity in the wake of Wakefield. *BMJ.* 2011;342:179–180.

49. Poland GA, Ovsyannikova IG, Kennedy RB. Personalized vaccinology: A review. *Vaccine.* 2018;36:5350–5357.

CHAPTER 4

PHARMACOGENOMICS RESOURCES

Roseann S. Gammal and Kelly E. Caudle

INTRODUCTION

Pharmacogenomics is a rapidly evolving field. The science behind gene/drug associations and its clinical utility has outpaced educational efforts; health care providers currently receive limited, if any, formal training in pharmacogenomics.[1,2] In spite of this, with the decline in the cost of genetic testing and the rise of direct-to-consumer genetic testing, clinicians will increasingly be called upon to incorporate pharmacogenomic test results into prescribing decisions. Fortunately, there are many freely available, evidence-based resources that clinicians can reference when faced with these challenges. Clinical practice guidelines exist that provide clinicians with actionable prescribing recommendations based on genetics. Online databases are also available that characterize and curate available pharmacogenomics

literature, alleles, genetic testing laboratories, and educational resources. Implementation resources from clinical decision support to gene/drug implementation guides are also available online. When faced with a pharmacogenomics clinical question or implementation challenge, understanding the nature and scope of these diverse resources will be an asset. Leveraging these key resources will facilitate the appropriate use of pharmacogenomic data in patient care (Table 4-1).

PHARMACOGENOMIC INFORMATION IN DRUG LABELS

The U.S. Food and Drug Administration (FDA) incorporates pharmacogenomic data into over 250 drug labels. A list of these drugs can be found in the FDA's "Table of

TABLE 4-1. Key Pharmacogenomics Resources

Resource	Description	Website
U.S. Food and Drug Administration (FDA) Resource		
FDA Table of Pharmacogenomic Biomarkers	Contains a list of drugs with pharmacogenomic information in their FDA-approved labeling.	https://www.fda.gov/drugs/science-research-drugs/table-pharmacogenomic-biomarkers-drug-labeling
Clinical Practice Guidelines		
Clinical Pharmacogenetics Implementation Consortium (CPIC) guidelines	Gene/drug pair guidelines that provide guidance on how to use existing pharmacogenomic test results to optimize medication therapy.	https://cpicpgx.org
Dutch Pharmacogenetics Working Group (DPWG) guidelines	Gene/drug pair guidelines that provide guidance on how to use existing pharmacogenomic test results to optimize medication therapy.	https://www.knmp.nl/producten/gebruiksrecht-g-standaard/informatie-over-de-g-standaard/the-g-standaard-the-medicines-standard-in-healthcare
The Canadian Pharmacogenomics Network for Drug Safety (CPNDS) guidelines	Gene/drug pair guidelines that provide guidance on when to order pharmacogenomic tests and how to use the results to optimize medication therapy.	https://cpnds.ubc.ca
Online Databases		
Pharmacogenomics Knowledgebase (PharmGKB)	Searchable database of curated pharmacogenomic literature and information. Also includes very important pharmacogene summaries and pharmacogenomic pathway diagrams.	https://pharmgkb.org
Pharmacogene Variation Consortium (PharmVar)	Online repository for pharmacogene nomenclature.	https://pharmvar.org
ClinVar and ClinGen	ClinVar is a submission-driven database of genomic variation from primary (e.g., clinical testing labs and researchers) and expert-curated submissions (e.g., expert panels and professional societies). ClinGen is a central database of genes and variants with standardized annotations for clinical relevance for clinical and research use that relies on ClinVar for variant data.	https://www.ncbi.nlm.nih.gov/clinvar/ https://clinicalgenome.org
Genetic Testing Registry (GTR)	Centralized database of genetic testing labs worldwide and their test offerings created via voluntary submissions.	https://www.ncbi.nlm.nih.gov/gtr/
Genetics/Genomics Competency Center (G2C2)	Online repository of curated, peer-reviewed genomics education materials for health care providers, including discipline-specific genomic competencies.	https://genomicseducation.net/
Implementation Resources		
CPIC Informatics Resources	Drug-agnostic gene information tables and guideline-specific tables, including allele definition tables, genotype to phenotype translation tables, allele functionality tables, and allele frequency tables. Also includes sample language for clinical decision support.	CPIC guideline supplements https://www.pharmgkb.org/page/pgxGeneRef
Clinical Decision Support Knowledgebase (CDS-KB)	Online repository of shared CDS implementation artifacts and design considerations for genomic medicine programs, including CDS architecture diagrams, usage scenarios, CDS images from their institution, workflow diagrams, mapping and translation tables, patient materials, and implementation guides.	https://cdskb.org

TABLE 4-1. Key Pharmacogenomics Resources (*Continued*)

Resource	Description	Website
IGNITE Spark Toolbox and Implementation Guides	Collection of genomic medicine resources for clinicians and researchers pertaining to special considerations, standard approaches, and best practices. Implementation guides outline key steps in the implementation process and link to freely available resources.	https://ignite-genomics.org
St. Jude Children's Research Hospital's "Implementation Resources for Professionals"	Website that contains links to pharmacogenomics publications, presentations, and competencies for specific genes.	https://www.stjude.org/research/clinical-trials/pg4kds-pharmaceutical-science/implementation-resources-for-professionals.html

Pharmacogenomic Biomarkers in Drug Labeling" online.[3] Pharmacogenomic information is located in many different sections of the drug label, including Adverse Reactions, Boxed Warning (also commonly referred to as "Black Box Warning"), Clinical Pharmacology, Clinical Studies, Contraindications, Dosage and Administration, Drug Interactions, Indications and Usage, Patient Counseling Information, Use in Specific Populations, and Warnings and Precautions. It is important to note that the FDA label only provides clear guidance on how to adjust drug dosing based on genetic information (e.g., 50% dose reduction in CYP2D6 poor metabolizers) for some drugs, whereas other information is merely informative and may simply summarize how certain genetic variants may affect drug exposure based on observations from clinical studies. Gene/drug pairs with pharmacogenomic information in the Boxed Warning section of the drug label, the FDA's highest level of warning for serious or life-threatening risks, include *HLA-B*57:01*/abacavir, *HLA-B*15:02*/carbamazepine, *CYP2C19*/clopidogrel, *CYP2D6*/codeine, *G6PD*/rasburicase, and *CYP2D6*/tramadol.

Although the FDA labeling is an authoritative and trustworthy resource for clinical pharmacogenomics information, there are important limitations to note. First, the FDA drug labeling may not reflect the current state of evidence for gene/drug associations and their clinical utility. Pharmacogenomic studies are ongoing, and the collective body of evidence for gene/drug associations is growing. There may be a significant lag between when the evidence supporting a particular gene/drug association crosses the threshold for clinical utility and when that information is updated in the drug label. At this time, it is not mandatory for drug manufacturers to provide genetic information in the drug label. Second, the FDA labeling may not clearly elucidate how a clinician could use clinically relevant pharmacogenomic information to improve patient care. This leaves interpretation up to individual clinicians, who are likely not well versed in this emerging field and therefore will not understand how to appropriately integrate what may be clinically important pharmacogenomic information into their clinical decision-making. For example, the FDA labels for tricyclic antidepressants (TCAs) state:

"The biochemical activity of the drug metabolizing isozyme cytochrome P450 2D6 (debrisoquin hydroxylase) is reduced in a subset of the Caucasian population (about 7% to 10% of Caucasians are so called 'poor metabolizers'); reliable estimates of the prevalence of reduced P450 2D6 isozyme activity among Asian, African, and other populations are not yet available. Poor metabolizers have higher than expected plasma concentrations of tricyclic antidepressants when given usual doses. Depending on the fraction of drug metabolized by P450 2D6, the increase in plasma concentration may be small, or quite large (8 fold increase in plasma AUC of the TCA)."[3]

Although the label mentions an actionable gene/drug association between CYP2D6 and TCAs, the label does not provide a specific dose adjustment or alternative therapy to consider in CYP2D6 poor metabolizers. To address the need for gene/drug clinical practice guidelines that are user friendly for clinicians and provide detailed, up-to-date instruction on how available pharmacogenomic test results could or should be used to guide prescribing decisions, international consortia such as the Clinical Pharmacogenetics Implementation Consortium, the Dutch Pharmacogenetics Working Group, and the Canadian Pharmacogenomics Network for Drug Safety were created.

CLINICAL PRACTICE GUIDELINES

Clinical Pharmacogenetics Implementation Consortium Guidelines

The Clinical Pharmacogenetics Implementation Consortium (CPIC; www.cpicpgx.org) was formed in

2009 to provide evidence-based guidelines describing how to interpret pharmacogenomic test results and use that information to guide prescribing.[4] CPIC is an international consortium funded by the National Institutes of Health (NIH) with more than 350 members (clinicians and scientists) from over 240 institutions and 33 countries including 10 observers from the FDA and NIH. As of October 2020, there are currently 25 published guidelines which encompass 20 genes and over 60 drugs across several therapeutic areas (see https://cpicpgx.org/guidelines/ for a list of current guidelines). New CPIC guidelines are published each year, and previously written guidelines are updated at least every five years or sooner to account for new evidence. These guidelines are used worldwide to translate pharmacogenomic information into clinical practice. A key assumption underlying CPIC guidelines is that pharmacogenomic test information is available at the point of prescribing. CPIC guidelines do not provide guidance on whether to order a particular pharmacogenomic test, but rather what to do if that information is available to the clinician (an increasingly common scenario with the decreasing cost of sequencing and the rise of direct-to-consumer genetic testing).

CPIC guidelines are freely available on the CPIC website (www.cpicpgx.org/guidelines) and in PubMed Central (https://www.ncbi.nlm.nih.gov/pmc). CPIC guidelines are being endorsed by professional societies, such as the American Society for Clinical Pharmacology and Therapeutics and by the American Society of Health-System Pharmacists.[5,6] Furthermore, the Association for Molecular Pathology has endorsed CPIC's Term Standardization for Clinical Pharmacogenetics Test Results Project,[7] and the College of American Pathologists (CAP) has stated "CAP applauds and supports the objectives, processes and work completed as of December 2018 by the Clinical Pharmacogenetics Implementation Consortium (CPIC®). These efforts will help clinicians, laboratories, health care providers and vendors."[8]

CPIC guidelines are written by an international team of clinicians and scientists who are experts in the field. CPIC follows a standard process for guideline development,[9] and these guidelines largely adhere to the National Academy of Medicine's Standards for Developing Trustworthy Clinical Practice Guidelines.[10] CPIC maintains a strict conflict-of-interest policy for authors in order to maintain the integrity of the guidelines.[11] Guideline authors conduct a systematic review and evaluation of the literature for a given gene/drug pair and grade the available evidence as high, moderate, or

weak. Based on the body of evidence available to support a gene/drug association, the author group derives clinical recommendations based on phenotype, which is based on genotype. Generally, the "Table 1" in a CPIC guideline describes the genotype-to-phenotype translation, and the "Table 2" describes the phenotype-to-recommendation translation. Each guideline follows a standard format and includes sections about the gene, including genetic test interpretation; the drug; evidence linking genetic variability to variability in drug-related phenotypes; therapeutic recommendations, including a section on pediatric considerations; and incidental findings, if applicable.

Each gene-based prescribing recommendation is assigned a strength of strong, moderate, or optional, based on the quality of available evidence to support a gene/drug association and the availability of viable alternative agents or alternative dosing strategies. In some cases, guideline authors may also assign a "no recommendation" option to a particular phenotype if there is insufficient evidence, confidence, or agreement to provide a recommendation to guide clinical practice at the time the guideline is written. Each guideline also contains detailed supplemental information, which includes a summary of the evidence review and resources pertaining to integrating pharmacogenomic test results into electronic health records (EHRs) with clinical decision support (see the CPIC Informatics Resources in the Implementation Resources section for more detail). To date, all CPIC guidelines are for clinically actionable gene/drug pairs. However, CPIC has plans to also develop guidelines for gene/drug pairs without clinical utility at this time. This guidance is also valuable to clinicians, particularly for those genetic tests that are currently offered by commercial laboratories but lack sufficient evidence to change drug selection or dosing.

In addition to the guidelines, the CPIC website has a "Genes-Drugs" page (https://cpicpgx.org/genes-drugs/) that assigns a level of A, B, C, or D to each gene/drug pair. This web page is one of the most highly accessed pages on the CPIC website with more than 52,000 page views in 2018.[12] CPIC level A indicates that genetic information *should* be used to change prescribing of the affected drug (strong or moderate prescribing recommendation); CPIC level B indicates that genetic information *could* be used to change prescribing of the affected drug because alternative therapies/dosing are extremely likely to be as effective and as safe as nongenetically based dosing (optional prescribing recommendation); CPIC level C indicates that although the gene is commonly tested, there are published studies at varying levels of evidence, some with mechanistic rationale, but no prescribing actions are recommended because (1) dosing based on genetics makes no convincing difference; or (2) alternatives are unclear, possibly less effective, more toxic, or otherwise impractical; or (3) few published studies or mostly weak evidence and clinical actions are unclear; and CPIC level D indicates that there are few published studies, clinical actions are unclear, there is little mechanistic basis, there is mostly weak evidence, or substantial conflicting data and testing for the gene are rare (no prescribing recommendations). Unless a gene/drug pair has a corresponding guideline, these levels are considered provisional until a CPIC guideline author group has systematically evaluated the evidence. CPIC uses these levels to prioritize the order of writing guidelines for particular gene/drug pairs. In addition to assessing the prescribing actionability, CPIC considers the following questions when prioritizing guidelines to write: (1) What is the severity of the clinical consequences (adverse effects, lack of response) if genetics are not used to inform prescribing? (2) Is the gene already subject to other CPIC guidelines? (3) Is there an available genetic test for that gene? (4) How commonly used are the affected drugs? (5) How common are the high-risk genetic variants? (6) Is there mention of genetic testing in drug labeling? (7) Are there pharmacogenetically based prescribing recommendations from professional organizations or others?[13]

Dutch Pharmacogenetics Working Group Guidelines

The Dutch Pharmacogenetics Working Group (DPWG) was established in 2005 by the Royal Dutch Association for the Advancement of Pharmacy (KNMP; https://www.knmp.nl/producten/gebruiksrecht-g-standaard/informatie-over-de-g-standaard/the-g-standaard-the-medicines-standard-in-healthcare). The DPWG is a multidisciplinary group that includes clinical pharmacists, physicians, clinical pharmacologists, clinical chemists, epidemiologists, and toxicologists. The objectives of the DPWG are (1) to develop pharmacogenetics-based therapeutic recommendations and (2) to assist drug prescribers and pharmacists by integrating the recommendations into computerized systems for drug prescription and automated medication surveillance. Similar to the CPIC method, the DPWG systematically evaluates the literature for gene/drug pairs, grades the evidence, and develops gene-based prescribing recommendations. In addition, the DPWG does not provide recommendations about ordering pharmacogenomic tests, but rather

how to optimize drug dosing in the growing population of patients with genotype data. DPWG guidelines were first published in English in 2008[14] and then updated in 2011.[15] Although not published, the most recent (2018) guidelines can be found online.[16] These recommendations are continuously updated and integrated into the G-standard, an extensive electronic drug database used in the Netherlands, which allows them to be available at the point of care through the nation's electronic prescribing system. In addition, the DPWG guidelines are the cornerstone of the Ubiquitous Pharmacogenomics (U-PGx) Consortium efforts to implement preemptive pharmacogenomic testing across health care institutions in seven European countries.[17,18]

DPWG assigns a level of evidence for each gene/drug interaction on a scale of 0 (lowest evidence) to 4 (highest evidence). Level 4 criteria include published controlled studies of good quality relating to phenotyped and/or genotyped patients or healthy volunteers and having relevant pharmacokinetic or clinical endpoints; level 3 criteria include published controlled studies of moderate quality relating to phenotyped and/or genotyped patients or healthy volunteers and having relevant pharmacokinetic or clinical endpoints; level 2 criteria include published case reports, well documented, and having relevant pharmacokinetic or clinical endpoints or well-documented case series; level 1 criteria include published incomplete case reports or product information; and level 0 criteria include data on file. The DPWG defines "good-quality" studies as those for which the use of a concomitant medication with a possible influence on the phenotype is reported in the manuscript; other confounders are reported (e.g., smoking status); the reported data are based on steady-state kinetics; and the results are corrected for dose variability. The quality of a study is deemed "moderate" whenever one or more of the "good-quality" criteria are missing. The DPWG also characterizes the clinical relevance of the gene/drug interaction using a 7-point scale.

CPIC and DPWG guidelines were formally compared in 2017 with respect to gene/drug pairs assessed, terminology, genotype-to-phenotype assignments, and clinical recommendations.[19] In general, there is a high rate of concordance between each consortium's clinical recommendations for the gene/drug pairs. The differences identified were attributed to differences in their applied methodologies for grading the evidence, differences with respect to when literature searches were conducted, and differences in clinical practice between the United States and the Netherlands. Identification of terminology and genotype-to-phenotype translation differences have led to efforts for harmonization between the two groups. For example, a recent effort to standardize *CYP2D6* genotype-to-phenotype translation was led by key stakeholders from both CPIC and DPWG leadership.[20]

Canadian Pharmacogenomics Network for Drug Safety Consortium Guidelines

The Canadian Pharmacogenomics Network for Drug Safety (CPNDS; http://cpnds.ubc.ca) is a national program whose mission is to reduce serious adverse drug reactions in children through the use of pharmacogenomic testing.[21] Their primary project objectives include (1) reducing the occurrence of permanent disability and deaths from severe adverse drug reactions and (2) developing cost-effect predictive pharmacogenomic tests for specific adverse drug reactions. The CPNDS employs surveillance clinicians in children's hospitals across Canada who collaborate with local health care professionals to identify and report adverse drug reactions, as well as collect clinical data and deoxyribonucleic acid (DNA) samples from patients. DNA samples are also collected from patients who received the same medication but did not experience the severe adverse drug reaction, and analyses are conducted to see if particular genetic variants increase the risk of these reactions.

In addition to publishing the findings of their studies, the CPNDS publishes pharmacogenomics clinical practice guidelines to improve the use of pharmacogenomic tests in the clinic.[22] To date, there are six CPNDS guidelines, the first of which was published in 2013. These guidelines focus on recommendations for genetic testing to reduce the incidence of anthracycline-induced cardiotoxicity[23]; managing and preventing cisplatin-induced hearing loss using pharmacogenomic markers[24]; genetic testing of *CYP2C9* and *VKORC1* variants in warfarin therapy[25]; recommendations for *HLA-B*15:02* and *HLA-A*31:01* genetic testing to reduce the risk of carbamazepine-induced hypersensitivity reactions[26]; *CYP2D6* genotyping for the safe and efficacious use of codeine[27]; and *CYP2D6* genotyping as a treatment decision aid for estrogen receptor–positive, nonmetastatic breast cancer patients.[28] A key difference between the CPNDS guidelines and the CPIC and DPWG guidelines is that the CPNDS guidelines address the question of whether the clinician should order genetic testing for particular groups of patients. These guidelines, along with the CPIC and DPWG guidelines, are annotated in the Pharmacogenomics Knowledgebase (PharmGKB).

ONLINE DATABASES

Pharmacogenomics Knowledgebase

The PharmGKB (www.pharmgkb.org) is an NIH-funded resource that was established in 2000. The mission of this publicly available online database is to collect, encode, and disseminate knowledge about the impact of human genetic variations on drug responses.[29] PharmGKB is maintained by a scientific curator team based out of Stanford University. The PharmGKB website contains many types of information and sections, including prescribing information, drug label annotations, curated pathways, very important pharmacogene (VIP) summaries, variant annotations, and clinical annotations. The website is easily searchable, with a main search box that can be used to find a gene, genetic variant, or drug of interest (or a combination of these).

PharmGKB curators work closely with CPIC staff to create CPIC guidelines, which users can find on the PharmGKB website. PharmGKB also provides links to other clinical guidelines, such as those written by DPWG and CPNDS, as well as other professional organizations. In addition, there are "Rx study annotations" in the prescribing information section of the website, which are prescribing recommendations from a publication not written by a professional society or consortium, but the study authors provide specific gene-based dosing recommendations. PharmGKB also keeps an updated list of drug labels that contain pharmacogenomic information, including American, Canadian, European, and Japanese medication labels.

Other resources that PharmGKB provides on their website include curated pathways and VIP summaries. The curated pathways are evidence-based diagrams depicting how a medication is metabolized or works in the body. These pathway diagrams are accompanied by a written description that explains how genetic variation affects the pathway based on available literature. The VIP summaries (https://www.pharmgkb.org/vips) provide a succinct overview of individual pharmacogenes that are particularly important for drug metabolism or response to one or several drugs. They review the gene structure, physiological role of the encoded protein, and relationship between genetic variants and drug response. Many of these summaries are published in the journal *Pharmacogenetics and Genomics*. To date, 66 VIP summaries are available on the PharmGKB website.

Variant and clinical annotations are core components of PharmGKB. Variant annotations describe the reported association between a variant (e.g., single-nucleotide polymorphism, indel, repeat, haplotype) and a drug phenotype, as described by a single published study.[30] Each variant annotation includes key study parameters, such as study size, population data, and statistics, that help put the annotation into context. PharmGKB curators combine multiple variant annotations into clinical annotations—a single summary of a gene/drug association. In these annotations, the phenotype for any given genotype is reported relative to the other genotypes. Each clinical annotation is assigned a level of evidence based on careful literature review: Level 1A, 1B, 2A, 2B, 3, or 4, with level 1 being the highest level of evidence and level 4 being the lowest. The levels are defined as follows: 1A—Annotation for a variant-drug combination in a CPIC or medication society–endorsed pharmacogenomic guideline or implemented at a Pharmacogenomics Research Network site or in another major health system; 1B—Annotation for a variant-drug combination where the preponderance of evidence shows an association. The association must be replicated in more than one cohort with significant p-values and preferably will have a strong effective size; 2A—Annotation for a variant-drug combination where the variant is within a VIP as defined by PharmGKB. These variants are in known pharmacogenes, so functional significance is more likely; 2B—Annotation for a variant-drug combination with moderate evidence of an association. The association must be replicated, but there may be some studies that do not show statistical significance and/or the effect size may be small; 3—Annotation for a variant-drug combination based on a single significant (not yet replicated) study or annotation for a variant-drug combination evaluated in multiple studies but lacking clear evidence of an association; 4—Annotation based on a case report; nonsignificant study; or in vitro, molecular, or functional assay evidence only.

For individuals interested in learning how to best use the PharmGKB resource or for educators interested in teaching their students about using PharmGKB, training exercises are provided on the PharmGKB website (https://www.pharmgkb.org/downloads).

Pharmacogene Variation Consortium

The Pharmacogene Variation Consortium (PharmVar; https://www.pharmvar.org/) is a recently created, NIH-supported online repository for pharmacogene nomenclature. Its mission is to catalog allelic variation of genes affecting drug disposition and response and to provide standard nomenclature for the global pharmacogenomics community, which will facilitate research

and clinical implementation efforts. PharmVar works closely with CPIC and PharmGKB, since their missions are aligned. PharmVar replaces and expands upon the widely regarded and used online resource, The Human Cytochrome P450 Allele Nomenclature Database.[31] The database is evolving from static CYP variation tables to an interactive, state-of-the-art database that encompasses important pharmacogenes beyond CYP, including other genes involved in drug metabolism, as well as genes involved in drug transport and response.[32] Gene expert panels review submissions, develop standard operating procedures, standardize the submission/review process, and designate haplotypes for various pharmacogenes. In addition, PharmVar will publish "GeneReviews," the first of which focuses on CYP2D6.[33]

ClinVar and ClinGen

Funded by the NIH and freely available, ClinVar (https://www.ncbi.nlm.nih.gov/clinvar/) is a submission-driven database that aims to aggregate information about genomic variation from primary (e.g., clinical testing labs and researchers) and expert-curated submissions (e.g., expert panels and professional societies like Clinical Genome Resource [ClinGen] and CPIC).[34] ClinVar reports the relationship between variants and conditions using standardized descriptions of variants, conditions, and terms for clinical significance.[35] ClinGen (https://clinicalgenome.org/) is a freely available, NIH-funded initiative with the aim to create a central database of genes and variants with standardized annotations for clinical relevance for clinical and research use. ClinGen relies on ClinVar for existing data on variants. ClinGen expert panels then review the data on these variants and submit interpretations to ClinVar as expert-reviewed reports. Features of ClinGen include sharing of genomic and phenotypic data, machine-learning algorithms for variant interpretation, and evidence-based expert consensus for curation of clinical validity.[34,36]

Genetic Testing Registry

The Genetic Testing Registry (GTR; https://www.ncbi.nlm.nih.gov/gtr/) was launched by the NIH due to the increasing number of available genetic tests and the lack of accessibility to this information to health care providers, researchers, and others. The GTR is a centralized database of genetic testing labs worldwide and their test offerings via voluntary submissions. To date, it includes information for over 18,000 tested genes and 500 laboratories.[37] Users can search by tests, conditions/phenotypes, genes, or labs. The information provided for each test includes the test's purpose, methodology, validity, evidence of the test's usefulness if available (e.g., CPIC guidelines), and laboratory contacts and credentials. Detailed instructions on how to use the GTR website are available at https://www.ncbi.nlm.nih.gov/gtr/docs/help/.

Genetics/Genomics Competency Center

The Genetics/Genomics Competency Center (G2C2; https://genomicseducation.net/) is a National Human Genome Research Institute–sponsored online repository of curated, peer-reviewed genomics education materials for health care providers. Resources are mapped to discipline-specific genomic competencies[38–42] for physicians, physician assistants, nurses, genetic counselors, and pharmacists. The competencies are written specifically for each discipline and provide knowledge and skills needed to perform specific functions in genomic medicine. For example, the competencies for pharmacists include basic genetic concepts; genetics and disease risk; pharmacogenomics; and ethical, legal, and social implications.

IMPLEMENTATION RESOURCES

CPIC Informatics Resources

Successful adoption of pharmacogenomics requires an efficient process to integrate pharmacogenomics test results into the EHR with clinical decision support (CDS) so genetic test results are available to clinicians at the point of care. Because EHR vendors do not yet provide a standard set of CDS functions for pharmacogenetics, CPIC provides vendor-agnostic resources to support the adoption of CPIC guidelines within an EHR. These resources include gene information tables and guideline-specific tables. The gene information tables provide a crosswalk from genotype to interpreted phenotype and include the gene definition table, gene functionality table, and genotype-to-phenotype translation table. These tables can be found on the CPIC guideline pages[43] and are available on PharmGKB at https://www.pharmgkb.org/page/pgxGeneRef. These tables also include a gene-specific frequency table reporting population-based allele frequencies and calculated diplotype and phenotype frequencies and a table containing gene codes from standard nomenclatures and knowledge bases (e.g., HGNC, NCBI, Ensebl, PharmGKB). Included with these tables is a figure outlining the steps to entering a genetic test result into the EHR (see Figure 4-1) and example consult (i.e., genetic test interpretation) language.

Each guideline is accompanied by guideline-specific tables and a figure containing the workflow and required data to couple the genetic test result with a drug-specific clinical recommendation. An example point-of-care CDS (i.e., interruptive alert) is provided based on the CPIC guideline for each phenotype group for each drug covered in the guideline, along with a list of drug codes from standard terminologies (e.g., RxNorm, DrugBank, ATC) and databases such as PharmGKB. These tables can be found on each CPIC guideline page on the CPIC website.[43]

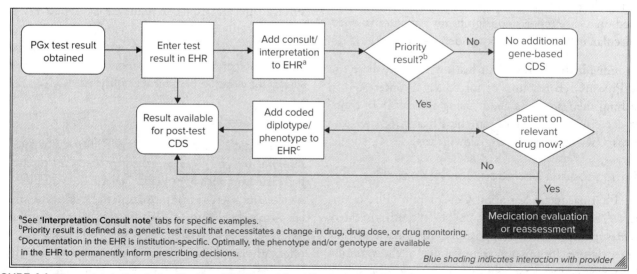

FIGURE 4-1 • Example electronic health record (EHR) workflow diagram provided with Clinical Pharmacogenetics Implementation Consortium guidelines. CDS, clinical decision support. PGx, pharmacogenetic. (Reproduced from Clinical Pharmacogenetics Implementation Consortium, U.S. Department of Health and Human Services.)

Clinical Decision Support Knowledgebase

The Clinical Decision Support Knowledgebase (CDS-KB; https://cdskb.org/) is a shared project between the two NIH-funded consortia: the Electronic Medical Records and Genomics (eMERGE) and Implementing Genomics in Practice (IGNITE) network. The goal of CDS-KB is to enable rapid translation and implementation of genomic medicine by cataloging and sharing CDS implementation artifacts and design considerations for genomic medicine programs. A broad community of institutions have shared institution-specific elements such as CDS architecture diagrams, usage scenarios, CDS images from their institution, workflow diagrams, mapping and translation tables, patient materials, and implementation guides. Although a free tool, to access the artifacts, a user account and acceptance of terms of use to restrict re-dissemination is required. Additionally, recorded webinars are available from a "Learning" section of the repository intended to focus on lessons learned from implementation strategies across the community (e.g., eMERGE, IGNITE, and others).

IGNITE Spark Toolbox and Implementation Guides

The Implementing GeNomics In practice (IGNITE) Pragmatic Clinical Trials Network is an NIH-funded network dedicated to implementing genomic medicine in clinical practice (https://ignite-genomics.org). As part of its work, the IGNITE network disseminates methods and best practices for genomics implementation through their website. The IGNITE Spark Toolbox is a collection of genomic medicine resources for clinicians and researchers pertaining to special considerations; standard approaches; and best practices in the design, conduct, and reporting of genomic medicine. Given the rapid pace of change in this field, this toolbox will continue to be added to and updated. IGNITE also provides "implementation guides" for select gene/drug pairs (e.g., *CYP2C19/clopidogrel*, *CYP2D6/opioids*) that outline key steps in the implementation process and link to freely available resources (https://gmkb.org/implementation-guides). These implementation guides were created by genomic medicine experts who have real-world experience in implementing the particular gene/drug pair into the clinical workflow of a health system.

St. Jude Children's Research Hospital Resources

St. Jude Children's Research Hospital is a global leader in the implementation of preemptive pharmacogenomic testing into routine clinical care through their PG4KDS ("Pharmacogenetics for Kids") protocol.[44] St. Jude pharmacists who lead this effort maintain an "Implementation Resources for Professionals" website that contains links to PG4KDS publications, PG4KDS presentations, videos of pharmacogenomics presentations, and pharmacogenomics competencies for specific genes that they have implemented.[45]

CONCLUSION

A number of pharmacogenomics resources are available to help clinicians interpret and apply pharmacogenomic test results to patient care. A working knowledge of the type of information contained in these resources is vital for any clinician who is actively implementing pharmacogenomics into clinical practice.

CASE SCENARIOS

Case 1

Patient A is a 48-year-old female with newly diagnosed depression who was referred to your pharmacogenomics clinic for testing to help choose optimal antidepressant therapy. You use a third-party commercial laboratory for genotyping, which tests for a standard panel of genes: *CYP2B6*, *CYP2C9*, *CYP2C19*, *CYP2D6*, *GRIK4*, *SLCO1B1*, and *TPMT*.

1. Which genes have associated CPIC guidelines for antidepressants?

Answer: CYP2D6 and CYP2C19 (for selective serotonin reuptake inhibitors [SSRIs] and TCAs).

2. The patient's psychiatrist would like to start the patient on citalopram. The patient's pharmacogenomic test results indicate the following: *CYP2B6 *1/*1, CYP2C9 *1/*3, CYP2C19 *17/*17, CYP2D6 *1/*2, GRIK4* rs1954787 TT, *SLCO1B1 *1/*5,* and *TPMT *1/*1.* Is citalopram an appropriate choice based on these results?

Answer: Citalopram is metabolized by CYP2C19 into inactive metabolites. CPIC's guideline for SSRIs indicates that it *would be best to avoid citalopram in CYP2C19 ultrarapid metabolizers due to the risk of subtherapeutic plasma concentrations and treatment failure. The patient is a CYP2C19 ultrarapid metabolizer (CYP2C19 *17/*17), so citalopram would not be the optimal choice of antidepressant.*

3. The psychiatrist asks you about the patient's *GRIK4* result, as she has heard that *GRIK4* can influence response to antidepressant therapy. Are there any evidence-based prescribing recommendations for *GRIK4* and antidepressants?

   Answer: GRIK4 is not included in the FDA labeling for any antidepressant, nor is there a clinical guideline for GRIK4 and antidepressants. CPIC rates this gene/drug association as level D, indicating that it is not actionable at this time.

Case 2

You are interested in implementing CYP2C19/clopidogrel at your health system for patients who receive percutaneous coronary interventions.

1. What resource provides a step-by-step implementation guide for CYP2C19/clopidogrel?

   Answer: The IGNITE Spark Toolbox

2. Your hospital's clinical laboratory is not equipped to offer CYP2C19 genotyping at this time. What resource can you use to identify genetic testing labs that test for CYP2C19?

   Answer: The Genetic Testing Registry

3. You would like to integrate CYP2C19 test results into the EHR with CDS so that patients who are CYP2C19 intermediate and poor metabolizers can be flagged at the point of prescribing. Which resources provide sample CDS language for CYP2C19/clopidogrel?

   Answer: CPIC Informatics resources (supplemental information from the CYP2C19/clopidogrel CPIC guideline); the Clinical Decision Support Knowledgebase (CDS-KB); and the IGNITE SPARK Toolbox

Case 3

Patient B is a 7-year-old female with acute lymphoblastic leukemia who requires treatment with mercaptopurine as part of her chemotherapy regimen.

1. Which gene(s) is/are included in the FDA labeling for mercaptopurine, and is this information actionable?

   Answer: TPMT and NUDT15 are both included in the FDA labeling for mercaptopurine. This information is actionable. Specifically, the labeling states that dose reduction may be necessary in patients who have TPMT or NUDT15 deficiency.

2. Which online resource provides a pharmacogenomic pathway diagram for thiopurines?

   Answer: PharmGKB

3. Which organization(s) provide evidence-based guidelines for genotype-guided mercaptopurine dosing?

   Answer: The CPIC and the DPWG

PHARMACOGENOMICS CLINICAL PEARLS

- Pharmacogenomic information can be found in many sections of an FDA-approved drug label, which may or may not be actionable.

- In addition to providing resources to facilitate genotype-to-phenotype to recommendation translation, the CPIC provides many informatics resources, including sample language for clinical consults and interruptive alerts.

- In addition to CPIC, the DPW and the CPNDS provide pharmacogenomics guidelines.

- PharmGKB is a searchable database of curated pharmacogenomics literature and information, but also includes other resources such as VIP summaries and pharmacogenomic pathway diagrams.

- PharmVar is a recently created online resource that houses allele definitions for pharmacogenes using standard nomenclature.

- The IGNITE Spark Toolbox provides "implementation guides" for select gene/drug pairs that outline key steps in the implementation process.

ABBREVIATIONS AND ACRONYMS

CAP: College of American Pathologists

CDS: clinical decision support

CDS-KB: Clinical Decision Support Knowledge-base

ClinGen: Clinical Genome Resource

CPIC: Clinical Pharmacogenetics Implementation Consortium

CPNDS: Canadian Pharmacogenomics Network for Drug Safety

CYP: cytochrome P450

DPWG: Dutch Pharmacogenetics Working Group

EHR: electronic health record

eMERGE: Electronic Medical Records and Genomics

FDA: Food and Drug Administration

G2C2: Genetics/Genomics Competency Center

GTR: Genetic Testing Registry

HLA: Human Leukocyte Antigen Complex

IGNITE: Implementing Genomics in Practice

NIH: National Institutes of Health

PG4KDS: Pharmacogenetics for Kids

PharmGKB: Pharmacogenomics Knowledgebase

PharmVar: Pharmacogene Variation Consortium

TCA: tricyclic antidepressant

VIP: very important pharmacogene

Acknowledgments

This work was supported by the National Cancer Institute (CA 21765); the National Institutes of Health for CPIC (R24GM115264 and U24HG010135); and the American Lebanese Syrian Associated Charities (ALSAC).

REFERENCES

1. Campion M, Goldgar C, Hopkin RJ, Prows CA, Dasgupta S. Genomic education for the next generation of health-care providers. *Genet Med.* 2019;21(11):2422–2430.

2. Weitzel KW, Aquilante CL, Johnson S, Kisor DF, Empey PE. Educational strategies to enable expansion of pharmacogenomics-based care. *Am J Health Syst Pharm.* 2016;73(23):1986–1998.

3. Table of Pharmacogenomic Biomarkers in Drug Labeling. Available at https://www.fda.gov/drugs/science-research-drugs/table-pharmacogenomic-biomarkers-drug-labeling. Accessed June 26, 2019.

4. Relling MV, Klein TE. CPIC: Clinical Pharmacogenetics Implementation Consortium of the Pharmacogenomics Research Network. *Clin Pharmacol Ther.* 2011;89(3):464–467.

5. Tools and Resources. Available at https://www.ascpt.org/Resources/Knowledge-Center/Tools-and-resources. Accessed September 1, 2019.

6. Endorsed Documents. Available at https://www.ashp.org/pharmacy-practice/policy-positions-and-guidelines/browse-by-document-type/endorsed-documents. Accessed September 1, 2019.

7. Caudle KE, Dunnenberger HM, Freimuth RR, et al. Standardizing terms for clinical pharmacogenetic test results: Consensus terms from the Clinical Pharmacogenetics Implementation Consortium (CPIC). *Genet Med.* 2017;19(2):215–223.

8. Clinical Pharmacogenetics Implementation Consortium. Available at https://cpicpgx.org/. Accessed September 1, 2019.

9. Caudle KE, Klein TE, Hoffman JM, et al. Incorporation of pharmacogenomics into routine clinical practice: The Clinical Pharmacogenetics Implementation Consortium (CPIC) guideline development process. *Curr Drug Metab.* 2014;15(2):209–217.

10. Huddart R, Sangkuhl K, Whirl-Carrillo M, Klein TE. Are randomized controlled trials necessary to establish the value of implementing pharmacogenomics in the clinic? *Clin Pharmacol Ther.* 2019; 106(2):284–286.

11. Authorship on CPIC Guidelines. Available at https://cpicpgx.org/authorship-on-cpic-guidelines/. Accessed September 1, 2019.

12. Relling MV, Klein TE, Gammal RS, Whirl-Carrillo M, Hoffman JM, Caudle KE. The Clinical Pharmacogenetics Implementation Consortium: 10 years later. *Clin Pharmacol Ther.* 2019; 107(1):171–175.

13. Prioritization of CPIC Guidelines. Available at https://cpicpgx.org/prioritization-of-cpic-guidelines/. Accessed September 1, 2019.

14. Swen JJ, Wilting I, de Goede AL, et al. Pharmacogenetics: From bench to byte. *Clin Pharmacol Ther.* 2008;83(5):781–787.

15. Swen JJ, Nijenhuis M, de Boer A, et al. Pharmacogenetics: From bench to byte—An update of guidelines. *Clin Pharmacol Ther.* 2011;89(5):662–673.

16. Dutch Pharmacogenetics Working Group November 2018 Pharmacogenetic Recommendations. Available at https://www.knmp.nl/downloads/pharmacogenetic-recommendations-november-2018.pdf. Accessed July 10, 2019.

17. Manson LE, van der Wouden CH, Swen JJ, Guchelaar HJ. The Ubiquitous Pharmacogenomics Consortium: Making effective treatment optimization accessible to every European citizen. *Pharmacogenomics.* 2017;18(11):1041–1045.

18. van der Wouden CH, Cambon-Thomsen A, Cecchin E, et al. Implementing pharmacogenomics in Europe: Design and implementation strategy of the Ubiquitous Pharmacogenomics Consortium. *Clin Pharmacol Ther.* 2017;101(3):341–358.

19. Bank PCD, Caudle KE, Swen JJ, et al. Comparison of the guidelines of the Clinical Pharmacogenetics Implementation Consortium and the Dutch Pharmacogenetics Working Group. *Clin Pharmacol Ther.* 2018;103(4):599–618.

20. Caudle KE, Sangkuhl K, Whirl-Carrillo M, et al. Standardizing CYP2D6 genotype to phenotype translation: Consensus recommendations from the Clinical Pharmacogenetics Implementation Consortium and Dutch Pharmacogenetics Working Group. *Clin Transl Sci.* 2019; 13(1):116–124.

21. Tanoshima R, Khan A, Biala AK, et al. Analyses of adverse drug reactions-Nationwide Active Surveillance Network: Canadian

Pharmacogenomics Network for Drug Safety Database. *J Clin Pharmacol*. 2019;59(3):356–363.

22. Amstutz U, Carleton BC. Pharmacogenetic testing: Time for clinical practice guidelines. *Clin Pharmacol Ther*. 2011;89(6):924–927.

23. Aminkeng F, Ross CJ, Rassekh SR, et al. Recommendations for genetic testing to reduce the incidence of anthracycline-induced cardiotoxicity. *Br J Clin Pharmacol*. 2016;82(3):683–695.

24. Lee JW, Pussegoda K, Rassekh SR, et al. Clinical practice recommendations for the management and prevention of cisplatin-induced hearing loss using pharmacogenetic markers. *Ther Drug Monit*. 2016;38(4):423–431.

25. Shaw K, Amstutz U, Kim RB, et al. Clinical practice recommendations on genetic testing of CYP2C9 and VKORC1 variants in warfarin therapy. *Ther Drug Monit*. 2015;37(4):428–436.

26. Amstutz U, Shear NH, Rieder MJ, et al. Recommendations for HLA-B*15:02 and HLA-A*31:01 genetic testing to reduce the risk of carbamazepine-induced hypersensitivity reactions. *Epilepsia*. 2014;55(4):496–506.

27. Madadi P, Amstutz U, Rieder M, et al. Clinical practice guideline: CYP2D6 genotyping for safe and efficacious codeine therapy. *J Popul Ther Clin Pharmacol*. 2013;20(3):e369–396.

28. Drogemoller BI, Wright GEB, Shih J, et al. CYP2D6 as a treatment decision aid for ER-positive non-metastatic breast cancer patients: A systematic review with accompanying clinical practice guidelines. *Breast Cancer Res Treat*. 2019;173(3):521–532.

29. McDonagh EM, Whirl-Carrillo M, Garten Y, Altman RB, Klein TE. From pharmacogenomic knowledge acquisition to clinical applications: The PharmGKB as a clinical pharmacogenomic biomarker resource. *Biomark Med*. 2011;5(6):795–806.

30. Whirl-Carrillo M, McDonagh EM, Hebert JM, et al. Pharmacogenomics knowledge for personalized medicine. *Clin Pharmacol Ther*. 2012;92(4):414–417.

31. Gaedigk A, Ingelman-Sundberg M, Miller NA, et al. The Pharmacogene Variation (PharmVar) Consortium: Incorporation of the Human Cytochrome P450 (CYP) Allele Nomenclature Database. *Clin Pharmacol Ther*. 2018;103(3):399–401.

32. Gaedigk A, Sangkuhl K, Whirl-Carrillo M, et al. The evolution of PharmVar. *Clin Pharmacol Ther*. 2019;105(1):29–32.

33. Nofziger C, Turner AJ, Sangkuhl K, et al. PharmVar GeneReview: CYP2D6. *Clin Pharmacol Ther*. 2019;107(1):154–170.

34. ClinGen & ClinVar Partnership. Available at https://clinicalgenome.org/about/clingen-clinvar-collaboration/. Accessed September 1, 2019.

35. Landrum MJ, Lee JM, Benson M, et al. ClinVar: Improving access to variant interpretations and supporting evidence. *Nucleic Acids Res*. 2018;46(D1):D1062–D1067.

36. Rehm HL, Berg JS, Brooks LD, et al. ClinGen—The Clinical Genome Resource. *N Engl J Med*. 2015;372(23):2235–2242.

37. Genetic Testing Registry. Available at https://www.ncbi.nlm.nih.gov/gtr/. Accessed September 1, 2019.

38. Goldgar C, Michaud E, Park N, Jenkins J. Physician assistant genomic competencies. *J Physician Assist Educ*. 2016;27(3):110–116.

39. Roederer MW, Kuo GM, Kisor DF, et al. Pharmacogenomics competencies in pharmacy practice: A blueprint for change. *J Am Pharm Assoc (2003)*. 2017;57(1):120–125.

40. Korf BR, Berry AB, Limson M, et al. Framework for development of physician competencies in genomic medicine: Report of the Competencies Working Group of the Inter-Society Coordinating Committee for Physician Education in Genomics. *Genet Med*. 2014;16(11):804–809.

41. Essentials of Genetic and Genomic Nursing: Competencies, Curricula Guidelines and Outcome Indicators, 2nd ed. Available at https://www.genome.gov/Pages/Careers/HealthProfessionalEducation/geneticscompetency.pdf. Accessed August 1, 2019.

42. Practice-Based Competencies for Genetic Counselors. Available at https://www.gceducation.org/wp-content/uploads/2019/02/ACGC-Core-Competencies-Brochure_15_Web.pdf. Accessed August 1, 2019.

43. Guidelines, Clinical Pharmacogenetics Implementation Consortium (CPIC), US Department of Health and Human Services. Available at https://cpicpgx.org/guidelines/. Accessed September 1, 2019.

44. Hoffman JM, Haidar CE, Wilkinson MR, et al. PG4KDS: A model for the clinical implementation of pre-emptive pharmacogenetics. *Am J Med Genet C Semin Med Genet*. 2014;166C(1):45–55.

45. Implementation Resources for Professionals. Available at https://www.stjude.org/research/clinical-trials/pg4kds-pharmaceutical-science/implementation-resources-for-professionals.html. Accessed September 2, 2019.

CARDIOLOGY PHARMACOGENOMICS

Whitney D. Maxwell

LEARNING OBJECTIVES

1. Identify key variants associated with the metabolism and clearance of antiplatelets, beta blockers, statins, and vitamin K antagonists.

2. Evaluate literature describing the clinical impact of pharmacogenetic variants on safety, efficacy, and patient outcomes when recommending cardiology pharmacotherapy.

3. Review Clinical Pharmacogenetics Implementation Consortium (CPIC) guidelines and other relevant guidelines for pharmacogenetics-guided dosing recommendations.

ANTIPLATELET PHARMACOGENOMICS

Clopidogrel and CYP2C19

Antiplatelet therapies are utilized to prevent the glycoprotein IIb/IIIa receptor on platelets from becoming activated by adenosine diphosphate (ADP) binding to the platelet at the $P2Y_{12}$ portion of the ADP receptor on the platelet surface. In the absence of antiplatelet therapy, activation of the glycoprotein IIb/IIIa receptor enables fibrinogen binding and platelet aggregation. By inhibiting ADP binding to the platelet, $P2Y_{12}$ inhibitors prevent glycoprotein IIb/IIIa activation and resultant platelet aggregation.[1,2] $P2Y_{12}$ inhibitors, including clopidogrel, prasugrel, and ticagrelor, are used for treatment of acute coronary syndrome (ACS), as well as prevention of recurrent thrombosis following ACS.[3,4] Of these options, only clopidogrel and prasugrel must be converted from prodrug to active drug to metabolites to provide optimal therapeutic efficacy, as ticagrelor does not require biotransformation for pharmacologic efficacy.[3] Clopidogrel is converted to its active metabolite by CYP1A2, 2B6,

2C19, 2C9, 3A4, and 3A5, with CYP2C19 being the most clinically important.[2] Prasugrel is primarily converted to its active metabolite by CYP2B6 and 3A5. CYP2C19, 2C9, 2D6, and 3A4 isoenzymes are also involved in its metabolism to a lesser extent.[2]

Mechanism of Drug-Gene Interaction

Several pharmacogenomic variants exist that are associated with lower serum concentrations of clopidogrel's active metabolite, including the *CYP2C19*2* allele (rs4244285, c.681G>A), which is the most prevalent no-function allele found in approximately 15% of Caucasians and individuals of African descent and approximately one-third of Asians.[5] The serum concentration of clopidogrel's active metabolite is 30% lower when this variant is present.[6] The *CYP2C19*3* (rs4986893, c.636 G>A) as well as **4, *5, *6, *7*, and **8* alleles occur less commonly, but also have detrimental effects on serum concentrations of clopidogrel's active metabolite, thus reducing the antiplatelet activity and efficacy of the drug. The mean absolute reduction in platelet aggregation is reported to

TABLE 5-1. Commonly Occurring CYP450 2C19 Allele Examples

Allele	Nucleotide Variation	dbSNP (RefSNP) #	CYP2C19 Protein Effects	Function
*1	None	None	None	Normal function
*2	c.681G>A	rs4244285	Splicing defect	No function
*3	c.636G>A	rs4986893	Trp212Xaa	No function
*17	c.-806C>T	rs12248560	Increased transcription	Increased function

TABLE 5-2. CYP2C19 Alleles with Known Function

Allele Functional Status	CYP2C19 Star Alleles
Normal function	*1, *11, *13, *15, *18, *28
Decreased function	*9, *10, *16, *19. *25, *26
No function	*2, *3, *4, *5, *6, *7, *8. *22, *24, *35, *36, *37
Increased function	*17

be significantly lower in both intermediate (−9.1) and poor (−28.7) metabolizers compared to normal metabolizers ($p < 0.05$).[7-9] A variant that increases the antiplatelet activity of clopidogrel has also been identified. The CYP2C19*17 (rs12248560, c.806 C>T) allele actually enhances transcription of the gene encoding CYP2C19 and is therefore an increased-function allele, as it enables conversion of a higher percentage of inactive clopidogrel parent drug to active clopidogrel metabolites.[8] The presence of CYP2C19 variants has not been shown to decrease serum concentrations or efficacy of prasugrel.[10] Since ticagrelor does not require conversion to an active metabolite and CYP2C19 variants do not affect prasugrel efficacy, currently the only antiplatelet with efficacy concerns related to genetic variation in CYP2C19 is clopidogrel. A summary of commonly occurring CYP2C19 allele examples is provided in Table 5-1, and the functional status of the currently known CYP2C19 alleles is provided in Table 5-2.[11,12] Table 5-3 provides a summary of CYP2C19 phenotypes resulting from various genotypes. For example, the combination of two no-function CYP2C19 alleles is associated with the poor metabolizer phenotype.[5] Intermediate metabolizers may have one normal-function allele plus one no-function allele. The presence of one increased-function allele does not fully overcome the effects of a nonfunctional allele, so individuals with both no-function and increased-function alleles (e.g., *2/*17) are considered to have intermediate metabolizer phenotypes as well. One increased-function allele with one normal-function allele produces the rapid metabolizer phenotype, and ultrarapid metabolizers have two increased-function alleles.[5,13]

Consequence of Drug-Gene Interaction

Large meta-analyses have demonstrated an increase in major adverse cardiovascular (CV) events (HR: 1.55) and in-stent thrombosis (HR: 2.67) in CYP2C19*2 heterozygote variants and homozygote variants (CV event HR: 1.76, in-stent thrombosis HR: 3.97) compared to wild-type, but no significant attenuation of response or increase in clinical risk has been identified in individuals with these variants when taking prasugrel or ticagrelor.[7,14,15] A variety of observational studies, as well as a recently published prospective multisite study, have demonstrated significantly higher rates of major adverse cardiovascular events (MACEs) within the 12 months following percutaneous coronary intervention (PCI) in carriers of no-function CYP2C19 alleles when receiving clopidogrel therapy versus alternative antiplatelet therapy (HR: 2.26, 95% CI: 1.18–4.32, $p = 0.013$).[16,17] A 42% reduction in the incidence of a composite of cardiovascular death, nonfatal myocardial infarction (MI), nonfatal stroke, or major bleeding has also been noted among patients with ACS and either a *2 or *17 CYP2C19 variant allele receiving pharmacogenetic-guided antiplatelet therapy versus standard care in a randomized trial ($p < 0.001$).[18] Conflicting studies exist, but suggest that rapid (e.g., *1/*17 genotype) and ultrarapid metabolizer phenotypes may be (e.g., *17/*17 genotype) associated with increased bleeding risk.[8]

The package label for clopidogrel contains a Black Box Warning alerting clinicians of the diminished antiplatelet effects in patients homozygous for nonfunctional CYP2C19 variants, with instructions for clinicians to consider use of another P2Y$_{12}$ inhibitor in patients with the CYP2C19 poor metabolizer phenotype.[19] Currently, the package label does not specifically recommend preemptive pharmacogenetic testing, and there are limited data evaluating clinical implementation of pharmacogenetics-guided antiplatelet therapy. However, some experts have found the existing data evaluating outcomes from clopidogrel use in poor or intermediate metabolizers with ACS undergoing PCI sufficiently compelling to begin implementing genotype-guided treatment in clinical settings,

TABLE 5-3. Summary of Guideline Recommendations for Clopidogrel Therapy Adjustments Based on CYP2C19 Phenotype

Genotypes	Diplotype Examples	Likely Phenotype	CPIC Recommendation for Antiplatelet Therapy for Patients with ACS undergoing PCI	DPWG Recommendation for Antiplatelet Therapy
Two increased-function alleles or one normal-function + one increased-function allele	*17/*17, *1/*17	Ultrarapid metabolizer	Consider clopidogrel, prasugrel, or ticagrelor	No action is required
Two normal-function alleles	1/*1	Normal metabolizer	Consider clopidogrel, prasugrel, or ticagrelor	—
One normal-function allele + one no-function allele or One no-function allele + one increased-function allele	*1/*2, *1/*3, *2/*17	Intermediate metabolizer	Use alternative to clopidogrel; consider prasugrel or ticagrelor	PCI, Stroke, or TIA: choose an alternative to clopidogrel or double dose to 150 mg/day (600 mg loading dose)
Two no-function alleles	*2/*2, *2/*3, *3/*3	Poor metabolizer	Use alternative to clopidogrel; consider prasugrel or ticagrelor	PCI, Stroke, or TIA: avoid clopidogrel

and several institutions have genotype-guided antiplatelet therapy programs in place.[20] The 2011 American College of Cardiology (ACC)/American Heart Association (AHA) guidelines on PCI provide a Class IIb, level of evidence C recommendation for clopidogrel genetic testing in patients at high risk for poor clinical outcomes, stating that it might be considered to identify patients undergoing PCI who are at risk for reduced clopidogrel efficacy, with substitution of prasugrel or ticagrelor in these patients. However, this guideline recommends against routine genetic screening of all patients undergoing PCI to identify poor candidates for clopidogrel therapy.[21] No recommendations were provided regarding genetic screening in the 2015 focused update to this guideline.[22] Ongoing randomized trials could provide evidence to inform more widespread implementation of personalized antiplatelet therapy in the future.[23,24]

Treatment Recommendation

The Clinical Pharmacogenomics Implementation Consortium (CPIC) and Dutch Pharmacogenetics Working Group (DPWG) guidelines provide therapeutic recommendations based on CYP2C19 phenotype categories.[5,25] According to CPIC, clinicians should consider prasugrel or ticagrelor instead of clopidogrel for patients undergoing PCI with CYP2C19 poor metabolizer and intermediate metabolizer phenotypes. Extensive (normal) and ultrarapid metabolizers are considered candidates for clopidogrel, prasugrel, or ticagrelor.[5] The CPIC and DPWG guideline recommendations are compared side by side in Table 5-3.[5,25]

Clinical reasons other than pharmacogenomics may supplant the use of clopidogrel in some patients undergoing PCI. While ticagrelor and prasugrel are considered higher-intensity antiplatelet therapy options, they have also been associated with higher bleeding risk compared to clopidogrel. Nonetheless, efforts to provide higher-intensity antiplatelet therapy to patients who are at greatest risk for recurrent thrombosis may lead to preferential use of ticagrelor or prasugrel, eliminating the need for clopidogrel pharmacogenetics analysis in those instances.[26] However, side effects such as dyspnea and bradycardia may limit the use of ticagrelor in some patients.[3] Concerns regarding bleeding risk associated with prasugrel also prevents its use in the management of some patients with ACS, such as those with history of prior transient ischemic attack (TIA) or stroke.[3]

BETA BLOCKER PHARMACOGENOMICS

Metoprolol and CYP2D6

Beta blockers are a diverse class of cardiovascular agents that inhibit beta receptors, providing negative inotropy, decreasing cardiac output, and lowering blood pressure by decreasing peripheral vascular resistance.[27] The variability within this class relates to impact on alpha receptors, cardioselectivity, vasodilatory effects, and intrinsic sympathomimetic activity.[28] The elimination pathways are also variable, typically including hepatic metabolism and renal excretion. Atenolol, sotalol, and nadolol are hydrophilic and are primarily renally excreted.[29] Propranolol is metabolized by a variety of pathways, including CYP1A2.[27] Labetalol undergoes extensive first-pass metabolism, and its primary mode of hepatic elimination is glucuronide conjugation.[30] Carvedilol is metabolized by CYP1A1, 1A2, 2C9, 2D6 (minimally), 2E1, and 3A4, while metoprolol and nebivolol are primarily eliminated by CYP2D6.[27] Although bisoprolol is partially metabolized by CYP2D6, CYP3A4 metabolism and renal excretion appear to be the primary methods of bisoprolol elimination.[31]

Mechanism of Drug-Gene Interaction

While CYP2D6 is not a primary metabolic pathway for most beta blockers, as shown in Table 5-4, since it is the primary metabolic pathway for metoprolol and nebivolol, the impact of pharmacogenetic variants on pharmacokinetics should be considered.[27,29–33] As is the case with most CYP450 isoenzymes, there are a variety of variant alleles for CYP2D6. Some examples of the most commonly occurring CYP2D6 alleles, the single nucleotide polymorphisms (SNPs) present, and their functional status of the alleles are provided in Table 5-5.[34,35] Over 100 CYP2D6 variant alleles have currently been identified.[35] While the functional level of many of these alleles has not yet been determined, the functional status of currently known CYP2D6 alleles

is provided in Table 5-6.[35,36] The presence of decreased- and no-function CYP2D6 alleles has been associated with significantly higher plasma concentrations, are under the curve (AUC), and significantly longer half-life of metoprolol.[37–40]

Consequence of Drug-Gene Interaction

Significant associations between CYP2D6 poor metabolizers and greater reductions in heart rate and bradycardia have been identified in several studies, particularly in the initial titration phase of therapy with metoprolol.[39–42] The package

TABLE 5-4. Relative Extent of Beta Blocker Metabolism by CYP2D6

Beta Blocker	Extent of Metabolism by CYP450 2D6
Atenolol	None
Bisoprolol	Minimal
Carvedilol	Minimal
Labetalol	Minimal
Metoprolol	Primary
Nebivolol	Primary
Propranolol	Minimal
Timolol	Minimal

TABLE 5-5. Selected Commonly Occurring CYP2D6 Allele Examples

Allele	Nucleotide Variation	dbSNP (RefSNP) ID #	CYP2D6 Protein Effects	Function
*1	None	None	"Wild type"	Normal function
*2	2850C>T	rs16947	Arg296Cys	Normal function
	4180G>C	rs1135840	Ser486Thr	
*3	2549delA	rs35742686	Frameshift mutation	No function
*4	1846G>A	rs3892097	Splicing defect	No function
*5	CYP2D6 Gene deletion	No function		
*6	1707delT	rs5030655	Frameshift mutation	No function
*9	2615_2617delAAG	rs5030656	Deletion mutation	Decreased function
*10	100 C>T	rs1065852	Pro34Ser	Decreased function
*17	1023C>T	rs28371706	Thr107Ile	Decreased function
	2850 C>T	rs16947	Arg296Cys	
*29	1659G>A; 1661G>C; 2850C>T; 3183G>A; 4180G>C	rs61736512 rs1058164	Val136Met	Decreased function
		rs16947 rs59421388 rs1135840	Arg296Cys	
			Val338Met	
			Ser486Thr	
*41	2850C>T	rs16947	Arg296Cys	Decreased function
	2988G>A	rs28371725	Splicing defect	
	4180G>C	rs1135840	Ser486Thr	
*1xN	Copy Number Variation	N/A	Increased protein production	Increased function

TABLE 5-6. CYP2D6 Alleles with Known Function

Allele Functional Status	CYP 2D6 Star Alleles
Normal function	*1,*2, *27, *33, *34,*35, *39, *45, *46, *48, *53
Decreased function	*9†, *10†, *14, *17†, *29†, *41†, *49, *50, *54, *55, *59, *72, *84
No function	*3†, *4†, *5†, *6†, *7, *8, *11, *12, *13, *15, *18, *19, *20, *21, *31, *36, *38, *40, *42, *44, *47, *51, *56, *57, *60, *62, *68. *69, *92, *96, *99, *100, *101, *114

† Most commonly occurring alleles.

label for metoprolol provides a summary of the pharmacokinetic impacts of *CYP2D6* variants, but states that the safety and tolerability of metoprolol do not appear to be affected in variants. Additionally, the package label does not provide any recommendations regarding pharmacogenetic testing. At this time, the ACC/AHA guidelines do not provide formal dosing recommendations for *CYP2D6* variants or any pharmacogenetic testing recommendations in patients for whom metoprolol therapy is being considered.[43]

Treatment Recommendation

Currently, CPIC does not have a guideline available to address *CYP2D6* variants and metoprolol use but may consider developing one in the future if a review of the evidence warrants. The DPWG published a guideline in 2018 that addresses beta blocker therapy in patients with *CYP2D6* variant alleles. Table 5-7 summarizes the recommendations provided in this guideline.[25,36,44,45] This guideline provides no recommendations for modifying drug therapy in patients taking atenolol because of the absence of gene–drug interactions, since it is primarily renally excreted. Although bisoprolol undergoes some degree of CYP2D6 metabolism, the CYP2D6 enzyme is considered a small contributor to the overall elimination of bisoprolol. Studies evaluating the impact of genetic variation within *CYP2D6* on bisoprolol pharmacokinetics and pharmacodynamics have failed to indicate a substantial effect.[38] Thus, the 2018 DPWG guideline indicates the absence of a gene–drug interaction for bisoprolol. Similarly, although carvedilol levels can be elevated in patients who are CYP2D6 poor metabolizers, DPWG does not recommend any therapy adjustments in patients with *CYP2D6* variants who take carvedilol. However, DPWG recommends that patients with an intermediate metabolizer phenotype taking metoprolol in whom gradual heart rate reduction is desired, or in whom symptomatic bradycardia occurs, should receive

no more than half of the standard dose or undergo slower-than-usual dose titration.[25] Similarly, the DPWG recommends that patients with a poor metabolizer phenotype taking metoprolol should receive no more than one-fourth of the standard dose, with slow titration of doses to enable gradual reduction in heart rate either preemptively or if patients with this phenotype experience symptomatic bradycardia while taking metoprolol.[25] Since individuals with the ultrarapid metabolizer phenotype have been noted to have reduced efficacy with regard to heart rate or blood pressure reduction when taking the target dose of metoprolol 200 mg/day, DPWG recommends using the maximum daily dose of metoprolol as an adjusted target dose. Since there are a variety of maximum daily dose recommendations for metoprolol based on indication for use, the adjusted target dose will vary based on indication for use. DPWG recommends that if metoprolol efficacy is still insufficient at the recommended maximum daily dose for a particular indication, the dose can be increased to 2.5 times the standard dose, or the patient can be switched to an alternative beta blocker that is not extensively metabolized by CYP2D6 (e.g., bisoprolol or carvedilol in patients with heart failure, since there are patient outcomes data with these beta blockers in the heart failure population). According to DPWG, alternative beta blocker therapy for patients with other indications for beta blocker use could include bisoprolol or atenolol.[25] However, many clinicians may hesitate to use atenolol due to concerns regarding its efficacy and safety in patients with renal impairment.[46] Although a primary mechanism for nebivolol elimination is CYP2D6 metabolism, in studies evaluating both pharmacokinetics and pharmacodynamics, nebivolol safety and efficacy were not significantly different in normal metabolizers versus poor metabolizers. Thus, nebivolol is not subject to the same pharmacogenetic variant-related concerns as metoprolol. This may possibly be related to the therapeutic effects provided by the active metabolites of nebivolol in normal metabolizers or to the almost doubling of renal clearance seen in poor metabolizers.[47,48] Since beta blocker therapy management is typically driven by clinical response, as it is dosed and titrated to effect based on a patient's heart rate, the clinical utility of pharmacogenetics-guided metoprolol therapy is yet to be fully understood.

HMG-COA REDUCTASE INHIBITORS ("STATIN") PHARMACOGENOMICS

Simvastatin and SLCO1B1

Statins or HMG-CoA reductase inhibitors comprise one of the most frequently prescribed drug classes in outpatient settings.[49] They are used primarily for

TABLE 5-7. Summary of DPWG Guideline Recommendations for Metoprolol Therapy Adjustments Based on CYP2D6 Phenotype

Genotypes	Diplotype Examples	Likely Phenotype	DPWG Recommendations for Metoprolol Therapy
An individual carrying more than two copies of normal-function alleles	*1/*1xN, *1/*2xN	Ultrarapid metabolizer	*Initially*: Use maximum daily dose of metoprolol recommended based on indication for use
			If efficacy insufficient on maximum daily dose: Increase metoprolol dose to 2.5 times the standard dose or switch patient to alternate beta blocker therapy
An individual carrying two normal-function or two reduced-function alleles-or-one normal-function allele + either one no-function* or one decreased-function allele	*1/*1, *1/*2, *2/*2	Normal metabolizer	—
An individual carrying one decreased-function and one no-function allele	*4/*10, *5/*41	Intermediate metabolizer	If a gradual reduction in heart rate is desired, or if symptomatic bradycardia occurs, use 50% of standard dose or increase the dose in smaller steps
An individual carrying only no-function alleles	*4/*4, *4/*5, *5/*5	Poor metabolizer	If a gradual reduction in heart rate is desired, or if symptomatic bradycardia occurs, use 25% of standard dose or increase the dose in smaller steps

* Individuals with one normal allele and one no-function allele may have previously been described as intermediate metabolizers in the literature.

secondary and primary CV event risk reduction and cholesterol lowering.[50] They are a fairly homogeneous class of drugs; however, the agents within this class do have some differences with regard to pharmacokinetics and pharmacogenomics. Pravastatin and rosuvastatin are hydrophilic statins that are not metabolized to a great extent by the CYP450 enzyme family and are instead metabolized by a variety of pathways, mostly by excretion as unchanged drug in the feces. Otherwise, most statins are metabolized by CYP450 enzymes.[51] Simvastatin is a statin of particular interest because it has been associated with muscle-related toxicity in patients with pharmacogenetic variants. Simvastatin is metabolized to active and inactive metabolites by CYP3A4 and CYP3A5 in the intestines. The organic anion transporting polypeptide 1B1 (OATP1B1) transporter protein is required to facilitate the uptake of simvastatin and its metabolites into the liver. CYP2C8 and CYP3A4 further metabolize simvastatin to active and inactive metabolites in the liver. Ultimately, the ATP Binding Cassette Subfamily B Member 1 (ABCB1) protein transporter facilitates the elimination of simvastatin through return of these metabolites from the liver to the gut for elimination.[52]

Mechanism of Drug-Gene Interaction

Up to one-fifth of the general population carries a decreased-function allele (rs4149056, c.521 T>C) for the SLCO1B1 gene that encodes the OATP1B1 protein that facilitates hepatic uptake of simvastatin. The SLCO1B1*5 variant allele can also be found as haplotypes along with rs2306283 (SLCO1B1*15) or rs4149015 (SLCO1B1*17), as shown in Table 5-8.[53,54] Individuals carrying at least one decreased-function allele or haplotype (*5, *15, or *17) have significantly higher serum concentrations of simvastatin compared to noncarriers, with homozygous variant genotypes being associated with a doubling of the AUC and C_{max} concentrations compared to individuals with wild-type genotypes.[55]

Consequence of Drug-Gene Interaction

The odds ratio for muscle-related adverse events in patients taking simvastatin with one copy of the rs4149015 variant allele has been shown to range between 1.7 and 4.5 in studies, and homozygous variants may have a nearly 17-fold increase in risk for simvastatin-related myopathy. No association between the SLCO1B1 variant and simvastatin's therapeutic impact on patient outcomes, such as reducing cardiovascular morbidity or mortality, has been

TABLE 5-8. Haplotypes Associated with Reduced SLCO1B1 Transporter Function

Ref SNP ID #s	Nucleotide Change	Amino Acid Change	Phenotypes	Haplotype		
rs4149056						
	c.521T>C	Valine to alanine (174th codon) p.Val174Ala	TT: Normal activity, reduced statin [plasma]	*5		
			TC: Intermediate activity, slightly increased statin [plasma]			
			CC: Low activity, increased statin [plasma]		*15	
rs2306283						*17
	c.388A>G	Asparagine to aspartic acid (130th codon) p.Asn130Asp	AA: Normal activity, reduced statin [plasma]			
			AG: Intermediate activity, slightly increased statin [plasma]			
			GG: Low activity, increased statin [plasma]			
rs4149015						
	c.-910G>A	Promoter variant	GG: Normal activity, reduced statin [plasma]			
			AG: Intermediate activity, slightly increased statin [plasma]			
			AA: Low activity, increased statin [plasma]			

identified to date.[56] This may be related to the relationship between hepatic statin concentrations and efficacy, as well as the relationship between serum concentrations and side effects, such as myalgia or myopathy.

The package label for simvastatin does not contain information about pharmacogenetic variants or recommendations regarding pharmacogenetic testing.[57] Additionally, the 2018 AHA/ACC guideline on the management of blood cholesterol does not provide recommendations for pharmacogenetic testing.[58]

Treatment Recommendation

CPIC provides a guideline addressing simvastatin use in patients with known *SLCO1B1* variants. Based on this guideline, there are three SLCO1B1 phenotypes: normal function, intermediate function, and low function. According to the guideline, individuals with one decreased-function allele and one normal-function allele (heterozygotes) (e.g., *1/*5) are considered to have an intermediate-function phenotype. Individuals with two decreased-function alleles (e.g., *5/*5) are considered to have a low-function phenotype. CPIC guidelines recommend that individuals with intermediate- or low-function phenotypes either receive an alternative statin such as pravastatin or rosuvastatin or receive lower doses of simvastatin. Consideration of routine creatine kinase monitoring for individuals with intermediate- or low-function phenotypes is also recommended in the CPIC guidelines.[53]

Available studies evaluating the impact of *SLCO1B1* carrier status on musculoskeletal adverse effects (AEs) in patients taking a variety of statins are summarized in Table 5-9.[59–63] Rosuvastatin is transported into the liver by *SLCO1B1*, and its pharmacokinetic parameters, including AUC and C_{max} concentrations, are increased in rs4149056 carriers.[64] Thus, it seems that rosuvastatin tolerability would be substantially affected in rs4149056 carriers. However, *SCLO1B1*5* carrier status was not significantly associated with musculoskeletal AE in an adequately powered subgroup of the JUPITER trial (HR 0.95, 95% CI 0.79 to 1.15).[59] Although the sample size was very small, another study published by Puccetti et al. failed to find a statistically significant association between the incidence of musculoskeletal AE and rosuvastatin therapy in carriers of the rs4149056 allele. However, a significant association was found between atorvastatin use and musculoskeletal AE in rs4149056 carriers.[62] Thus, rosuvastatin is currently considered a viable therapeutic option in patients with rs4149056 carrier status.[53] Of note, emerging data in Asian populations are calling this into question. Preliminary findings from a small study demonstrated significantly higher rates of musculoskeletal AE in Asian subjects taking rosuvastatin who are rs4149056 carriers compared to noncarrier Asian subjects, suggesting that the lower dose requirements in Asian patients may be related to this polymorphism.[65–67]

Data evaluating the safety of atorvastatin use in rs4149056 carriers are equivocal. Some studies, although typically underpowered, have failed to identify an association between rs4149056 carrier status and musculoskeletal AE in patients taking atorvastatin, while others have

TABLE 5-9. Associations Between Other Statins and Musculoskeletal Adverse Events in Studies Evaluating Carriers of *SCLO1B1*5*

Statin	Study Population	Findings	Limitations/Discussion
Rosuvastatin 20 mg	8782 patients from JUPITER study (n = 2484 musculoskeletal AE)	No statistically significant association between musculoskeletal AE and rosuvastatin	Manuscript states, "we anticipate sufficient power among 417 cases of myalgia among those on rosuvastatin to detect a relationship..."
Atorvastatin 10–80 mg	45 patients taking atorvastatin (n = 10 musculoskeletal AE)	No statistically significant association between myopathy and atorvastatin	Not adequately powered: 44%–52% power to detect an association between atorvastatin and myopathy, with an effect size of 3–3.5.
Atorvastatin 20–80 mg	143 Brazilian patients taking atorvastatin (n = 14 musculoskeletal AE)	No statistically significant association between myopathy and atorvastatin ($p = 0.30$)	Unclear if study met power for rs4149056 analysis/endpoint
Atorvastatin or Rosuvastatin	88 patients taking atorvastatin or rosuvastatin (n = 76 musculoskeletal AE)	No statistically significant association between rosuvastatin and myopathy. There was a statistically significant association between atorvastatin and myopathy (OR = 2.7, 95% CI: 1.3–4.9); p <0.001).	Preliminary data from case-control study; small sample size.
Atorvastatin 10 mg, 80 mg and Pravastatin 10 mg, 40 mg	509 patients (n = 99 musculoskeletal AE)	No statistically significant association between pravastatin and muscular AE; nonstatistically significant increase in musculoskeletal AE with atorvastatin.	Atorvastatin 10 mg is equipotent to pravastatin 40 mg and simvastatin 20 mg, so a relatively lower pravastatin dose was used when considering simvastatin and atorvastatin potencies

identified a significant association.[60–63] Thus, the CPIC guidelines do not list atorvastatin as a viable therapeutic option in patients with the rs4149056 allele.[53]

The STRENGTH (Statin Response Examined by Genetic Haplotype Markers) study evaluated patients randomized to either atorvastatin, simvastatin, or pravastatin and the incidence of musculoskeletal AE. Compared to noncarriers, study subjects with at least one rs4149056 allele had numerically higher musculoskeletal AE with atorvastatin and significantly higher musculoskeletal AE with simvastatin. The risk of musculoskeletal AE in carriers compared to noncarriers who were taking pravastatin, a relatively less myotoxic statin, was negligible. However, it should be noted that a relatively lower pravastatin dose was used when considering simvastatin and atorvastatin potencies.[63] The commonality between rosuvastatin and pravastatin, which are the two statins recommended by CPIC for use in individuals who are homozygous or carriers of rs4149056, is that they are both hydrophilic statins that are eliminated by way of multiple metabolic pathways with minimal CYP450

metabolism and a large percentage of drug being excreted in the feces.[53,68,69] The generally increased tolerability of rosuvastatin and pravastatin compared to other statins that have been noted in some studies has been attributed to these common characteristics.[70]

ANTICOAGULANT PHARMACOGENOMICS

Warfarin and CYP2C9, VKORC1, and CYP4F2

Hemostasis occurs by way of activated vitamin K–dependent clotting factors. These clotting factors become activated through a multistep process that begins with oxidized vitamin K (typically consumed in the diet) being converted by the vitamin K epoxide reductase enzyme complex subunit 1 (VKORC1) to reduced vitamin K. Reduced vitamin K subsequently facilitates the carboxylation of inactive clotting factors, leading to their activation.[71] This process is shown in Figure 5-1. CYP4F2 prevents overactivation of clotting factors by metabolizing reduced vitamin K.[72–74]

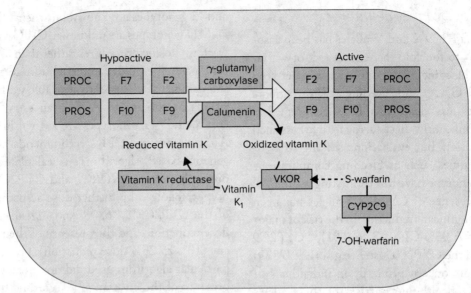

FIGURE 5-1 • Activation of vitamin K-dependent clotting factors. (Reproduced, with permission, from DiPiro JT, Yee GC, Posey LM, Haines ST, Nolin TD, Ellingrod VL, eds. *Pharmacotherapy: A Pathophysiologic Approach.* 11th ed. New York: McGraw-Hill; 2020.)

As seen in Figure 5-1, warfarin is a potent anticoagulant that works by inhibiting the VKORC1 enzyme subunit to prevent vitamin K from being converted to the reduced form that is needed for clotting factor activation.[71] Warfarin is a racemic structure composed of two enantiomers. The R-warfarin enantiomer is metabolized by CYP3A4. On the other hand, the S-warfarin enantiomer is the most clinically active enantiomer and is metabolized by CYP2C9 to inactive metabolites.[75] Thus, variants in the genes encoding the VKORC1, CYP4F2, and CYP2C9 enzymes that affect their function are obvious causes of altered warfarin pharmacokinetics, efficacy, and safety.[76]

Mechanism of Drug-Gene Interaction

An SNP in the *VKORC1* promoter region c.-1639 G>A (rs9923231) occurs more commonly in Caucasians and has been associated with increased warfarin efficacy, with carriers requiring lower warfarin doses than noncarriers, due to reduced VKORC1 function at baseline in patients with this variant.[75] Additionally, *2 (c.430 C>T, p.Arg144Cys, rs1799853) and *3 (c.1075 A>C, p.Ile359Leu, rs1057910) alleles of *CYP2C9* occur commonly in Caucasians and are decreased-function alleles that have also been associated with lower warfarin dose requirements due to impaired metabolism of the S-warfarin enantiomer.[77] Table 5-10 summarizes the *CYP2C9* alleles with known functional status.[78] *CYP2C9* *5, *6, *8, and *11, as well as rs12777823 which is a noncoding variant in the *CYP2C* gene cluster, are variants that account for lower warfarin dose requirements in patients of African ancestry.[76,79] Conversely, the *CYP4F2*3* (c.1297 G>A, p.Val433Met, rs2108622) variant allele has

TABLE 5-10. CYP2C9 Alleles with Known Function

Allele Functional Status	CYP2C9 Star Alleles
Normal function	*1, *9
Decreased function	*2, *3
No function	*6, *15, *25
Possibly decreased function	*4, *5, *8, *11, *12, *13, *31

been associated with increased warfarin requirements due to decreased metabolism of reduced vitamin K, leading to increased availability of reduced vitamin K and therefore increased activation of vitamin K–dependent clotting factors at baseline.[72]

Because they primarily affect vitamin K recycling and metabolism rather than warfarin metabolism, the *VKORC1* and *CYP4F2* polymorphisms confer primarily pharmacodynamic effects affecting warfarin sensitivity and dosing requirements, rather than directly affecting pharmacokinetic parameters such as warfarin plasma concentrations.[80] On the other hand, individuals carrying the *CYP2C9*2* allele experience reduced S-warfarin metabolism and have higher serum warfarin concentrations, particularly of the potent S-warfarin enantiomer.[81] Carriers of the *CYP2C9*2* allele require an approximate 15% to 20% dose reduction per allele, with homozygotes requiring an approximately 30% to 40% dose reduction, and individuals carrying the *3 allele require approximately 80% to 90% dose reductions.[82] The *CYP2C* cluster (e.g., rs12777823) has also been associated with lower warfarin clearance compared to nonvariants.[79]

Consequence of Drug-Gene Interaction

The presence of CYP2C9*2 and *3 alleles has been associated with a two- to fourfold increase in risk of warfarin-related major bleeding.[77,83] The relationship between VKORC1 (-1639 G>A) and bleeding risk in patients taking warfarin is less clear. VKORC1 genotype has been shown to significantly affect surrogate markers such as overanticoagulation, but evaluations seeking to associate patient outcomes such as bleeding complications with VKORC1 genotype have had conflicting results.[84,85] Conversely, the presence of CYP4F2*3 alleles has been associated with a significant reduction in the risk of major bleeding (OR: 0.62; 95% CI: 0.43 to 0.91).[86] CYP2C9 *5, *6, *8, *11, and the CYP2C cluster (e.g., rs12777823) are also variants of concern primarily in individuals of African ancestry, and although carriers of these alleles have lower warfarin dose requirements, their impact on therapy-related patient outcomes such as bleeding or thrombosis remains unclear.[76]

Specific recommendations regarding pharmacogenomic testing in patients taking warfarin therapy have not been provided by ACC/AHA.[43] The package label of warfarin provides recommendations regarding expected maintenance doses of warfarin when VKORC1 and CYP2C9 *2 and *3 genotypes are known, but suggests standard dose titration and monitoring recommendations in patients whose CYP2C9 and VKORC1 genotypes are unknown.[87]

Treatment Recommendation

CPIC guidelines recommend that patients with known VKORC1 and CYP2C9*2 and *3 genotypes first be stratified according to ancestry to determine if a pharmacogenomic-based warfarin dosing algorithm should be used to calculate the initial weekly warfarin dose. Two pharmacogenetic-based warfarin dosing algorithms, the International Warfarin Pharmacogenetics Consortium (IWPC) and an algorithm discovered by Gage et al., exist and have been used in clinical studies.[88,89] Compared to the table from the warfarin package label that addresses only VKORC1 and CYP2C9*2 and *3 genotypes, pharmacogenetic-based warfarin dosing algorithms have been shown to be more accurately predictive of warfarin dose than the table from the warfarin package label.[90] The CPIC guidelines provide more information on these algorithms, but it is important to note that while the algorithm available at www.warfarin-dosing.org includes VKORC1, CYP 2C9*2,*3,*5, *6, and CYP4F2 genotypes, it is still not inclusive of all clinically relevant genotypes for patients of African descent, such as CYP2C9*8,*11, and rs12777823.[91-94] If the patient is of African ancestry and only their VKORC1 and CYP2C9*2 and *3 genotypes are known but their CYP2C9*5, *6, *8, and *11 genotypes are unknown, CPIC recommends usual warfarin dosing procedures rather than using an algorithm for a genotype-guided approach due to the inaccuracy of standalone use of currently available warfarin dosing algorithms in patients of African ancestry.[76] If CYP2C9*5, *6, *8, and *11 genotypes are known in an individual of African ancestry, CPIC recommends using pharmacogenetics-based algorithms to calculate initial warfarin dosing based on VKORC1 and CYP2C9*2 and *3 genotypes, followed by further dose adjustments for carriers of the CYP2C9*5, *6, *8, and *11 alleles (15% to 30% dose reduction) and the presence of the rs12777823 variant (10% to 25% dose reduction), presumably when the particular algorithm used did not already account for the presence of these variants.[76] According to CPIC, in individuals of non-African ancestry, pharmacogenetics-based algorithms should be used to calculate initial warfarin dosing when VKORC1 and CYP2C9*2 and *3 genotypes are known. Dose reductions of 15% to 30% may be considered (as an optional CPIC recommendation) in individuals of non-African ancestry who are carriers of CYP2C9*5, *6, *8, and *11 alleles. CPIC also provides as an optional recommendation that slight increases (5% to 10%) in warfarin dose can be considered in individuals of non-African ancestry who are carriers of the CYP4F2*3 allele. These optional dose changes should presumably be applied when the algorithm selected for use does not already account for the presence of the associated variants. CPIC guidelines also recommend considering an alternative therapy to warfarin when patients are CYP2C9 poor metabolizers or when they are both VKORC1 variant carriers and CYP2C9 poor metabolizers. All of this information is synthesized by CPIC in a dosing recommendation algorithm, which is available at https://cpicpgx.org/guidelines/guideline-for-warfarin-and-cyp2c9-and-vkorc1/.[76]

The CPIC guidelines provide recommendations on how to manage patients with known pharmacogenomic variants, but do not necessarily address the utility of prospective screening of patients who are candidates for warfarin therapy.[76] However, several clinical trials conducted over the last decade have sought to provide information regarding the utility of pharmacogenetics-guided warfarin dosing based on the use of algorithms. The outcomes associated with pharmacogenetic algorithm–guided warfarin dosing versus usual warfarin dosing are summarized in Table 5-11.[95-99] The results from these studies are somewhat conflicting regarding the primary outcome of out-of-range international normalized ratio (INR) values, which is a surrogate marker.

However, the recently published Genetic Informatics Trial (GIFT) study does provide positive support for proactive, pharmacogenetic algorithm–guided warfarin therapy. The GIFT study demonstrates improved patient safety outcomes with pharmacogenetic-guided warfarin dosing, with a significant reduction in the primary outcome of combined risk of major bleeding, INRs $\geq$4, or death compared to usual warfarin dosing.[99] The cost-effectiveness of pharmacogenetic algorithm–guided warfarin dosing remains unclear.

TABLE 5-11. Studies Evaluating Pharmacogenetic Algorithm–Guided Warfarin Dosing vs. Usual Care

Trial Name and Study Population	Intervention	Key Outcomes
COUMA-GEN Trial: 206 (~90% Caucasian) patients genotyped for *CYP2C9*2*, *CYP2C9*3*, and *VKORC1* variants	PGx algorithm–guided dosing vs. usual warfarin dosing (Algorithm generated by study authors)	• 1°: Per-patient % Out-of-range INRs: p = NS • 2°: Time to 1st supratherapeutic INR: p = NS • 2°: INR TTR: p = NS • 2°: % Patients reaching therapeutic INR on days 5 and 8: p = NS • 2°: # INR measurements and dose adjustments: INRs (p = NS), dose adjust (p = 0.035) • 2°: serious adverse drug events (major bleeding, INR$\geq$4, use of vit k): p = NS
COUMA-GEN II Trial: 504 (~90% Caucasian) patients genotyped for *CYP2C9*2*, *CYP2C9*3*, and *VKORC1* (c.-1639 G>A) variants	PGx algorithm–guided dosing vs. usual warfarin dosing Algorithms: IWPC and modified IWPC	• 1°: % OOR INRs and % TTR: p <0.001 for both ↓ OOR INRs & ↑ TTR @ 30d & 3m • 2°: Time to 1st therapeutic INR: p = NS • 2°: Avg. % INR $\geq$4 or $\leq$1.5: ↓ in PGx group vs. no PGx (p<0.001) • 2°: Avg. % INR $\geq$ 4: p = NS • 2°: Avg. % INR $\leq$1.5: ↓ in PGx group vs. no PGx (p<0.001) • 2°: 90-day incidence of serious adverse events: ↓ in PGx group vs. no PGx (p = 0.001) • 2°: Time to 1st therapeutic INR: p = NS
COAG Trial: 1015 (~67% Caucasian) patients genotyped for *CYP2C9*2*, *CYP2C9*3*, and *VKORC1* (c.-1639 G>A) variants	PGx algorithm–guided dosing vs. usual warfarin dosing Algorithms: Gage	• 1°: % TTR through week 12: p = NS • 2°: % TTR in black subgroup: ↓ in PGx group vs. non PGx group (p = 0.01) • 2°: % TTR in non-black subgroup: p = NS • 2°: % TTR in male and female subgroups: p = NS • 2°: % TTR in # genetic variants present subgroups: p = NS • 2°: % TTR in first 2 weeks of study subgroup: p = NS • 2°: % TTR in second 2 weeks of study subgroup: p = NS
EU-PACT Trial: 455 (>95% Caucasian) patients genotyped for *CYP2C9*2*, *CYP2C9*3*, and *VKORC1* (c.-1639 G>A) variants	PGx algorithm–guided dosing vs. usual warfarin dosing Algorithms: modified IWPC	• 1°: % TTR through day 28: ↑ in PGx group (67.4%) vs. non PGx group (60.3%) (p<0.001) • 2° (post-hoc): % TTR week 1–4: ↑ in PGx group vs. non PGx group (p<0.001) • 2° (post-hoc): % TTR week 5–8: ↑ in PGx group vs. non PGx group (p<0.001) • 2° (post-hoc): % TTR week 9–12: p = NS • 2°: % patients with INR $\geq$4: ↓ in PGx group (27.0%) vs. non PGx group (36.6%) (p = 0.03) • 2°: % of time with INR $\geq$4: ↓ in PGx group (2.3%) vs. non PGx group (5.3%) (p<0.001) • 2°: % of time with INR<2: p = NS • 2°: Median time to TTR: ↓ in PGx group vs. non PGx group (p<0.001) • 2°: Median time to stable dose: ↓ in PGx group vs. non PGx group (p = 0.003) • 2°: # dose adjustments needed: ↓ in PGx group vs. non PGx group (p = 0.02) • 2°: Major bleeding events: p = NS

(Continued)

TABLE 5-11. Studies Evaluating Pharmacogenetic Algorithm–Guided Warfarin Dosing vs. Usual Care *(Continued)*

Trial Name and Study Population	Intervention	Key Outcomes
GIFT Trial: 1650 (~91% Caucasian) patients genotyped for *CYP2C9*2, CYP2C9*3, CYP4F2,* V433M, and *VKORC1* (c.-1639 G>A) variants	PGx algorithm–guided dosing vs. usual warfarin dosing Algorithms: Gage	• 1°: Composite of: major bleeding, INR ≥4, VTE, or death • 10.8% (Genotype) vs. 14.7% (Usual); RR(95%CI): 0.73 (0.56–0.95); $p = 0.02$ • 2°: Major bleeding: p = NS • 2°: INR ≥4: 6.9% (Genotype) vs. 9.8% (Usual); RR(95%CI): 0.71 (0.51–0.99); $p = 0.04$ • 2°: VTE: p = NS • 2°: Death: no deaths reported in study • 2°: % TTR: 54.7% (Genotype) vs. 51.3% (Usual); $p = 0.004$

OOR = out-of-range; TTR = time in therapeutic range; NS = not significant; INR = International normalized ratio.

CASE SCENARIOS

Case 1

History of Present Illness: BK is a 76-year-old male who experienced nausea, vomiting, coughing, shortness of breath, and "feeling like his chest was on fire" when finishing up his workout at the gym early this morning. Upon presentation to the emergency department, his oxygen saturation levels were 86%, electrocardiogram (ECG) showed mild ST-segment elevation in lead V1 through V6, and troponin level was elevated. BK was taken to the cardiac catheterization lab, where it was discovered that he had proximal left anterior descending (LAD) artery and underwent PCI with placement of a drug-eluting stent. He is now recovering from PCI in the cardiac intensive care unit (ICU), where his wife informs the medical team that he has pharmacogenomic testing done recently and provides the wallet card with his genotype information. The medical team consults the pharmacogenomics specialist for assistance in medication therapy optimization using his pharmacogenomics data.

- Genotype data:

  - *CYP2C19 *1/*3*

  - *VKORC1* c.-1639 GG

  - *CYP2C9*1/*1*

  - *CYP2D6*3/*4*

  - *SLCO1B1 *1/*5*

Past Medical History (PMH): hypertension, dyslipidemia

Current medication list: ticagrelor 180 mg PO × 1, followed by 90 mg BID, aspirin 81 mg daily, metoprolol succinate 50 mg daily, lisinopril 10 mg daily, nitroglycerin 0.4 mg PRN chest pain, and atorvastatin 80 mg daily.

Question: As the pharmacogenomics specialist on the medical team, what pharmacotherapy recommendations would you make to optimize this patient's pharmacotherapy plan based on his pharmacogenomics data?

Answer: Because of the need for higher-intensity antiplatelet effects, the patient's CYP2C19 intermediate metabolizer status, and the unfavorability of using prasugrel in a patient >75 years of age, ticagrelor therapy is appropriate. Because of the CYP2D6 poor metabolizer phenotype, consideration could be given to reducing the metoprolol tartrate dose to 12.5 mg BID, with careful monitoring for signs of bradycardia. Switching from atorvastatin 80 mg daily to another high-intensity statin therapy with less myalgia risk in *SLCO1B1*5* allele carriers such as rosuvastatin 40 mg daily could help improve the likelihood of statin tolerability.

Case 2

History of Present Illness: RD is a 73-year-old, nonsmoking, Caucasian male with hypertension, dyslipidemia, and stage 4 chronic kidney disease (estimated CrCl 21 mL/min) who was recently admitted for treatment of a deep vein thrombosis (DVT). The medical team would like to initiate warfarin therapy to treat his DVT, but your health system's pharmacogenomics-integrated clinical decision support tool flagged the warfarin order for consultation from a pharmacogenomics specialist based on the patient's pharmacogenomic data housed in the electronic medical record:

- Current medications

  - Atorvastatin 10 mg daily

  - Lisinopril 40 mg daily

- Physical exam data

    - Weight = 186 lb

    - Height = 5 feet, 9 inches

    - LFTs = WNL

    - Baseline INR = 1.1

- Genotype data:

    - CYP2C19 *1/*2

    - VKORC1 c.-1639 GG

    - CYP2C9*3/*3 (homozygous mutant)

    - CYP2D6*1/*2

    - SLCO1B1 *1/*1

Question: What warfarin dosing recommendation would you make to optimize this patient's anticoagulation therapy based on his pharmacogenomics data?

Answer: Per CPIC guidelines, patients of non-African ancestry whose VKORC1 and CYP2C9 *2 and *3 genotype data are available should have their initial warfarin dose calculated based on a validated published pharmacogenetic algorithm such as www.warfarindosing.org. According to this algorithm, the weekly warfarin dose should be approximately 20 mg/week. A reasonable starting dose might be 5 mg now, then 2.5 mg daily, with an anticipated maintenance dose of 2.5 mg daily except 5 mg one day per week. CPIC also recommends consideration of alternative agents in patients with CYP2C9 poor metabolism, but this patient is most likely being prescribed warfarin instead of Direct Oral Anticoagulants for this indication due to his renal dysfunction.

PHARMACOGENOMICS CLINICAL PEARLS

- Pharmacogenetic variants may affect the safety and efficacy of cardiovascular pharmacotherapy options in a variety of ways depending on the activity of the drug and resultant metabolites. Prospective pharmacogenomic testing is not yet the standard of care for most cardiovascular pharmacotherapy options, but when genotypes are known there are several gene–drug pairs with clinical evidence available to guide therapy adjustments.

- When patients with available pharmacogenomic data are prescribed the following cardiovascular pharmacotherapy options, clinical guidelines are available to provide pharmacogenomics-based dosing recommendations: clopidogrel, metoprolol, simvastatin, and warfarin.

ABBREVIATIONS AND ACRONYMS

CPIC: Clinical Pharmacogenetics Implementation Consortium

DPWG: Dutch Pharmacogenetic Working Group

SNP: Single nucleotide polymorphism

ACS: Acute coronary syndrome

ADP: Adenosine diphosphate

PCI: Percutaneous coronary intervention

NSTEMI: Non-ST-Elevation Myocardial Infarction

TIA: Transient ischemic attack

OATP1B1: Organic Acid-Transporting Polypeptide 1B1

AUC: Area under the curve

C$_{max}$: Maximum serum drug concentration

SLCO1B1: Solute Carrier Organic Anion Transporter Family Member 1B1

VKORC1: Vitamin K Epoxide Reductase Enzyme Complex Subunit 1

REFERENCES

1. Clappers N, Brouwer MA, Verheugt FW. Antiplatelet treatment for coronary heart disease. *Heart.* 2007;93:258–265.

2. Paikin JS, Eikelboom JW, Cairns JA, Hirsh J. New antithrombotic agents—I nsights from clinical trials. Nat Rev Cardiol. 2010;7:498–509.

3. Amsterdam EA, Wenger NK, Brindis RG, et al. 2014 AHA/ACC guideline for the management of patients with non–ST-elevation acute coronary syndromes. *J Am Coll Cardiol.* 2014;64(24): e139–e228.

4. O'Gara PT, Kushner FG, Ascheim DD, et al. 2013 ACCF/AHA guideline for the management of ST-elevation myocardial infarction. *J Am Coll Cardiol.* 2013;61(4):e78–e140.

5. Scott SA, Sangkuhl K, Stein CM, et al. Clinical Pharmacogenetics Implementation Consortium guidelines for CYP2C19 genotype and clopidogrel therapy: 2013 update. *Clin Pharmacol Ther.* 2013;94:317–323.

6. Liang Y, Hirsh J, Weitz JI, et al. Active metabolite concentration of clopidogrel in patients taking different doses of aspirin: Results of the interaction trial. *J Thromb Haemost.* 2015;13:347–352.

7. Mega JL, Close SL, Wiviott SD, et al. Cytochrome p-450 polymorphisms and response to clopidogrel. *N Engl J Med.* 2009;360:354–362.

8. Sorich MJ, Polasek TM, Wiese MD. Systematic review and meta-analysis of the association between cytochrome P450 2C19 genotype and bleeding. *J Thromb Haemost*. 2012;108:199–200.

9. Sibbing D, Koch W, Gebhard D, et al. Cytochrome 2C19*17 allelic variant, platelet aggregation, bleeding events, and stent thrombosis in clopidogrel-treated patients with coronary stent placement. *Circulation*. 2010;121:512–518.

10. Effient [package insert]. Indianapolis, IN: Eli Lilly & Co; 2009.

11. CYP2C19 Allele Nomenclature. PharmVar Pharmacogene Variation Consortium. Available at https://www.pharmvar.org/htdocs/cyp2c19.htm. Accessed September 29, 2019.

12. CYP2C19. PharmVar Pharmacogene Variation Consortium. Available at https://www.pharmvar.org/gene/CYP2C19. Accessed September 29, 2019.

13. Dean L. Clopidogrel therapy and CYP2C19 genotype. In: Pratt V, McLeod H, Rubinstein W, et al., eds. *Medical Genetics Summaries* [Internet]. Bethesda, MD: National Center for Biotechnology Information (US); 2012. Available at https://www.ncbi.nlm.nih.gov/pubmed/28520346. Accessed September 29, 2019.

14. Mega JL, Simon T, Collect JP, et al. Reduced-function CYP2C19 genotype and risk of adverse clinical outcomes among patients treated with clopidogrel predominantly for PCI: A meta-analysis. *JAMA*. 2010;304:1821–1830.

15. Chen S, Zhang Y, Wang L, et al. Effects of dual-dose clopidogrel, clopidogrel combined with tongxinluo capsule, and ticagrelor on patients with coronary heart disease and CYP2C19*2 gene mutation after percutaneous coronary interventions (PCI). *Med Sci Monit*. 2017;23:3824–3830.

16. Holmes DR, Dehmer GJ, Kaul S, et al. ACCF/AHA clopidogrel clinical alert: Approaches to the FDA "boxed warning." *J Am Coll Cardiol*. 2010;56(4):321–341.

17. Cavallari LH, Lee CR, Beitelshees AL, et al. Multisite investigation of outcomes with implementation of CYP2C19 genotype-guided antiplatelet therapy after percutaneous coronary intervention. *JACC Cardiovasc Interv*. 2018;11(2):181–191.

18. Notarangelo FM, Maglietta G, Bevilacqua P, et al. Pharmacogenomic approach to selecting antiplatelet therapy in acute coronary syndromes: PHARMCLO trial. *J Am Coll Cardiol*. 2018;71:1869–1877.

19. Plavix [package insert]. Bridgewater, NJ: Bristol-Myers Squibb/Sanofi Pharmaceuticals Partnership. Revised 2019.

20. Lewis JP. Implementation of genotype-guided antiplatelet therapy: Feasible but not without obstacles. *Circ Genom Precis Med*. 2018;11(4):1–5.

21. Levine GN, Bates ER, Blankenship JC, et al. 2011 ACCF/AHA/SCAI guideline for percutaneous coronary intervention. *J Am Coll Cardiol*. 2011;58(24):e44–e122.

22. Levine GN, Bates ER, Blakenship JC, et al. 2015 ACC/AHA/SCAI focused update on primary percutaneous coronary intervention for patients with ST-elevation myocardial infarction: An update of the 2011 ACCF/AHA/SCAI guideline for percutaneous coronary intervention and the 2013 ACCF/AHA guideline for the management of ST-elevation myocardial infarction. *J Am Coll Cardiol*. 2016;67(10):1235–1250.

23. NIH/NLM ClinicalTrials.gov. Available at https://clinicaltrials.gov/ct2/show/NCT01742117. Accessed January 17, 2020.

24. Bergmeijer TO, Janssen PWA, Schipper JC, et al. CYP2C19 genotype–guided antiplatelet therapy in ST-segment elevation myocardial infarction patients—Rationale and design of the patient

25. 2018 Pharmacogenetic Recommendation Text. Dutch Pharmacogenetic Working Group Guidelines. Available at https://www.knmp.nl/patientenzorg/medicatiebewaking/farmacogenetica/pharmacogenetics-1. Accessed February 17, 2020.

26. Baber U, Leisman DE, Cohen DJ, et al. Tailoring antiplatelet therapy intensity to ischemic and bleeding risk. *Circ Cardiovasc Qual Outcomes*. 2019:12; 1–12.

27. Zisaki A, Miskovic L, Hatzimanikatis V. Antihypertensive drugs metabolism: An update to pharmacokinetic profiles and computational approaches. *Curr Pharm Des*. 2015;21(6):806–822.

28. Ram CVS. Beta-blockers in hypertension. *Am J Cardiol*. 2010;106(12):1819–1825.

29. Mehvar R, Brocks DR. Stereospecific pharmacokinetics and pharmacodynamics of beta-adrenergic blockers in humans. *J Pharm Pharm Sci*. 2001;4(2):185–200.

30. Trandate [package insert]. San Diego, CA: Prometheus Laboratories; 2010.

31. Nozawa T, Taguchi M, Tahara K, et al. Influence of CYP2D6 genotype on metoprolol plasma concentration and beta-adrenergic inhibition during long-term treatment: A comparison with bisoprolol. *J Cardiovasc Pharmacol*. 2005;46(5):713–720.

32. Zisaki A, Miskovic L, Hatzimanikatis V. Antihypertensive drugs metabolism: An update to pharmacokinetic profiles and computational approaches. *Curr Pharm Des*. 2015;21(6):806–822.

33. Shin J, Johnson JA. Pharmacogenetics of beta-blockers. *Pharmacotherapy*. 2007;27(6):874–887.

34. CYP2D6 Allele Nomenclature. PharmVar Pharmacogene Variation Consortium. Available at https://www.pharmvar.org/htdocs/cyp2d6.htm. Accessed September 30, 2019.

35. CYP2D6. PharmVar Pharmacogene Variation Consortium. Available at https://www.pharmvar.org/gene/CYP2D6. Accessed September 30, 2019.

36. Dean L. Metoprolol therapy and CYP2D6 genotype. In: Pratt V, McLeod H, Rubinstein W, et al., eds. *Medical Genetics Summaries* [Internet]. Bethesda, MD: National Center for Biotechnology Information (US); 2012. Available at https://www.ncbi.nlm.nih.gov/books/NBK425389/. Accessed September 30, 2019.

37. Lennard MS, Silas JH, Freestone S, et al. Oxidation phenotype—A major determinant of metoprolol metabolism and response. *N Engl J Med*. 1982;307(25):1558–1560.

38. Nozawa T, Taguchi M, Tahara K, et al. Influence of CYP2D6 genotype on metoprolol plasma concentration and β-adrenergic inhibition during long-term treatment: A comparison with bisoprolol. *J Cardiovasc Pharmacol*. 2005;46:713–720.

39. Rau T, Wuttke H, Michels LM, et al. Impact of the CYP2D6 genotype on the clinical effects of metoprolol: A prospective longitudinal study. *Clin Pharmacol Ther*. 2009;85(3):269–272.

40. Batty JA, Hall AS, White HL, et al. An investigation of CYP2D6 genotype and response to metoprolol CR/XL during dose titration in patients with heart failure: A MERIT-HF substudy. *Clin Pharmacol Ther*. 2014;95(3):321–330.

41. Hamadeh IS, Langaee TY, Dwivedi R, et al. Impact of CYP2D6 polymorphisms on clinical efficacy and tolerability of metoprolol tartrate. *Clin Pharmacol Ther*. 2014;96(2):175–181.

42. Bijl MJ, Visser LE, van Schaik RH, et al. Genetic variation in the CYP2D6 gene is associated with a lower heart rate and

outcome after primary PCI (POPular) Genetics study. *Am Heart J*. 2014;168(1):16–22.

blood pressure in beta-blocker users. *Clin Pharmacol Ther.* 2009;85(1):45–50.

43. Guidelines and Clinical Documents. American College of Cardiology website. Available at https://www.acc.org/guidelines. Accessed September 30, 2019.

44. Crews KR, Gaedigk A, Dunnenberger HM, et al. Clinical Pharmacogenetics Implementation Consortium guidelines for cytochrome P450 2D6 genotype and codeine therapy: 2014 update. *Clin Pharmacol Ther.* 2014;95(4):376–382.

45. CYP2D6. SNPedia. Available at https://www.snpedia.com/index.php/CYP2D6. Accessed October 1, 2019.

46. Wiysonge CS, Bradley HA, Volmink J, et al. Beta-blockers for hypertension. *Cochrane Database Syst Rev.* 2012;15(8):CD002003.

47. Lefebvre J, Poirier L, Poirier P, et al. The influence of CYP2D6 phenotype on the clinical response of nebivolol in patients with essential hypertension. *Br J Clin Pharmacol.* 2007;63(5):575–582.

48. Wojciechowski D, Papademetriou V. β-blockers in the management of hypertension: Focus on nebivolol. *Expert Rev Cardiovasc Ther.* 2008;6(4):471–479.

49. CDC. Available at https://www.cdc.gov/nchs/fastats/drug-use-therapeutic.htm. Accessed January 17, 2020.

50. Grundy SM, Stone NJ, Bailey AL, et al. 2018 AHA/ACC/AACVPR/AAPA/ABC/ACPM/ADA/AGS/APhA/ASPC/NLA/PCNA guideline on the management of blood cholesterol. *J Am Coll Cardiol.* 2019;73(24):e285–e350.

51. Chong PH, Seeger JD, Franklin C. Clinically relevant differences between the statins: Implications for therapeutic selection. *Am J Med.* 2001;111(5):390–400.

52. Mangravite LM, Thorn CF, Krauss RM. Clinical implications of pharmacogenomics of statin treatment. *Pharmacogenomics J.* 2006;6(6):360–374.

53. Ramsey LB, Johnson SG, Caudle KE, et al. The clinical pharmacogenetics implementation consortium guideline for SLCO1B1 and simvastatin-induced myopathy: 2014 update. *Clin Pharmacol Ther.* 2014;96(4):423–428.

54. Johnson JA, et al. *Pharmacogenomics: Applications to Patient Care.* 3rd ed. Lenexa, KS: ACCP; 2015:102–113.

55. Pasanen MK, Neuvonen M, Neuvonen PJ, Niemi M. *SLCO1B1* polymorphism markedly affects the pharmacokinetics of simvastatin acid. *Pharmacogenet Genomics.* 2006;12:873–879.

56. Maxwell WD, Ramsey LB, Johnson SG, et al. Impact of pharmacogenetics on efficacy and safety of statin therapy for dyslipidemia. *Pharmacotherapy.* 2017;37(9):1172–1190.

57. Zocor [package insert]. Whitehouse Station, NJ: Merck & Co., Inc. Revised 2019.

58. Grundy SM, Stone NJ, Bailey AL, et al. 2018 AHA/ACC/AACVPR/AAPA/ABC/ACPM/ADA/AGS/APhA/ASPC/NLA/PCNA guideline on the management of blood cholesterol: A report of the American College of Cardiology/American Heart Association Task Force on Clinical Practice Guidelines. *JACC.* 2019;73(24):e285–e350.

59. Danik JS, Chasman DI, MacFadyen JG, et al. Lack of association between SLCO1B1 polymorphisms and clinical myalgia following rosuvastatin therapy. *Am Heart J.* 2013;6:1008–1014.

60. Brunham LR, Lansberg PJ, Zhang L, et al. Differential effect of the rs4149056 variant in SLCO1B1 on myopathy associated with simvastatin and atorvastatin. *Pharmacogenomics J.* 2012;12(3):233–237.

61. Santos PC, Gagliardi AC, Miname MH, et al. SLCO1B1 haplotypes are not associated with atorvastatin-induced myalgia in Brazilian patients with familial hypercholesterolemia. *Eur J Clin Pharmacol.* 2012;68(3):273–279.

62. Puccetti L, Ciani F, Auteri A. Genetic involvement in statins induced myopathy. Preliminary data from an observational case-control study. *Atherosclerosis.* 2010;211(1):28–29.

63. Voora D, Shah SH, Spasojevic I, et al. The SLCO1B1*5 genetic variant is associated with statin-induced side effects. *J Am Coll Cardiol.* 2009;54(17):1609–1616.

64. Statin Pathway—Generalized, Pharmacokinetics. PharmGKB. Available at https://www.pharmgkb.org/pathway/PA145011108. Accessed October 1, 2019.

65. Bai X, Zhang B, Wang P. Effects of SLCO1B1 and GATM gene variants on rosuvastatin-induced myopathy are unrelated to high plasma exposure of rosuvastatin and its metabolites. *Acta Pharmacol Sin.* 2019;40(4):492–499.

66. Liu JE, Liu XY, Chen S, et al. SLCO1B1 521T > C polymorphism associated with rosuvastatin-induced myotoxicity in Chinese coronary artery disease patients: a nested case-control study. *Eur J Clin Pharmacol.* 2017;73(11):1409–1416.

67. Wu HF, Hristeva N, Chang J, et al. Rosuvastatin pharmacokinetics in Asian and white subjects wild type for both OATP1B1 and BCRP under control and inhibited conditions. *J Pharm Sci.* 2017;106(9):2751–2757.

68. Crestor [package insert]. Wilmington, DE: Astra Zeneca Pharmaceuticals LP. Revised 2003.

69. Pravachol [package insert]. Princeton, NJ: Bristol-Myers Squibb Company. Revised 2016.

70. Khine H, Yuet WC, Adams-Huet B, Ahmad Z. Statin-associated muscle symptoms and SLCO1B1 rs4149056 genotype in patients with familial hypercholesterolemia. *Am Heart J.* 2016;179:1–9.

71. Stafford DW. The vitamin K cycle. *J Thromb Haemost.* 2005;3(8):1873–1878.

72. Danese E, Montagnana M, Johnson JA, et al. Impact of the CYP4F2 p.V433M polymorphism on coumarin dose requirement: Systematic review and meta-analysis. *Clin Pharmacol Ther.* 2012;92(6):746–756.

73. McDonald MG, Rieder MJ, Nakano M, et al. CYP4F2 is a vitamin K1 oxidase: An explanation for altered warfarin dose in carriers of the V433M variant. *Mol Pharmacol.* 2009;75(6):1337–1346.

74. Edson KZ, Prasad B, Unadkat JD, et al. Cytochrome P450-dependent catabolism of vitamin K: ω-hydroxylation catalyzed by human CYP4F2 and CYP4F11. *Biochemistry.* 2013;52(46):8276–8285.

75. Owen RP, Gong L, Sagreiya H, et al. VKORC1 pharmacogenomics summary. *Pharmacogenet Genomics.* 2010;20(10):642–644.

76. Johnson JA, Caudle KE, Gong L, et al. Clinical Pharmacogenetics Implementation Consortium (CPIC) guideline for pharmacogenetics-guided warfarin dosing: 2017 update. *Clin Pharmacol Ther.* 2017;102(3):397–404.

77. Aithal GP, Day CP, Kesteven PJ, Daly AK. Association of polymorphisms in the cytochrome P450 CYP2C9 with warfarin dose requirement and risk of bleeding complications. *Lancet.* 1999;353(9154):717–719.

78. CYP2C9. PharmVar Pharmacogene Variation Consortium. Available at https://www.pharmvar.org/gene/CYP2C9. Accessed October 2, 2019.

79. Perera MA, Cavallari LH, Limdi NA, et al. Genetic variants associated with warfarin dose in African-American individuals: A genome-wide association study. *Lancet*. 2013;382(9894):790–796.

80. Luxembourg B, Schneider K, Sittinger K, et al. Impact of pharmacokinetic (CYP2C9) and pharmacodynamic (VKORC1, F7, GGCX, CALU, EPHX1) gene variants on the initiation and maintenance phases of phenprocoumon therapy. *Thromb Haemost*. 2011;105(1):169–180.

81. Redman AR. Implications of cytochrome P450 2C9 polymorphism on warfarin metabolism and dosing. *Pharmacotherapy*. 2001;21(2):235–242.

82. Johnson JA, Gong L, Whirl-Carrillo M, et al. Clinical Pharmacogenetics Implementation Consortium Guidelines for CYP2C9 and VKORC1 genotypes and warfarin dosing. *Clin Pharmacol Ther*. 2011;90(4):625–629.

83. Higashi MK, Veenstra DL, Kondo LM, et al. Association between CYP2C9 genetic variants and anticoagulation-related outcomes during warfarin therapy. *JAMA*. 2002;287(13):1690–1698.

84. Sridharan K, Modi T, Bendkhale S, et al. Association of genetic polymorphisms of CYP2C9 and VKORC1 with bleeding following warfarin: A case-control study. *Curr Clin Pharmacol*. 2016;11(1):62–68.

85. Yang J, Chen Y, Li X, et al. Influence of CYP2C9 and VKORC1 genotypes on the risk of hemorrhagic complications in warfarin-treated patients: A systematic review and meta-analysis. *Int J Cardiol*. 2013;168(4):4234–4243.

86. Roth JA, Boudreau D, Fujii MM, et al. Genetic risk factors for major bleeding in patients treated with warfarin in a community setting. *Clin Pharmacol Ther*. 2014;95(6):636–643.

87. Coumadin [package insert]. Princeton, NJ: Bristol-Myers Squibb Company. Revised 2017.

88. International Warfarin Pharmacogenetics Consortium, Klein TE, Altman RB, et al. Estimation of the warfarin dose with clinical and pharmacogenetic data. *N Engl J Med*. 2009;360:753–764.

89. Gage BF, Eby C, Johnson JA, et al. Use of pharmacogenetic and clinical factors to predict the therapeutic dose of warfarin. *Clin Pharmacol Ther*. 2008;84:326–331.

90. Finkelman BS, Gage BF, Johnson JA, et al. Genetic warfarin dosing: Tables versus algorithms. *J Am Coll Cardiol*. 2011;57:612–618.

91. WarfarinDosing. Available at http://www.warfarindosing.org/Source/Home.aspx. Accessed October 8, 2019.

92. IWPC Dose Calculator. Available at https://cpicpgx.org/content/guideline/publication/warfarin/2011/IWPC_dose_calculator.xls. Accessed October 8, 2019.

93. Nagai R, Ohara M, Cavallari LH, et al. Factors influencing pharmacokinetics of warfarin in African-Americans: Implications for pharmacogenetic dosing algorithms. *Pharmacogenomics*. 2015;16(3):217–225.

94. Drozda K, Wong S, Patel SR, et al. Poor warfarin dose prediction with pharmacogenetic algorithms that exclude genotypes important for African Americans. *Pharmacogenet Genomics*. 2015;25(2):73–81.

95. Anderson JL, Horne BD, Stevens SM, et al. Randomized trial of genotype-guided versus standard warfarin dosing in patients initiating oral anticoagulation. *Circulation*. 2007;116(22):2563–2570.

96. Anderson JL, Horne BD, Stevens SM, et al. A randomized and clinical effectiveness trial comparing two pharmacogenetic algorithms and standard care for individualizing warfarin dosing (CoumaGen-II). *Circulation*. 2012;125(16):1997–2005.

97. Kimmel SE, French B, Kasner SE, et al. A pharmacogenetic versus a clinical algorithm for warfarin dosing. *N Engl J Med*. 2013;369(24):2283–2293.

98. Pirmohamed M, Burnside G, Eriksson N, et al. A randomized trial of genotype-guided dosing of warfarin. *N Engl J Med*. 2013;369(24):2294–22303.

99. Gage BF, Bass AR, Lin H, et al. Effect of genotype-guided warfarin dosing on clinical events and anticoagulation control among patients undergoing hip or knee arthroplasty: The GIFT randomized clinical trial. *JAMA*. 2017;318(12):1115–1124.

CHAPTER 6

INFECTIOUS DISEASES PHARMACOGENOMICS

Jerika T. Lam

LEARNING OBJECTIVES

1. Recognize and interpret common pharmacogenomic relationships that affect adverse events and efficacy of medications used in infectious diseases.

2. Discuss the clinical utility of pharmacogenomics in the management of infectious diseases, particularly antiprotozoal, antifungal, and antiviral agents.

INTRODUCTION

Applying pharmacogenomics in infectious diseases requires consideration of the genomes of the pathogen (e.g., bacteria and virus) and the human host. The pathogen's genome could be used to identify the antigen, specific infecting organism, and factors that could contribute to antimicrobial resistance. Development of diagnostic microbiology tools and effective vaccines could be enhanced by knowing the portions of a pathogen that are important antigenic determinants. For instance, important genes that confer resistance to antimicrobials can be detected with these assay tests. The information subsequently can be used to select the appropriate antimicrobial treatment for the infection.[1] Similarly, the human host's genome may have susceptibility genes and new drug targets that may be used in the treatment of infectious diseases. Genetic polymorphisms in the human immune system have also been associated with susceptibility to infections and response to antimicrobial treatments.[2] Understanding human genomics could lead to informed infectious disease management by knowing how each individual's genomic variation affects his or her response to the pathogen, antimicrobial agent, or vaccine.

Pharmacogenomics in infectious diseases could provide more accurate results than phenotypic assays that are subject to significant intrinsic variation caused by a large number of external factors that affect bacterial growth and the intrinsic biological variation in the organisms themselves.[2] With regard to diagnostic tools, there are nucleic acid testing assays that directly detect resistant bacteria and viral pathogens from clinical samples.[1] In infectious diseases, comparative genomics is used to determine the available genome sequences to perform either interspecies or intraspecies comparisons of bacterial genome content or to compare the human genome with those of other model organisms. Furthermore, comparative genomics includes the powerful tools of bioinformatics and microarray technology to identify virulence determinants, antimicrobial drug targets, vaccine targets, and new markers for diagnostics.[2] For example, the study of the genome content of Bacillus Calmette-Guérin strains using *Mycobacterium tuberculosis* was achieved by using microarray-based comparative genomics.[3]

As was mentioned in Chapter 1, pharmacogenomics involves genes that encode drug-metabolizing enzymes, drug transporters, and drug targets—proteins that might influence drug response. Furthermore, variation in drug response and effects could be associated with pharmacokinetic (PK) factors that influence the concentration of a drug that will reach the therapeutic target. Among the PK factors, genetic variation in the expression and function of drug-metabolizing enzymes (primarily the cytochrome P450 system) can influence the plasma drug concentrations and therapeutic effects. Another genetic factor that may affect individual drug response is the variation in human leukocyte antigen genes,[4] such as observed in individuals receiving abacavir, carbamazepine, phenytoin, and allopurinol. For the content of this chapter, only particular anti-infectives and antivirals will be discussed based on the scientific and clinical evidence, as well as recommendations from the U.S. Food and Drug Administration (FDA), Clinical Pharmacogenetics Implementation Consortium (CPIC), and PharmGKB.

ANTI-INFECTIVES

Dapsone and Primaquine

Dapsone is a diaminodiphenyl sulfone antibiotic that is FDA-approved to treat dermatological conditions, including acne, dermatitis herpetiformis, and leprosy. Dapsone is also used off-label for many conditions, including malaria, and as a second-line antibiotic to prevent *Pneumocystis jirovecii* pneumonia and toxoplasmosis in individuals with HIV-1 infection who have a sulfur allergy and cannot take trimethoprim-sulfamethoxazole. Primaquine phosphate is an 8-aminoquinoline antiprotozoal agent that is FDA-approved for prophylaxis and prevention of relapse to malaria caused by *Plasmodium vivax* and *Plasmodium ovale*. Both of these medications have been reported to cause hemolytic anemia in individuals who are deficient or do not have the glucose-6-phosphate dehydrogenase (G6PD) enzyme.[5-8]

G6PD is a cytoplasmic protein and has two essential roles within the cell: production of nicotinamide adenine dinucleotide phosphate hydrogen (NADPH) and ribose-5-phosphate.[6] This enzyme is expressed in all cells, and it plays a critical role in the red blood cells (RBCs). The RBCs do not have mitochondria and depend solely on G6PD as the sole source of NADPH to relieve oxidative stress and protect the hemoglobin β chain from oxidation.[6,7,9] The levels of G6PD decrease over the lifespan of the RBCs, which is approximately 3 months. When the required levels of NADPH cannot be maintained, the amount of reduced glutathione decreases and leads to oxidative damage. The overall result is lysis of the RBCs.[5-7] Therefore, G6PD is critical in preserving the integrity of the RBC and defending it against oxidative damage.[10]

Globally, an estimated 400 million people carry a mutation in the G6PD gene that is associated with deficient enzyme function, particularly in certain racial groups such as individuals of African, Asian, and Mediterranean descent.[5] G6PD deficiency is inherited as an X-linked recessive genetic disorder and most often affects males.[7,8] It is difficult to predict the clinical course of a patient by G6PD activity, reduced glutathione content, or the presence/absence of severe neonatal jaundice because most patients with G6PD deficiency are asymptomatic. The problem arises when a patient with G6PD deficiency takes a medication that requires metabolism via the G6PD pathway. This could result in jaundice and/or hemolytic anemia in the patient.

Mechanism and Consequence of Drug–Gene Interaction

Numerous factors contribute to drug-induced hemolytic anemia in G6PD-deficient individuals, including dosage, concomitant medications, concurrent infections, and possible genetic variants.[7] For dapsone, the hemolytic activity is most likely dose-related and associated with dapsone's N-hydroxy metabolites.[11,12] Furthermore, a study comparing the safety of two different antimalarial regimens for *Plasmodium falciparum* showed that patients with G6PD deficiency who received dapsone experienced significantly lower hemoglobin and hematocrit values.[13] On the other hand, hemolysis associated with primaquine is thought to be from its metabolism by CYP450 enzymes, where the metabolites induce the formation of methemoglobin and reactive oxygen intermediates.[14]

Treatment Recommendation

The World Health Organization (WHO) and FDA have issued warnings and precautions for the use of dapsone and primaquine because of the risk of hemolytic anemia in individuals deficient in G6PD.[15] Furthermore, the WHO recommends testing individuals to predict risk of hemolysis in G6PD when prescribing dapsone and primaquine, especially in areas of high prevalence of G6PD deficiency.[9,16] Caution should be taken when administering dapsone to G6PD-deficient individuals, although it is not contraindicated. Close monitoring of the complete blood count and reticulocyte count is recommended for patients receiving dapsone. In contrast, there is solid evidence associating primaquine with hemolytic anemia in G6PD-deficient individuals.[8,17,18] Consequently, primaquine should be avoided in G6PD-deficient individuals for safety concerns.

Voriconazole

Voriconazole is a second-generation triazole antifungal agent that has enhanced spectrum of activity against invasive fungal infections caused by molds (i.e., *Aspergillus* spp.) and yeasts (i.e., *Candida* spp.). Voriconazole is primarily used to treat invasive aspergillosis and other fungal infections found in immunocompromised patients. It inhibits CYP450-dependent 14α-lanosterol demethylation, thereby disrupting the synthesis of ergosterol, an essential compound of the fungal cell membranes. As a result, voriconazole damages the fungal cell membrane leading to the inhibition of fungal cell growth for yeasts (fungistatic activity) or fungal cell death for molds (fungicidal activity).[19,20]

Voriconazole is extensively metabolized by the liver primarily by CYP2C19, CYP2C9, and CYP3A4 enzymes. It is also an inhibitor of CYP2C19, 2C9, and 3A4 substrates. The CYP2C19 enzymatic pathway serves as the main metabolic pathway for voriconazole and contributes to the wide interpatient variability in voriconazole trough concentrations due to the enzyme's genetic polymorphisms. There are also nongenetic factors that could affect voriconazole serum concentrations such as the person's age, gender, liver condition, and concomitant medications.[21]

Mechanism of Drug–Gene Interaction

The *CYP2C19* gene is highly polymorphic, and the majority of people carry the *1, *2, *3, or *17 alleles. CYP2C19 normal functioning is associated with the *CYP2C19*1* allele compared to *CYP2C19*2* (rs4244285; 19154G>A) and *3 (rs4986892; 17948G>A) alleles, which are associated with loss of enzymatic functioning.[22] Interestingly, the *CYP2C19*17* allele (rs12248560; c.-806C>T) is associated with increased enzymatic activity. The frequency of the *2 allele varies between populations, where it is prevalent in approximately 15% of Caucasians, 18% of African Americans, and between 29% and 34% of Asians.[23] The frequency of the *3 allele is much smaller and is prevalent in approximately 0.6% of Caucasians, 0.3% of African Americans, and between 2% and 9% of Asians. In contrast, the frequency of the *CYP2C19*17* allele is found in approximately 22% of Caucasians, 19% of African Americans, 2% of East Asians, and 17% of South or Central Asians.[23]

Individuals could be placed into various categories based on their CYP2C19 polymorphisms. Ultrarapid metabolizers (UMs) and rapid metabolizers (RMs) are characterized by the *CYP2C19*17* allele (*17/*17 and *1/*17, respectively) and have an increased CYP2C19 enzyme activity. Several studies have reported that those with the *1/*17 genotype had significantly increased clearance compared to normal metabolizers (NMs).[24–26] The NM phenotype is expressed by the homozygous *CYP2C19*1* allele. In contrast, the intermediate metabolizers (IMs) could carry one *1 allele and a loss-of-function allele, such as *1/*2, which produces a reduced enzyme function.[22] IMs could also carry a loss-of-function allele and a gain-of-function allele such as *2/*17.[23,27] Poor metabolizers (PMs), on the other hand, carry two loss-of-function alleles (i.e., *2/*2), resulting in deficient or low CYP2C19 enzyme activity and increased concentrations of voriconazole compared to NMs.[22] At present, there is insufficient evidence to support the probable influence of CYP3A4 polymorphisms on the trough concentrations of voriconazole.[28]

Consequence of Drug–Gene Interaction

Since voriconazole is primarily metabolized by CYP2C19, its trough concentrations could be affected by the enzymatic polymorphisms, which could lead to the development of serious adverse effects or subtherapeutic antifungal effect. For instance, PMs could have high voriconazole serum concentrations and experience visual disturbances (e.g., altered color discrimination, blurred vision, photophobia, the appearance of bright spots and wavy lines), visual hallucinations, other neurologic disorders, and hepatotoxicity.[29–31] These adverse reactions are reversible if caught early and after discontinuation of voriconazole. Other adverse effects have also been reported for voriconazole, such as rash and photosensitivity; however, these may not be related to trough concentrations.[19] Theoretically, UMs may have low voriconazole serum concentrations and could experience suboptimal clinical efficacy, treatment failure, and risk of azole resistance.

Treatment Recommendation

Since there are no consistent studies demonstrating an association between *CYP2C19* genotype and adverse effects, there are no alternative dosage recommendations for voriconazole, particularly for patients who express the RM, NM, and IM phenotypes. These patients could benefit from the recommended standard voriconazole dosage. Monitoring of their liver function tests will need to be performed throughout voriconazole therapy. On the other hand, patients who express the UM phenotype may have subtherapeutic concentrations of voriconazole

TABLE 6-1. Dosing Recommendations for Voriconazole Based on CYP2C19 Phenotype for Adults and Pediatric Patients (Children and Adolescents <18 years old)

CYP2C19 Phenotype	Implications for Voriconazole Pharmacologic Measures	Recommendations	Classification of Recommendations
Ultrarapid metabolizer (*17/*17)	In patients for whom an ultrarapid metabolizer genotype (*17/*17) is identified, the probability of attainment of therapeutic concentrations is small	Choose an alternative agent that is not dependent on CYP2C19 metabolism as primary therapy in lieu of voriconazole. Such agents include liposomal amphotericin B, and posaconazole.[a,b]	Moderate
Rapid metabolizer (*1/*17)	In patients for whom a rapid metabolizer genotype (*1/*17) is identified, the probability of attainment of therapeutic concentrations is variable	Initiate therapy with recommended standard of care dosing.[a] Use therapeutic drug monitoring to titrate dose to therapeutic trough concentrations.[b,c]	Moderate
Normal metabolizer (*1/*1)	Normal voriconazole metabolism	Initiate therapy with recommended standard-of-care dosing.[a]	Strong
Intermediate metabolizer	Higher dose-adjusted trough concentrations of voriconazole compared with normal metabolizers	Initiate therapy with recommended standard-of-care dosing.[a]	Moderate
Poor metabolizer	Higher dose-adjusted trough concentrations of voriconazole and may increase probability of adverse events	Choose an alternative agent that is not dependent on CYP2C19 metabolism as primary therapy in lieu of voriconazole. Such agents include liposomal amphotericin B and posaconazole.[a,d] In the event that voriconazole is considered to be the most appropriate agent, based on clinical advice, for a patient with poor metabolizer genotype, voriconazole should be administered at a preferably lower-than-standard dosage with careful therapeutic drug monitoring.	Moderate[d]

[a]Further dose adjustments or selection of alternative therapy may be necessary due to other clinical factors, such as drug interactions, hepatic function, renal function, species, site of infection, therapeutic drug monitoring (TDM), and comorbidities.

[b]Achieving voriconazole therapeutic concentrations in the pediatric population with ultrarapid and rapid metabolizer phenotypes in a timely manner is difficult. As critical time may be lost in achieving therapeutic concentrations, an alternative antifungal agent is recommended in order that the child receives effective antifungal therapy as soon as possible.

[c]Meticulous TDM is critical for rapid metabolizers. There is insufficient evidence to distinguish a CYP2C19*1/*17 and *1/*1 pediatric patient due to large variability in trough concentrations.

[d]Recommendation based upon data extrapolated from adults.

Source: Reproduced, with permission, from Moriyama B, Obeng AO, Barbarino J, et al. Clinical Pharmacogenetics Implementation Consortium (CPIC) guidelines for CYP2C19 and voriconazole therapy. Clin Pharmacol Ther. 2017;102(1):45–51.

and could benefit from receiving an alternative antifungal agent that has a similar spectrum of activity against the invasive mycosis, such as liposomal amphotericin B or posaconazole (Table 6-1).

The U.S. FDA and Health Canada include a warning in the voriconazole drug label for individuals who are PMs of CYP2C19 that they could experience a fourfold higher drug exposure compared to UMs and NMs.[32] In order to reduce the risk of drug toxicity, PMs should receive another antifungal agent for treatment if clinically appropriate. However, if voriconazole is strongly indicated for the treatment of the invasive mycosis in a patient with PM phenotype, then the treatment approach is to administer a lower dosage with therapeutic drug monitoring of voriconazole concentrations and close monitoring of clinical symptoms.[33]

ANTIVIRALS

The addition of protease inhibitors with other antiretroviral agents in the mid-1990s marked the era of highly active antiretroviral therapy (HAART), which enhanced the treatment armamentarium against HIV-1 infection. The advent of HAART significantly helped to reduce deaths associated with AIDS-related malignancies and opportunistic infections. In spite of improved efficacy against HIV in the early millennium, HAART regimens were associated with intolerable adverse effects and toxicities for patients. Moreover, these complex regimens were associated with high pill burden and increased administration frequency that affected the patient's medication adherence. Nowadays, combination antiretroviral therapies are much better tolerated and simplified to mainly single-tablet regimens administered once a day to ensure better medication adherence. However, the individual antiretroviral agents still possess certain adverse drug reactions, characterized by short- and long-term toxicities, depending on the particular agent used. In this setting, pharmacogenomics plays a very important role in predicting adverse effects caused by certain antiretroviral agents that will be further discussed in the sections that follow.

Abacavir

Abacavir sulfate is a nucleoside analogue of the nucleoside reverse transcriptase inhibitor (NRTI) class. The NRTI class is an essential part of the antiretroviral backbone to treat HIV-1 infection. Abacavir inhibits the viral reverse transcriptase enzyme and causes chain termination of the HIV replication process. It is available as a single-drug tablet and widely used in combination with other antiretroviral agents to achieve viral suppression and improve the immunological status in patients living with HIV-1 infection. It is also co-formulated with other antiretroviral agents as fixed-dose combination pills to reduce pill burden and improve medication adherence for patients. Abacavir is hepatically metabolized by glucuronidation enzymes and does not affect the CYP450 system.[34] However, it has been associated with life-threatening hypersensitivity reactions (HSRs), such as Stevens-Johnson syndrome and toxic epidermal necrolysis, in HIV-positive children and adults from clinical trials and case reports.[35–39] Over 90% of HSRs could occur in the first six weeks after starting abacavir.[40,41]

Mechanism of Drug–Gene Interaction

The HSR is an extreme form of adaptive immune response occurring when the immune system reacts inappropriately to certain antigens, leading to inflammatory reactions and tissue organ damage.[42] The HSR process is driven by the interaction between the major histocompatibility complex (MHC) Class I, the human leukocyte antigen B (*HLA-B*) gene, and its variant allele *57:01. The HLA-B protein and other Class I group members (HLA-A and HLA-C) are cell-surface molecules responsible for the presentation of endogenous peptides to immune system cells.[43] As a brief background of the HLA nomenclature, the first set of digits describes the "type" or "antigen" designation of the HLA allele. The second set of digits describes the "subtype" of the HLA allele. The combination of the first and second set of digits describes the HLA allele and its nucleotide polymorphisms associated with changes in the amino acid sequence of the protein or nonsynonymous substitution. For instance, *HLA-B*57:01* is of B57 "type" and 01 "subtype."[44]

The MHC Class I antigen presentation and activation of *HLA-B*57: 01* on the cell surface, in turn, elicit T-cell activation (Figure 6-1).[45] Furthermore, activation of *HLA-B*57:01*–restricted CD8+ T cells results in the secretion of inflammatory mediators, tumor necrosis factor alpha (TNF-alpha) and interferon gamma (IFN-gamma), that lead to the induction of a delayed-type HSR.[46] In other words, abacavir is thought to induce HSR by binding to an antigen-presenting cleft unique to *HLA-B*57:01* and altering the self-peptides presented to T cells, which result in an immune response. The likelihood for abacavir to cause an HSR is heightened in patients carrying the *HLA-B*57:01* allele only and not in carriers of other *HLA-B* alleles, as well as why compounds similar to abacavir do not react with *HLA-B*57:01*.[46] With regard to the prevalence of *HLA-B*57:01* allele expression among different populations, the allele occurs between a 5% and 8% frequency in European populations, 1% frequency in Asian populations, and less than 1% frequency in African populations. Of note, the allele occurs between 2% and 4% frequency in African Americans in the United States.[47]

Mallal and colleagues demonstrated that the presence of the *HLA-B*57:01* allele is indicative of HSR to abacavir in the PREDICT-1 study.[48] They performed a double-blind, prospective, randomized study involving 1956 patients from 19 countries who were infected with HIV-1 and had not previously received abacavir. The study patients were randomly assigned into two groups: control group (patients who received abacavir without *HLA-B*57:01* screening) and prospective-screening group (*HLA-B*57:01* positive patients who did not receive abacavir treatment). All patients who received abacavir were observed for six weeks. The clinical diagnosis of abacavir-associated HSR was immunologically confirmed via performing epicutaneous patch testing with the use of abacavir. Patients who developed an HSR were identified as having a positive result on the epicutaneous patch testing and carried the *HLA-B*57:01* allele. Among the patients who received abacavir without undergoing screening (control group), 7.8% were clinically diagnosed with HSR; however, only

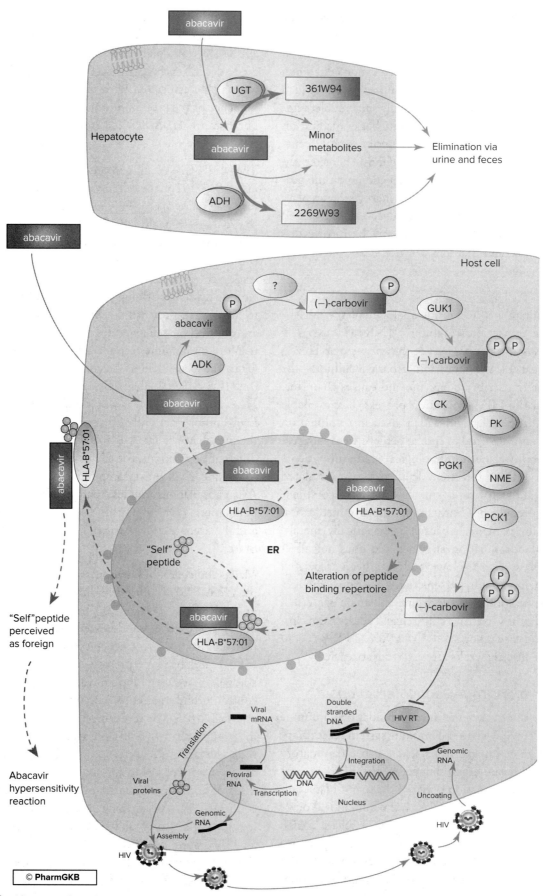

© PharmGKB

FIGURE 6-1 • *(Continued)*

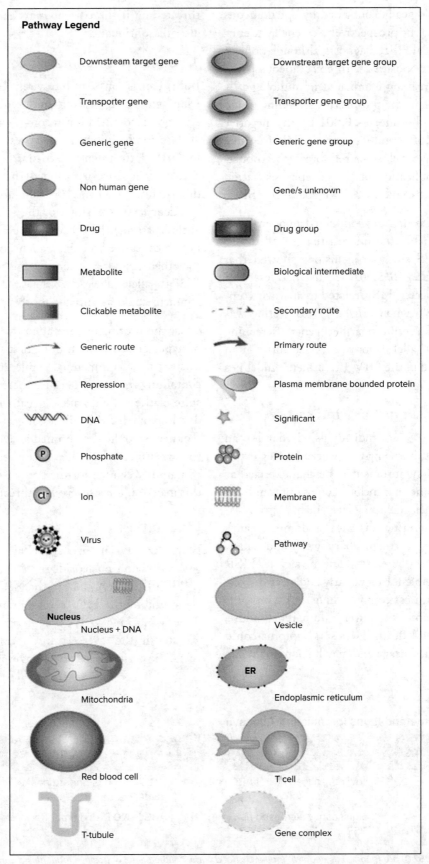

FIGURE 6-1 • Abacavir HSR pathway. (Reprinted with permission from Whirl-Carrillo M, McDonagh EM, Hebert JM, et al. (2012), Pharmacogenomics Knowledge for Personalized Medicine. Clinical Pharmacology & Therapeutics, 92: 414-417.)

2.7% were immunologically confirmed by epicutaneous patch testing. Among the prospectively screened patients, 3.4% received a clinical HSR diagnosis, although none of the clinical cases were positive with epicutaneous patch testing. In short, screening eliminated immunologically confirmed HSR (0% in the prospective-screening group vs. 2.7% in the control group, $p < 0.001$), with a negative predictive value of 100% and a positive predictive value of 47.9%. The study conclusions reinforced the robustness and clinical application of the genetic association between HLA-B*57:01 and the risk for abacavir HSR.[48]

Similarly, Young and colleagues conducted an open-label, multicenter study in North America that enrolled 725 patients. The ARIES study's conclusions showed that patients who were HLA-B*57:01 negative had less than 1% of clinically suspected HSR related to abacavir compared with 4% to 8% when HLA-B*57:01 testing was not performed.[49] As a result, pharmacogenetic screening for the HLA-B*57:01 allele prior to abacavir initiation in patients was included in the HIV-1 treatment guidelines in 2008.

Consequence of Drug–Gene Interaction

Approximately 5% to 8% of individuals will develop an HSR to abacavir within the first six weeks of drug exposure. Abacavir HSR symptoms may be characterized as a multiorgan syndrome that includes one symptom from two or more categories, including fever, rash, gastrointestinal (i.e., nausea, vomiting, diarrhea, abdominal pain), respiratory (i.e., dyspnea, cough, pharyngitis), and constitutional (i.e., malaise, fatigue, arthralgia, myalgia).[50] HSR symptoms are reversible if caught early and after discontinuation of abacavir. Less common signs and symptoms of HSR include hypotension, liver failure, renal failure, respiratory failure and death.[41] These symptoms could worsen with continued usage and may be potentially life

threatening if the patient is rechallenged with abacavir after discontinuation.[51,52]

Treatment Recommendation

Both Panels on Antiretroviral Therapy and Medical Management for Adult and Pediatric HIV Infection strongly recommend screening for the HLA-B*57:01 allele prior to initiating an abacavir-containing regimen for HIV-1 treatment. Fixed-dose combination regimens that contain abacavir include Triumeq (abacavir/lamivudine/dolutegravir) and Epzicom (abacavir/lamivudine). If a patient screens positive for the HLA-B*57:01 allele (the allele is present), then abacavir-containing regimens should not be considered for this patient to avoid HSR risk. On the other hand, if a patient screens negative for the HLA-B*57:01 allele (allele is absent), then abacavir-containing regimens could be initiated for this patient (Table 6-2).

Close monitoring of the patient for signs and symptoms of hypersensitivity within the first six weeks of initiation is strongly recommended while receiving an abacavir-containing treatment because there may still be a risk in spite of the patient's allele negativity.[48,53] A patient who develops an HSR while taking an abacavir-containing regimen should be immediately discontinued from that treatment. Rechallenge or restarting an abacavir-containing regimen for the patient should be avoided, as this may result in a severe, life-threatening abacavir HSR.

Efavirenz

Efavirenz is an antiretroviral agent of the first generation non-nucleoside reverse transcriptase inhibitor (NNRTI) class. Similar to the NRTI class, the NNRTI class inhibits the HIV reverse transcriptase enzyme by directly blocking DNA polymerization, which is a critical step in the reverse transcription process. For many years, the co-formulation of efavirenz with NRTI agents

TABLE 6-2. Recommendations for Initiating Abacavir

Test Result for HLA-B*57:01[a]	Implications for Phenotype	Recommendations for ABC Therapy	Classification of Recommendation
Negative	Low or reduced risk of ABC HSR	Use ABC per standard dosing guidelines	Strong
Positive	Significantly increased risk of ABC HSR	ABC is **NOT** recommended	Strong

[a] Genetic tests for HLA-B*57:01 are reported as negative (patient is not a carrier of the allele) or positive (patient is a carrier of the 57:01 allele).
HLA-B: human leukocyte antigen B; ABC: abacavir; HSR: hypersensitivity reaction.

Source: Adapted, with permission, from Martin MA, Klein TE, Dong BJ, et al. Clinical Pharmacogenetics Implementation Consortium guidelines for HLA-B genotype and abacavir dosing. Clin Pharmacol Ther. 2012;91(4):734–738.

(i.e., tenofovir disoproxil fumarate and emtricitabine) as a single-tablet regimen was the preferred standard of care treatment for HIV-1 infection because of its antiviral potency and efficacy. An efavirenz-containing regimen was also preferred because it was administered as a one-pill, once-a-day regimen (preferably taken at bedtime), which reduces the pill burden issue associated with other antiretroviral regimens. However, since the emergence of the integrase strand transfer inhibitors as a more potent and tolerable antiretroviral class, efavirenz was relegated to the "alternative" therapy category in 2015 for children and adults with HIV-1 infection.

Mechanism of Drug–Gene Interaction

Efavirenz is commonly known to cause central nervous system (CNS) and neuropsychiatric adverse effects such as somnolence, vivid dreams, impaired concentration, depression, psychosis, and suicidal ideation. These adverse effects could occur within the first couple of weeks of treatment initiation and typically resolve over time. However, the effects could persist in some individuals and affect their quality of life. Efavirenz is predominantly metabolized by CYP3A4 and 2B6, with minor metabolism by CYP2A6 to form inactive hydroxylated metabolites.[54,55] The major metabolite is 8-hydroxy-efavirenz, which is generated primarily by CYP2B6 and lacks antiviral activity (Figure 6-2).[56] It is also a mixed inhibitor and inducer of CYP3A4 substrates. One study has reported that chronic dosing of efavirenz can increase CYP2B6 expression via activation of the constitutive androstane receptor, which promotes its own metabolism or autoinduction.[57] The magnitude of efavirenz autoinduction and exposure varies among individuals and could be influenced by the polymorphisms of the CYP2B6 gene. Individuals with CYP2B6 *1/*1 and *1/*6 genotypes have considerable CYP2B6 induction, while those with CYP2B6 *6/*6 have minimal or no autoinduction.[58] In short, the CYP2B6 gene has polymorphisms that could lead to large variability in efavirenz plasma concentrations and exposure that exist between patients given the same dose of the medication.

Consequence of Drug–Gene Interaction

Multiple studies have linked the CYP2B6 gene with CNS and neuropsychiatric toxicities, particularly in individuals with the CYP2B6 *6/*6 genotype who are considered PMs of efavirenz. These individuals typically have high plasma efavirenz concentrations and reduced clearance of efavirenz.[59-61] Based on current evidence, CYP2B6 NMs are expected to have normal efavirenz metabolism at the standard daily dose of 600 mg. On the other hand,

the metabolism of efavirenz is reduced in CYP2B6 IMs, who may experience a 1.3-fold increased risk of adverse events and higher dose-adjusted trough concentrations compared with NMs.[62-66] Of note, CYP2B6 PMs may experience up to a 4.8-fold increased risk for adverse events because of higher plasma trough concentrations and exposure compared to NMs and IMs.[67-73]

Treatment Recommendation

There is guidance on dosing efavirenz based on an individual's CYP2B6 genotype. CYP2B6 UMs and RMs may have slightly lower dose-adjusted trough efavirenz concentrations comprised to NMs; however, current evidence does not suggest the effect to be clinically significant.[55,68,69] Efavirenz is available both as a stand-alone antiretroviral agent and as a single-tablet regimen at the standard dose of 600 mg/day. The current Department of Human Health and Services HIV-1 treatment guidelines recommend the administration of efavirenz co-formulated with other antiretroviral agents as a fixed-dose, single-tablet regimen. As such, efavirenz should be administered at the standard dose for patients who have the UM, RM, and NM phenotypes, since they are expected to have an overall normal efavirenz metabolism. There is a lower dose recommendation for individuals who are CYP2B6 IMs and should be initiated on efavirenz 400 mg/day because they may experience up to a 1.3-fold increased risk of adverse events.[62-66]

In 2018, the FDA approved a generic, co-formulated single-tablet regimen comprised of efavirenz 400 mg with tenofovir disoproxil fumarate and lamivudine (Symfi Lo) for individuals who could benefit from a reduced efavirenz dose. This stemmed from the ENCORE study, which randomized treatment-naïve patients to two treatment groups of efavirenz 600 mg/day and 400 mg/day regardless of their CYP2B6 genotype. Both groups were combined with tenofovir and emtricitabine as a complete antiretroviral treatment regimen. The study demonstrated that the efavirenz 400 mg/day group was non-inferior to the 600 mg/day group in virologic efficacy.[74] Of note, there is a similar recommendation for individuals with the CYP2B6 PM phenotype to be initiated at a lower daily dose of efavirenz 400 mg or 200 mg because of the increased efavirenz trough concentrations and exposure. Aside from the availability of efavirenz 600 mg and 400 mg single-tablet regimens, there is no co-formulated tablet with 200 mg efavirenz. Therefore, initiating an individual on a reduced efavirenz dose of 200 mg/day may increase his or her pill burden. Clinically, it is recommended for the CYP2B6 PM to be initiated

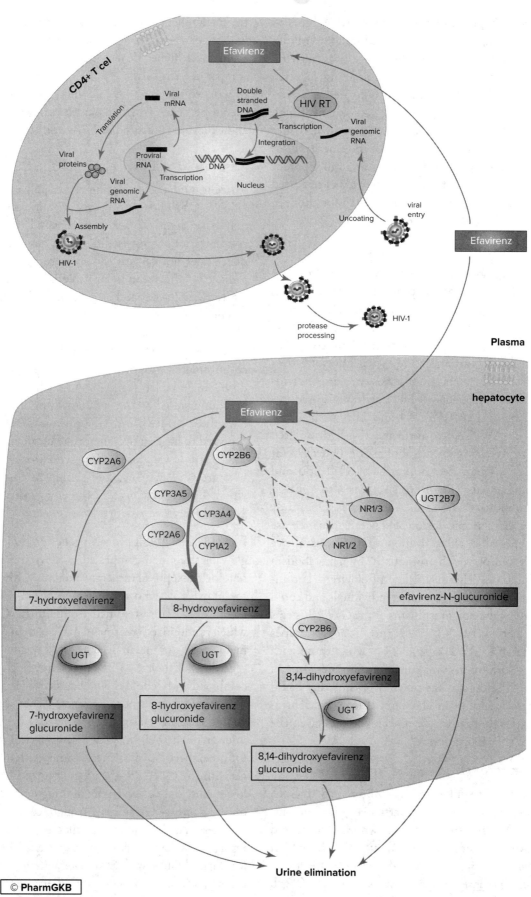

FIGURE 6-2 • (Continued)

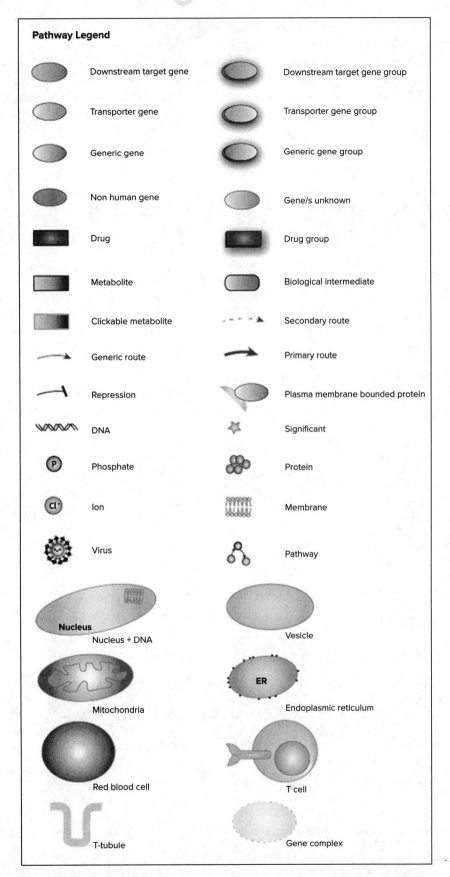

FIGURE 6-2 • Efavirenz pathway. (Reprinted, with permission, from Whirl-Carrillo M, McDonagh EM, Hebert JM, et al. (2012), Pharmacogenomics Knowledge for Personalized Medicine. Clinical Pharmacology and Therapeutics, 92: 414-417.)

on an efavirenz 400 mg single-tablet regimen for HIV-1 treatment to ensure adherence and virologic suppression. Furthermore, the individual should be closely monitored for bothersome CNS and neuropsychiatric adverse events and may need to be switched to another antiretroviral treatment regimen if he or she cannot tolerate the adverse events.[75] Table 6-3 summarizes the dosing recommendations for efavirenz for children weighing >40 kg and adults based on *CYP2B6* phenotype and genotype interpretations. By personalizing efavirenz dosages for HIV-1 treatment based on the individual's *CYP2B6* allele, this may help reduce efavirenz exposure and CNS and neuropsychiatric adverse effects without compromising antiviral efficacy.

TABLE 6-3 Recommendations for Efavirenz Dosing in Children (>40 kg) and Adults

CYP2B6 Phenotype	Genotypes	Examples of Diplotypes	Implications	Dosing Recommendations	Classification of Recommendation
Ultra-Rapid Metabolizer	An individual carrying two increased-function alleles	*4/*4, *22/*22, *4/*22	Slightly lower dose-adjusted trough concentrations of EFV compared with normal metabolizers	Initiate EFV with standard dosing (600 mg/day)	Strong
Rapid Metabolizer	An individual carrying one normal-function allele and one increased-function allele	*1/*4, *1/*22	Slightly lower dose-adjusted trough concentrations of EFV compared with normal metabolizers	Initiate EFV with standard dosing (600 mg/day)	Strong
Normal Metabolizer	An individual carrying two normal-function alleles	*1/*1	Normal EFV metabolism	Initiate EFV with standard dosing (600 mg/day)	Strong
Intermediate Metabolizer	An individual carrying one normal-function allele and one decreased-function allele, OR one normal-function allele and one no-function allele, OR one increased-function allele and one decreased-function allele, OR one increased-function allele and one no-function allele	*1/*6, *1/*18, *4/*6, *4/*18, *6/*22, *18/*22	Higher dose-adjusted trough concentrations of EFV compared with normal metabolizers; increased risk of CNS adverse events	Consider initiating EFV with decreased dose of 400 mg/day[a,b,c]	Moderate
Poor Metabolizer	An individual carrying two decreased-function alleles, OR two no-function alleles, OR one decreased-function allele and one no-function allele	*6/*6, *18/*18, *6/*18	Higher dose-adjusted trough concentrations of EFV compared with normal metabolizers; significantly increased risk of CNS adverse events and treatment discontinuation	Consider initiating EFV with decreased dose of 400 or 200 mg/day[a,b,c,d]	Moderate

[a] If therapeutic drug monitoring is available and a lower dose of EFV is prescribed, consider obtaining steady-state plasma EFV concentrations to ensure concentrations are within the therapeutic range of 1–4 µg/mL.

[b] EFV is available as a co-formulated single-tablet regimen at a decreased dose of 400 mg/day with tenofovir disoproxil fumarate and lamivudine (Symfi Lo).

[c] The ENCORE study showed that in treatment-naïve patients randomized to initiate EFV-based regimens (combined with tenofovir and emtricitabine), 400 mg/day was noninferior to 600 mg/day regardless of CYP2B6 genotype.

[d] To prescribe EFV at a decreased dose of 200 mg/day in a multidrug regimen may require prescribing more than one pill once daily. If so, the provider should weigh the potential benefit of reduced dose against the potential detrimental impact of increased pill number.

EFV: efavirenz.

Source: Adapted, with permission, from Desta Z, Gammal RS, Gong L, et al. Clinical Pharmacogenetics Implementation Consortium (CPIC) guideline for CYP2B6 and efavirenz-containing antiretroviral therapy. *Clin Pharmacol Ther.* 2019;106(4):726–733.

CASE SCENARIOS

Case 1

CV, a 33-year-old Caucasian woman, is diagnosed with HIV-1 infection. She also found out she is seven weeks pregnant and experiences daily morning sickness. She has NKDA. Her physical examination is normal. CV wants to receive antiretroviral therapy (ART). The prescriber wants to start her on Triumeq (dolutegravir/abacavir/lamivudine).

1. What laboratory test should be ordered before starting CV on this regimen?

*Answer: HLA-B*5701 allele test.*

*Rationale: If CV is HLA-B*57:01 negative, she can be considered for an abacavir-containing regimen (i.e., Triumeq). Triumeq is safe in pregnant women with HIV-1 infection with adequate folate supplementation.*

2. What is the risk of initiating CV on Triumeq before obtaining the laboratory test?

*Answer: The risk of developing an HSR associated with abacavir-containing regimens. The risk is high if she is positive for HLA-B*57:01.*

Case 2

A patient has been taking Atripla (efavirenz 600 mg/tenofovir disoproxil fumarate 300 mg/emtricitabine 200 mg) for two weeks and is complaining of having vivid nightmares. He also reports having difficulty concentrating at work and feeling depressed.

1. What pharmacogenomic test would you order for this patient?

Answer: CYP2B6 polymorphism to determine if the patient is an intermediate or poor metabolizer of this enzyme.

2. The pharmacogenomic test result is reported as CYP2B6 *6/*6. How do you interpret this result?

Answer: This patient is a CYP2B6 poor metabolizer and may experience higher plasma trough concentrations and exposure of efavirenz, resulting in having more CNS and neuropsychiatric side effects and adverse events.

3. What is your next plan of action for this patient?

Answer: Discontinue the Atripla regimen and initiate the patient on a lower efavirenz dose (400 mg) regimen. The patient could also be switched to another regimen that is preferred by the HIV-1 treatment guidelines, is not metabolized by the CYP2B6 enzyme, and is effective for him.

Case 3

A patient is receiving voriconazole for treatment of invasive aspergillosis in the hospital. Into the fourth day of therapy, he starts screaming of seeing the storm troopers in his room. He also complains of seeing bright spots and wavy lines. You suspect that the adverse effects the patient is experiencing are associated with voriconazole.

1. How is voriconazole metabolized?

Answer: Voriconazole is metabolized by the CYP2C19 enzyme.

Voriconazole is discontinued because of the bothersome adverse effects. An alternative antifungal agent is initiated to continue treatment of invasive aspergillosis. A pharmacogenomic test is obtained for this patient.

2. Based on the patient's drug-induced adverse effects, what result would you expect from the patient's pharmacogenomic report?

Answer: He is a CYP2C19 poor metabolizer. PMs could have high voriconazole serum concentrations and experience visual disturbances (e.g., altered color discrimination, blurred vision, photophobia, the appearance of bright spots and wavy lines), visual hallucinations, other neurologic disorders, and hepatotoxicity. These adverse reactions are reversible if caught early and after discontinuation of voriconazole.

PHARMACOGENOMICS CLINICAL PEARLS

■ G6PD-deficient individuals are at risk of hemolytic anemia. Before initiating dapsone and primaquine, individuals should be tested for the G6PD enzyme. Dapsone should be used with caution in G6PD-deficient individuals with close monitoring of their complete blood count (CBC) and reticulocyte count.

Primaquine should be avoided in G6PD-deficient individuals for safety concerns.

■ Voriconazole is a triazole antifungal that is a substrate and inhibitor of CYP2C19, CYP2C9, and CYP3A4 enzymes. It is mainly metabolized by CYP2C19. Poor metabolizers of CYP2C19 will have high voriconazole

- serum concentrations and could experience bothersome adverse effects such as visual disturbances, visual hallucinations, other neurological disorders, and hepatotoxicity.

- Alternative antifungal agents other than voriconazole are recommended for individuals with CYP2C19 UM (*17/*17) and PM (*2/*2) phenotypes because of possible treatment failure and bothersome adverse effects, respectively.

- Abacavir is associated with HSR, such as Stevens-Johnson syndrome and toxic epidermal necrolysis. The HLA-B*57:01 allele is associated with high incidence of HSR. Before initiating abacavir-containing regimens, an HLA-B*57:01 allele test should be performed. If an individual is HLA-B*57:01 negative, he or she could receive abacavir. If an individual is HLA-B*57:01 allele positive, he or she should not receive abacavir.

- An abacavir-containing regimen should not be resumed after it is discontinued for suspected rash or HSR due to a higher risk for the individual to develop serious, life-threatening adverse effects.

- Efavirenz is a substrate of CYP2B6 and CYP3A4. It is also a mixed inducer and inhibitor of CYP3A4. The magnitude of efavirenz autoinduction and exposure varies among individuals and could be influenced by the polymorphisms of the CYP2B6 gene.

- Intermediate and poor metabolizers of CYP2B6 (*1/*6 and *6/*6, respectively) should be initiated on low-dose efavirenz 400 mg (combined with other antiretroviral agents) to minimize the risk for the individual to develop CNS and neuropsychiatric adverse effects.

ABBREVIATIONS AND ACRONYMS

G6PD: Glucose-6-phosphate dehydrogenase

HIV: Human immunodeficiency virus

HLA: Human leukocyte antigen

HSR: Hypersensitivity reaction

MHC: major histocompatibility complex

NADPH: nicotinamide adenine dinucleotide phosphate hydrogen

NRTI: Nucleoside reverse transcriptase inhibitor

NNRTI: Non-nucleoside reverse transcriptase inhibitor

REFERENCES

1. Zhang R, Zhang CT. The impact of comparative genomics on infectious disease research. Microbes Infect. 2006;8(6):1613–1622.
2. Aceti A. Pharmacogenomics for infectious diseases. J Med Microb Diagn. 2016.5(1):1000223.
3. Behr MA, Wilson MA, Gill WP, et al. Comparative genomics of BCG vaccines by whole-genome DNA microarray. Science. 1999;284(5419):1520–1523.
4. The HLA Adverse Drug Reaction Database. Allele frequencies in worldwide populations. Available at http://www.allelefrequencies.net/default.asp. Accessed December 20, 2019.
5. Nkhoma ET, Poole C, Vannappagari V, et al. The global prevalence of glucose-6-phosphate dehydrogenase deficiency: A systematic review and meta-analysis. Blood Cells Mol Dis. 2009;42(3):267–278.
6. Mason PJ, Bautista JM, Gilsanz F. G6PD deficiency: The genotype-phenotype association. Blood Rev. 2007;21(5):267–283.
7. Cappellini MD, Fiorelli G. Glucose-6-phosphate dehydrogenase deficiency. Lancet. 2008;371(9606):64–74.
8. Beutler E. G6PD deficiency. Blood. 1994;84(11):3613–3636.
9. WHO Working Group. Glucose-6-phosphate dehydrogenase deficiency. Bull World Health Organ. 1989;67(6):601–611.
10. Youngster I, Arcavi L, Schechmaster R, et al. Medications and glucose-6-phosphate dehydrogenase deficiency: An evidence-based review. Drug Saf. 2010;33(9):713–726.
11. Grossman S, Budinsky R, Jollow D. Dapsone-induced hemolytic anemia: role of glucose-6-phosphate dehydrogenase in the hemolytic response of rat erythrocytes to N-hydroxydapsone. J Pharmacol Exp Ther. 1995;273(2):870–877.
12. Sheehy TW, Reba RC, Neff TA, et al. Supplemental sulfone (dapsone) therapy: Use in treatment of chloroquine-resistant falciparum malaria. Arch Intern Med. 1967;119(6):561–566.
13. Fanello CI, Karema C, Avellino P, et al. High risk of severe anaemia after chlorproguanil-dapsone+artesunate antimalarial treatment in patients with G6PD [A-] deficiency. PLoS ONE. 2008;3:e4031.
14. Ganesan S, Tekwani BL, Sahu R, et al. Cytochrome P(450)-dependent toxic effects of primaquine on human erythrocytes. Toxicol Appl Pharmacol. 2009;241(1):14–22.
15. FDA website with a table of Pharmacogenomic Biomarkers. Available at https://www.fda.gov/drugs/science-and-research-drugs/table-pharmacogenomic-biomarkers-drug-labeling. Accessed on June 10, 2020.
16. World Health Organization. Review of the safety of chlorproguanil-dapsone in the treatment of uncomplicated falciparum malaria in Africa: Report of a technical consultation convened by WHO, 1-2 July 2004, Geneva, 2005. [April 2011]; Available at http://www.who.int/malaria/publications/atoz/who_htm_mal_2005_1106/en/index.html. Accessed on June 10, 2020.
17. Greenberg MS, Wong H. Studies on the destruction of glutathione-unstable red blood cells: The influence of fava beans and primaquine upon such cells in vivo. J Lab Clin Med. 1961;57:733–746.

18. George JN, Sears DA, McCurdy PR, et al. Primaquine sensitivity in Caucasians: Hemolytic reactions induced by primaquine in G-6-PD deficient subjects. *J Lab Clin Med*. 1967;70:80–93.

19. Johnson LB, Kauffman CA. Voriconazole: A new triazole antifungal agent. *Clin Infect Dis*. 2003;36(5):630–637.

20. Mohr J, Johnson M, Cooper T, et al. Current options in antifungal pharmacotherapy. *Pharmacotherapy*. 2008;28(5):614–645.

21. Chu HY, Jain R, Xie H, et al. Voriconazole therapeutic drug monitoring: Retrospective cohort study of the relationship to clinical outcomes and adverse events. *BMC Infect Dis*. 2013;13:105.

22. Scott SA, Sangkuhl K, Shuldiner AR, et al. PharmGKB summary: Very important pharmacogene information for cytochrome P450, family 2, subfamily C, polypeptide 19. *Pharmacogenet Genomics*. 2012;22(2):159–165.

23. Hicks JK, Bishop JR, Sangkuhl K, et al. Clinical Pharmacogenetics Implementation Consortium (CPIC) guideline for CYP2D6 and CYP2C19 genotypes and dosing of selective serotonin reuptake inhibitors. *Clin Pharmacol Ther*. 2015;98(2):127–134.

24. Wang G, Lei HP, Li Z, et al. The CYP2C19 ultra-rapid metabolizer genotype influences the pharmacokinetics of voriconazole in healthy male volunteers. *Eur J Clin Pharmacol*. 2009;65(3):281–285.

25. Wang T, Zhu H, Sun J, et al. Efficacy and safety of voriconazole and CYP2C19 polymorphism for optimised dosage regimens in patients with invasive fungal infections. *Int J Antimicrob Agents*. 2014;44(5):436–442.

26. Weigel JD, Hunfeld NG, Koch BC, et al. Gain-of-function single nucleotide variants of the CYP2C19 gene (CYP2C19*17) can identify subtherapeutic voriconazole concentrations in critically ill patients: A case series. *Intensive Care Med*. 2015;41(11):2013–2014.

27. Scott SA, Sangkuhl K, Stein CM, et al. Clinical Pharmacogenetics Implementation Consortium guidelines for CYP2C19 genotype and clopidogrel therapy: 2013 update. *Clin Pharmacol Ther*. 2013;94(3):317–323.

28. Walsh TJ, Moriyama B, Penzak SR, et al. Response to "pharmacogenetics of voriconazole: CYP2C19 but also CYP3A4 need to be genotyped"— The pole of CYP3A4 and CYP3A5 polymorphisms in clinical pharmacokinetics of voriconazole. *Clin Pharmacol Ther*. 2017;102(2):190.

29. Hamada Y, Seto Y, Yago K, et al. Investigation and threshold of optimum blood concentration of voriconazole: A descriptive statistical meta-analysis. *J Infect Chemother*. 2012;18(4):501–507.

30. Pascual A, Calandra T, Bolay S, et al. Voriconazole therapeutic drug monitoring in patients with invasive mycoses improves efficacy and safety outcomes. *Clin Infect Dis*. 2008;46(2):201–211.

31. Tan K, Brayshaw, Tomaszewski K, et al. Investigation of the potential relationships between plasma voriconazole concentrations and visual adverse effects or liver function test abnormalities. *J Clin Pharmacol*. 2006;46(2):235–243.

32. Vfend [package insert]. New York, NY: Pfizer; 2019.

33. Moriyama B, Obeng AO, Barbarino J, et al. Clinical Pharmacogenetics Implementation Consortium (CPIC) guidelines for CYP2C19 and voriconazole therapy. *Clin Pharmacol Ther*. 2017;102(1):45–51.

34. McDowell JA, Chittick GE, Ravitch JR, et al. Pharmacokinetics of [^{14}C]abacavir, a human immunodeficiency virus type 1 (HIV-1) reverse transcriptase inhibitor, administered in a single oral dose to HIV-1-infected adults: A mass balance study. *Antimicrob Agents Chemother*. 1999;43(12):2855–2861.

35. Kumar PN, Sweet DE, McDowell JA, et al. Safety and pharmacokinetics of abacavir (1592U89) following oral administration of escalating single doses in human immunodeficiency virus type 1-infected adults. *Antimicrob Agents Chemother*. 1999;43(3):603–608.

36. Katlama C, Clotet B, Plettenberg A, et al. The role of abacavir (ABC, 1592) in antiretroviral therapy-experienced patients: Results from a randomized, double-blind, trial: CNA3002 European Study Team. *AIDS*. 2000;14(7):781–789.

37. Staszewski S, Katlama C, Harrer T. A dose ranging study to evaluate the safety and efficacy of abacavir alone or in combination with zidovudine and lamivudine in antiretroviral treatment naïve subjects. *AIDS*. 1998;12(16):F197–F202.

38. Kline MW, Blanchard S, Fletcher CV, et al. A phase I study of abacavir (1592U89) alone and in combination with other antiretroviral agents in infants and children with human immunodeficiency virus infection. *Pediatrics*. 1999;103(4):e47–000.

39. Khanna N, Klimkait T, Schiffer V, et al. Salvage therapy with abacavir plus a non-nucleoside reverse transcriptase inhibitor and a protease inhibitor in heavily pre-treated HIV-1 infected patients. Swiss HIV Cohort Study. *AIDS*. 2000;14(7):791–799.

40. Clay PG. The abacavir hypersensitivity reaction: A review. *Clin Ther*. 2002;24(10):1502–1514.

41. Hetherington S, McGuirk S, Powell G, et al. Hypersensitivity reactions during therapy with the nucleoside reverse transcriptase inhibitor abacavir. *Clin Ther*. 2001;23(10):1603–1614.

42. Roitt IM, Brostof J, Male DK. *Immunology*. London: Mosby; 1996.

43. Zhang Y, Mei H, Wang Q, et al. Peptide binding specificities of HLA-B*5701 and B*5801. *Sci China Life Sci*. 2012;55(9):818–825.

44. Martin MA, Klein TE, Dong BJ, et al. Clinical Pharmacogenetics Implementation Consortium. Clinical pharmacogenetics implementation consortium guidelines for HLA-B genotype and abacavir dosing. *Clin Pharmacol Ther*. 2012;91:734–738.

45. Watson M, Pimenta J, Spreen W, et al. HLA-B*5701 and abacavir hypersensitivity. *Pharmacogenetics*. 2004;14(11):783–784.

46. Chessman D, Kostenko L, Lethborg T, et al. Human leukocyte antigen class I-restricted activation of CD8+ T cells provides the immunogenetic basis of a systemic drug hypersensitivity. *Immunity*. 2008;28(6):822–832.

47. Small CB, Margolis DA, Shaefer MS, Ross LL. HLA-B*57:01 allele prevalence in HIV-infected North American subjects and the impact of allele testing on the incidence of abacavir-associated hypersensitivity reaction in HLA-B*57:01-negative subjects. *BMC Infect Dis*. 2017;17(1):256–261.

48. Mallal S, Phillips E, Carosi G, Molina JM, Workman C, Tomazic J, et al. HLA-B*5701 screening for hypersensitivity to abacavir. *N Engl J Med*. 2008;358(6):568–579.

49. Young B, Squires K, Patel P, et al. First large, multicenter, open-label study utilizing HLA-B*5701 screening for abacavir hypersensitivity in North America. *AIDS*. 2008;22(13):1673–1675.

50. Hewitt RG. Abacavir hypersensitivity reaction. *Clin Infect Dis*. 2002;34(8):1137–1142.

51. Frissen PH, de Vries J, Weigel HM, Brinkman K. Severe anaphylactic shock after rechallenge with abacavir without preceding hypersensitivity. *AIDS*. 2001;15(2):289.

52. Shapiro M, Ward KM, Stern JJ. A near-fatal hypersensitivity reaction to abacavir: Case report and literature review. *AIDS Read*. 2001;11(4):222–226.

53. Saag M, Balu R, Phillips E, et al. High sensitivity of human leukocyte antigen-b*5701 as a marker for immunologically confirmed abacavir hypersensitivity in white and black patients. *Clin Infect Dis.* 2008;46(7):1111–1118.

54. Ward BA, Gorski JC, Jones DR, et al. The cytochrome P450 2B6 (CYP2B6) is the main catalyst of efavirenz primary and secondary metabolism: Implication for HIV/AIDS therapy and utility of efavirenz as a substrate marker of CYP2B6 catalytic activity. *J Pharmacol Exp Ther.* 2003;306(1):287–300.

55. Desta Z, Saussele T, Ward B, et al. Impact of CYP2B6 polymorphism on hepatic efavirenz metabolism in vitro. *Pharmacogenomics.* 2007;8(6):547–558.

56. McDonagh EM, Lau JL, Alvarellos ML, et al. PharmGKB summary: Efavirenz pathway, pharmacokinetics. *Pharmacogenet Genomics.* 2015;25(7):363–376.

57. Meyer zu Schwabedissen HE, Oswald S, Bresser C, et al. Compartment-specific gene regulation of the CAR inducer efavirenz in vivo. *Clin Pharmacol Ther.* 2012;92(1):103–111.

58. Ngaimisi E, Mugusi S, Minzi OM, et al. Long-term efavirenz autoinduction and its effect on plasma exposure in HIV patients. *Clin Pharmacol Ther.* 2010;88(5):676–684.

59. Marzollini C, Telenti A, Decosterd LA, et al. Efavirenz plasma levels can predict treatment failure and central nervous system side effects in HIV-1-infected patients. *AIDS.* 2001;15(1):71–75.

60. Yilmer G, Amogne W, Habtewold A, et al. High plasma efavirenz level and CYP2B6*6 are associated with efavirenz-based HAART-induced liver injury in the treatment of naïve HIV patients from Ethiopia: A prospective cohort study. *Pharmacogenomics J.* 2012;12(6):499–506.

61. Abdelhady AM, Shugg T, Thong N, et al. Efavirenz inhibits the human ether-A-go-go related current (hERG) and induces QT interval prolongation in CYP2B6*6*6 allele carriers. *J Cardiovasc Electrophysiol.* 2016;27(10):1206–1213.

62. Dooley KE, Denti P, Martinson N, et al. Pharmacokinetics of efavirenz and treatment of HIV-1 among pregnant women with and without tuberculosis coinfection. *J Infect Dis.* 2015;211(2):197–205.

63. McIlleron HM, Schomaker M, Ren Y, et al. Effects of rifampin-based antituberculosis therapy on plasma efavirenz concentrations in children vary by CYP2B6 genotype. *AIDS.* 2013;27(12):1933–1940.

64. Robarge JD, Metzger IF, Lu J, et al. Population pharmacokinetic modeling to estimate the contributions of genetic and nongenetic factors to efavirenz disposition. *Antimicrob Agents Chemother.* 2017;61(1):e01813–e01816.

65. Mollan KR, Tierney C, Hellwege JN, et al. Race/ethnicity and the pharmacogenetics of reported suicidality with efavirenz among clinical trials participants. *J Infect Dis.* 2017;216(5):554–564.

66. Rotger M, Colombo S, Furrer H, et al. Influence of CYP2B6 polymorphism on plasma and intracellular concentrations and toxicity of efavirenz and nevirapine in HIV-infected patients. *Pharmacogenet Genomics.* 2005;15(1):1–5.

67. Ribaudo HJ, Liu H, Schwab M, et al. Effect of CYP2B6, ABCB1, and CYP3A5 polymorphisms on efavirenz pharmacokinetics and treatment response: An AIDS Clinical Trials Group study. *J Infect Dis.* 2010;202(5):717–722.

68. Rotger M, Tegude H, Colombo S, et al. Predictive value of known and novel alleles of CYP2B6 for efavirenz plasma concentrations in HIV-infected individuals. *Clin Pharmacol Ther.* 2007;81(4):557–566.

69. Ariyoshi N, Ohara M, Kaneko M, et al. Q172H replacement overcomes effects on the metabolism of cyclophosphamide and efavirenz caused by CYP2B6 variant with Arg262. *Drug Metab Dispos.* 2011;39(11):2045–2048.

70. Gross R, Bellamy SL, Ratshaa B, et al. CYP2B6 genotypes and early efavirenz-based HIV treatment outcomes in Botswana. *AIDS.* 2017;31(15):2107–2113.

71. Cummins NW, Neuhaus J, Chu H, et al. Investigation of efavirenz discontinuation in multi-ethnic populations of HIV-positive individuals by genetic analysis. *EBioMedicine.* 2015;2(7):706–712.

72. Leger P, Chirwa S, Turner M, et al. Pharmacogenetics of efavirenz discontinuation for reported central nervous system symptoms appears to differ by race. *Pharmacogenet Genomics.* 2016;26(10):473–480.

73. Johnson DH, Gebretsadik T, Shintani A, et al. Neuropsychiatric correlates of efavirenz pharmacokinetics and pharmacogenetics following a single oral dose. *Br J Clin Pharmacol.* 2013;75(4):997–1006.

74. ENCORE1 Study Group. Efficacy of 400 mg efavirenz versus standard 600 mg dose in HIV-infected, antiretroviral-naïve adults (ENCORE1): A randomised, double-blind, placebo-controlled, non-inferiority trial. *Lancet.* 2014;383(9927):1474–1482.

75. Desta Z, Gammal RS, Gong L, et al. Clinical Pharmacogenetics Implementation Consortium (CPIC) guideline for CYP2B6 and efavirenz-containing antiretroviral therapy. *Clin Pharmacol Ther.* 2019;106(4):726–733.

CHAPTER 7

ONCOLOGY PHARMACOGENOMICS

Amy L. Pasternak and Daniel L. Hertz

LEARNING OBJECTIVES

1. Define the difference between germline and somatic pharmacogenomics.

2. Recognize and be able to interpret common germline pharmacogenetic relationships that affect chemotherapy toxicity or efficacy.

3. Recognize and be able to interpret germline pharmacogenetic relationships that affect supportive care therapies.

INTRODUCTION

Pharmacogenomics in oncology is more complex than pharmacogenomics in other disease states because there can be clinical considerations for two different genomes: the tumor's somatic genome and the patient's germline genome. The somatic genome acquires genetic variation that causes oncogenic transformation, while the germline genome is the deoxyribonucleic acid (DNA) that is inherited; however, both can have implications for treatment decisions. Somatic genetic aberrations can be used to select a targeted agent for treatment. In some cancer types, these targeted therapies have now become the standard of care in first-line treatment, such as the use of imatinib in the treatment of Philadelphia chromosome–positive leukemia. Other examples of somatic pharmacogenomics include the use of epidermal growth factor receptor (EGFR) inhibitors, such as osimertinib, or B-rapidly accelerated fibrosarcoma (BRAF) inhibitors. The BRAF inhibitors, such as dabrafenib, are recommended as first-line treatment for patients with non–small cell lung cancer (NSCLC), with specific EGFR or BRAF mutations, respectively.[1] Historically, targeted therapies received approval for a specific cancer type harboring a specific genetic alteration; recently, however, the targeted therapy drug approval is shifting, where the indication for use is tied only to the genetic alteration. An example of this is the recent approval of the neurotrophic receptor tyrosine kinase (NTRK) inhibitor larotrectinib, which is indicated for the treatment of any metastatic solid tumor that harbors an NTRK gene fusion.[2] The clinical application of somatic pharmacogenomics is continuously evolving as new gene targets are discovered and new targeted therapies are developed.

The germline genome can provide information regarding cancer predisposition risk. This information can be used to identify patients who may benefit from enhanced cancer screening or cancer prevention interventions. Germline cancer predisposition genes may also have implications for treatment, such as the use of poly-ADP ribose polymerase (PARP) inhibitors (olaparib, rucaparib, and niraparib), which are specifically indicated for the treatment of patients who carry mutations in the breast cancer gene (*BRCA*). Additionally, germline pharmacogenomics can be used to predict the pharmacokinetics or pharmacodynamics of anticancer and supportive care therapies. A review of targeted therapies for somatic mutations and germline cancer predisposition genes is beyond the scope of this chapter, which will focus on the application of germline pharmacogenomics for anticancer and cancer supportive care therapies.

CHEMOTHERAPIES WITH GERMLINE PHARMACOGENETIC ASSOCIATIONS

There are multiple examples of germline pharmacogenetic relationships that can predict clinical outcomes associated with chemotherapies frequently used to treat patients with cancer. Associated clinical outcomes can be rates of adverse events related to the therapy or assessments of therapeutic efficacy. Additionally, new pharmacogenetics associations are continuing to be discovered, and this chapter will both discuss clinically actionable pharmacogenomic relationships and provide examples of investigational relationships that will likely be considered clinically actionable in the future.

Clinically Actionable Pharmacogenomic Relationships That Predict Medication Toxicity

Thiopurines and TPMT/NUDT15

Thiopurines are a standard therapy for treatment of acute lymphoblastic leukemia (ALL).[3,4] The thiopurines (azathioprine, mercaptopurine, thioguanine) are antimetabolite prodrugs that are bioactivated to the active metabolites, thioguanine nucleotides (TGNs). TGNs are incorporated into the DNA sequence, leading to disruption of cellular translation and subsequent apoptosis, which is associated with treatment-related adverse events. Mercaptopurine is the most frequently used thiopurine in the treatment of ALL.

Mechanism of Drug–Gene Interaction

Thiopurine methyltransferase (TPMT) and Nudix T hydrolase (NUDT15) are rate-limiting enzymes in the thiopurine metabolic pathway. TPMT prevents formation of TGNs through methylation of the parent compounds and upstream metabolites (Figure 7-1).[5,6] Approximately 10% of the population are TPMT intermediate metabolizers (IMs) (heterozygous for a *TPMT* no-function variant), while <1% of individuals are TPMT poor metabolizers (PMs) (carry two no-function variants for *TPMT*). Four alleles account for over 90% of all *TPMT* variation and are more common in individuals of European and African descent compared to other ethnicities (Table 7-1).[7,8]

TPMT activity can be determined via two testing methods. A genotype test can identify which genetic variants, if any, are present for an individual. Additionally, TPMT activity can be determined through an enzyme assay. TPMT is expressed in red blood cells (RBCs), so the incubation of RBCs with a thiopurine and subsequent measurement of the amount of a metabolite will also classify the phenotype of the individual.[9] Because TPMT enzyme activity is measured in RBCs, the results may not be accurate if the patient has recently had an RBC transfusion.[10]

NUDT15 is responsible for the inactivation of TGN (Figure 7-1).[6,11] The association between *NUDT15* genotype and thiopurines was first reported in 2014.[12] The most commonly studied no-function variant is 415C>T, which is found in both *NUDT15*2* and *NUDT15*3*. This single-nucleotide polymorphism (SNP) is significantly more common in individuals of Asian or Hispanic descent compared to other populations, with approximately 9% and 4% of individuals carrying this allele, respectively (Table 7-2).[13-15] Additional no-function variants continue to be discovered, which may be more common in other ethnicities.[11,16,17] Currently, NUDT15 phenotype can only be determined via a genotype test. Similar to TPMT, individuals are NUDT15 IMs if they are heterozygous for a

TABLE 7-1. Example TPMT Genetic Variants

Star Allele	Function	Allele Frequency (%)			
		European	African American	South/Central Asian	East Asian
*2	No function	0.2	0.5	0.02	0.01
*3A	No function	3.4	0.8	0.4	0.03
*3B	No function	0.2	0	0.2	0
*3C	No function	0.5	2.4	1.1	1.6

Source: Adapted from PharmGKB Gene Specific Information Tables for TPMT: TPMT Frequency Table. https://www.pharmgkb.org/page/tpmtRefMaterials.

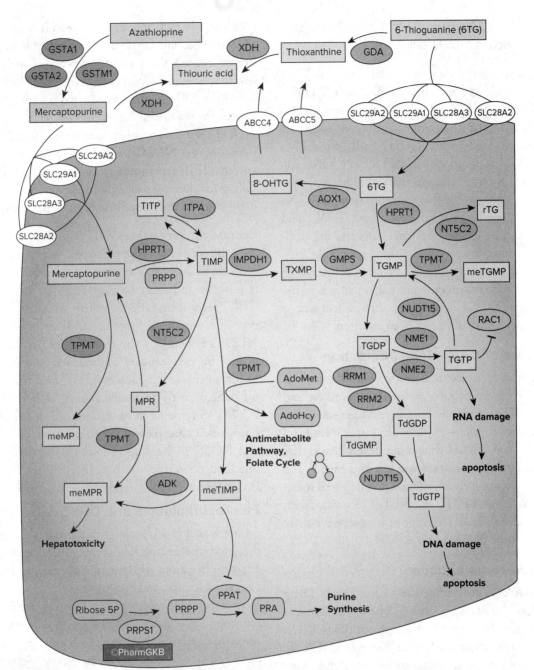

FIGURE 7-1 • Metabolism of azathioprine, thioguanine, and metcaptopurine. Source: Reprinted from PharmGKB Thiopurine Pathway, Pharmacokinetics/Pharmacodynamics. Summary. https://www.pharmgkb.org/pathway/PA2040.

TABLE 7-2. Example NUDT15 Genetic Variants

		Allele Frequency (%)			
Star Allele	Function	European	African American	South/Central Asian	East Asian
*2	No function	0	0	0	3.5
*3	No function	0	0	6.7	6.1

Source: Adapted from PharmGKB Gene Specific Information Tables for NUDT15: NUDT15 Frequency Table. https://www.pharmgkb.org/page/nudt15RefMaterials.

no-function *NUDT15* variant and NUDT15 PMs if they carry two no-function *NUDT15* variants.

Individuals who carry variants in either *TPMT* or *NUDT15* or both genes will have altered thiopurine metabolism. IMs and PMs of TPMT are unable to efficiently metabolize the thiopurine, leading to increased concentrations of TGN, while NUDT15 IMs and PMs have higher TGN accumulation in the DNA.[18–20] IMs will have higher TGN concentrations than an individual with no variant, and PMs have higher concentrations of TGNs than IMs. Although cases of variants in both *TPMT* and *NUDT15* are rare, current evidence suggests an additive effect of these genotypes on thiopurine tolerance. Individuals who are IMs of both TPMT and NUDT15 may have lower dose tolerance than a patient who is an IM for only one gene.[11,14,16] Thiopurine use in a patient who is a PM for both enzymes has never been reported.

Consequence of Drug–Gene Interaction

The dose-limiting side effects associated with thiopurines when used for cancer therapy are myelosuppression and hepatotoxicity. The development of myelosuppression frequently causes disruptions in thiopurine treatment, and in pediatric ALL decreased thiopurine dose intensity has been associated with poorer treatment response rates.[21] The rates and severity of myelosuppression secondary to toxicity are correlated with TPMT and NUDT15 activity, with 100% of PMs and ~35% of IMs experiencing severe toxicity requiring thiopurine dose reductions.[12,14,18]

Treatment Recommendation

Multiple sources, including the Food and Drug Administration (FDA) drug labeling, Clinical Pharmacogenetics Implementation Consortium (CPIC), and National Comprehensive Cancer Network (NCCN) guidelines provide recommendations for modifying thiopurine doses based on *TPMT* and/or *NUDT15* genetic results.[3,4,22,23]

Approximately 40% to 70% of patients who are IMs for TPMT or NUDT15 will not develop toxicity with standard doses of thiopurine; however, there is no method to identify which patients will tolerate full-dose treatment. CPIC recommends a dose reduction of 30% to 80% in TPMT and NUDT15 IMs to limit the risk for toxicity.[22] The NCCN guidelines include the CPIC dose recommendations; however, the FDA drug labeling recommends adjusting thiopurine doses based on tolerability for TPMT and NUDT15 IMs.[3,23] TPMT and NUDT15 PMs do not tolerate full doses of thiopurine medications and require substantial dose reductions to prevent toxicity.[14]

CPIC and FDA labeling recommend reducing the dose by at least 90%, and CPIC also recommends decreasing the dosing frequency to three times per week in TPMT PMs. Studies have demonstrated that these dose reductions based on TPMT phenotype have no adverse effects on treatment responses.[24] Because the relationship between *NUDT15* and thiopurines is relatively new, the exact dose tolerance of a NUDT15 PM is less well defined, but the current CPIC recommendation is similar to TPMT PM, calling for decreases of 75% to 90% of the standard dose depending on the thiopurine being administered.[22,23]

Because the prevalence of *TPMT* and *NUDT15* variants differs between populations, it is uncommon that individuals will carry variants in both genes; however, it is possible and must be considered in dosing decisions. CPIC recommendations follow an additive effect theory, where each no-function allele in either *TPMT* or *NUDT15* increases the risk for toxicity, which is supported by case reports of patients who carry variants in both genes.[11,14,16] However, the ideal thiopurine dose for patients with decreased activity in both TPMT and NUDT15 remains to be determined. It is currently recommended that patients with variants in both *TPMT* and *NUDT15* be dosed in accordance with their most impaired phenotype with reduced doses (either IM or PM recommendation) and close monitoring.[22]

Fluoropyrimidines and DPYD

5-fluorouracil (5-FU) and its oral prodrug capecitabine are the backbone in first-line combination chemotherapeutic regimens in various solid tumor malignancies, including colorectal, pancreatic, and breast cancer.[25–28] As with most chemotherapeutic agents, 5-FU treatment is administered at a maximum dose that is associated with an acceptable risk of severe toxicity, including myelotoxicity, diarrhea, mucositis, and hand–foot syndrome. In the general population treatment-related fatal toxicity occurs in <1% of patients.[29]

Mechanism of Drug–Gene Interaction

5-FU must be metabolically activated to cytotoxic metabolites for effectiveness, a process that accounts for relatively little of the overall disposition of 5-FU administered to a patient.

The majority of 5-FU is instead metabolically eliminated via dihydropyrimidine dehydrogenase (DPD), which is encoded by the *DPYD* gene. Many genetic variants in *DPYD* have been reported, some of which decrease a patient's enzymatic DPD activity. Reduced DPD activity leads to dramatically decreased elimination of 5-FU and increased systemic drug concentrations,[30] which can increase risk of severe toxicity and death.

Consequence of Drug–Gene Interaction

Increased risk of severe treatment-related toxicity has been well established for four diminished-activity *DPYD* variants (Table 7-3).[31,32] Though each variant is itself uncommon, a Caucasian patient has an approximate 7% chance of carrying a single variant (IM) and a 1/200 chance of carrying two variants, either as a homozygous or compound heterozygous diplotype (PM). A meta-analysis of >7000 patients found that DPYD IMs have a 60% to 340% relative increase in severe toxicity compared to a DPYD NM and an approximate 70% absolute risk of severe toxicity when treated with standard doses. Furthermore, the risk of treatment-related death in variant carriers who receive full doses is approximately 3%.[33] Precise estimates of the risk of toxicity and/or death for DPYD PMs are not known due to the relatively rare occurrence, but are generally accepted to be greater than the risk in carriers of a single variant.

Treatment Recommendation

It is well-established that DPYD IMs and PMs have increased toxicity risk, and it is generally accepted that patients who are known carriers should not receive full doses of 5-FU or capecitabine due to their unacceptable risk of severe treatment-related toxicity. CPIC has published evidence-based guidelines for translating *DPYD* genotype into DPD activity score and phenotype and has provided recommended dosing based on DPD activity scores (Table 7-4).[34] Patients who are DPD IMs (activity score 1.0 to 1.5) should receive a 50% dose reduction at treatment initiation, followed by dose escalation as tolerated. These recommendations are based primarily on two prospective single-arm studies of preemptive DPD genotype-guided treatment in which 50% dose reductions in DPD IMs normalized their toxicity rates and systemic drug concentrations, with wild-type patients receiving standard doses.[35,36]

TABLE 7-3. Example DPYD Genetic Variants

| Variant | Activity Score | Function | Allele Frequency | | | |
			European	African American	South/Central Asian	East Asian
c.1905+1G>A (*2A)	0	No function	0.8	0.3	0.5	0
c.1679T>G (*13)	0	No function	0.06	0	0	0
c.2846A>T	0.5	Decreased function	0.4	0.3	0.06	0
c.1129-5923C>G, c.1236G>A (HapB3)	0.5	Decreased function	2.4	0.3	1.9	0

Source: Adapted from PharmGKB Gene Specific Information Tables for DPYD: DPYD Frequency Table. https://www.pharmgkb.org/page/dpydRefMaterials.

TABLE 7-4. Clinical Pharmacogenetic Implementation Consortium Recommended Dosing of Fluoropyrimidines by DPD Phenotype

Phenotype	Activity Score	Dosing Recommendation	Classification of Recommendation
DPD normal metabolizer	2	Use label-recommended dosage and administration	Strong
DPD intermediate metabolizer	1–1.5	Reduce starting dose by 50%	Moderate–strong
DPD poor metabolizer	0.5	Avoid use of 5-FU or 5-FU prodrug regimens. In the event, based on clinical advice, alternative agents are not considered a suitable therapeutic option, 5-FU should be administered at a strongly reduced dose with early therapeutic drug monitoring.	Strong
	0	Avoid use of 5-FU or 5-FU prodrug regimens	Strong

Source: Adapted from CPIC Guideline for Fluoropyrimidines and DPYD, Clinical Pharmacogenetics Implementation Consortium (CPIC), Guideline for Dihydropyrimidine Dehydrogenase Genotype and Fluoropyrimidine Dosing: 2017 Update (October 2017). https://cpicpgx.org/guidelines/guideline-for-fluoropyrimidines-and-dpyd/. [Accessed February 4, 2020].

The prospective trials either did not enroll or excluded DPD PMs, and the appropriate doses for these patients are not well established. Current recommendations for patients who are DPD PMs with an activity score = 0.5 are to strongly reduce the doses (<25% of the normal dose), whereas there are no recommended safe doses in patients who are DPD PMs with an activity score = 0. As patients carrying these uncommon genotypes are treated, more information will be generated regarding optimal dosing.[37]

Irinotecan and UGT1A1

Irinotecan is a topoisomerase 1 inhibitor and is a component of multidrug combination regimens for several solid tumors, including lung, colon, gastric, rectal, and head and neck cancer. Irinotecan is a prodrug that must be bioactivated to SN-38. In addition to being responsible for treatment effectiveness, SN-38 is responsible for treatment-related toxicity, which includes neutropenia and diarrhea.

Mechanism of Drug–Gene Interaction

SN-38 is primarily eliminated via the hepatic phase II glucuronidation enzyme UDP-glucuronosyltransferase 1A1 (UGT1A1), which is encoded by UGT1A1. UGT1A1 has a common variant in its promoter region that affects the number of dinucleotide (TA) repeats in the TATA box. A typical patient has six TA repeats, but some patients have seven, which is referred to as UGT1A1*28 (rs8175347), or more. These additional TA repeats decrease the expression of UGT1A1 and its resultant enzymatic activity. Patients who carry UGT1A1*28 are IMs, and patients homozygous for UGT1A1*28 are PMs. Poor UGT1A1 metabolism leads to Gilbert syndrome, which is characterized by mild elevations of unconjugated bilirubin in the absence of liver disease. Other variants in UGT1A1 can cause Crigler-Najjar syndrome, which can cause life-threating elevations in unconjugated bilirubin. This same mechanism causes UGT1A1 IMs and PMs to have less efficient SN-38 glucuronidation, and consequently greater SN-38 concentrations during irinotecan treatment.[38–40]

Consequence of Drug–Gene Interaction

UGT1A1 IM and PM have been reported to have higher risk of irinotecan toxicity, but no corresponding increase in efficacy.[41,42]

Based on their greater SN-38 exposure, UGT1A1 IMs or PMs would be expected to benefit from lower irinotecan doses than wild-type patients. Indeed, genotype-guided dose-escalation studies have found that UGT1A1 PMs have lower maximum tolerated doses.[43–45] These doses are currently undergoing prospective testing in genotype-guided

studies to determine whether UGT1A1-guided dosing improves clinical outcomes. A randomized study in patients with colorectal cancer found that genotype-guided dose escalation in wild-type and heterozygous patients improved response without increasing toxicity, as compared to standard dosing.[46] Other studies in several cancer types have found that genotype-guided dosing normalizes efficacy and/or toxicity between genotype groups,[47–49] suggesting that optimal doses have been identified for patients within each genotype strata.

Treatment Recommendation

Similar to other pharmacogenetic associations, there is sufficient evidence to warrant personalized irinotecan dosing in patients with a known UGT1A1 genotype. Although CPIC has not published dosing recommendations, the FDA-approved labeling for irinotecan recommends UGT1A1 PM patients receive a 25% dose reduction. Similarly, the Dutch Pharmacogenomics Working Group (DPWG) recommends a 30% dose reduction for UGT1A1 PM patients scheduled to receive >250 mg/m². [50] Finally, NCCN recommends caution and more intense toxicity monitoring for patients with Crigler-Najjar or Gilbert syndrome receiving irinotecan due to the risk of hyperbilirubinemia.[51] The FDA has a similar warning for patients who are UGT1A1 PMs receiving treatment with drugs that cause hyperbilirubinemia due to inhibition of UGT1A1, such as the tyrosine kinase inhibitors nilotinib and pazopanib.[52–54]

Belinostat and UGT1A1

Mechanism of Drug–Gene Interaction

Belinostat is a histone deacetylase inhibitor that is FDA-approved for the treatment of relapsed or refractory peripheral T-cell lymphoma, although it is currently being studied for the treatment of other malignancies. Belinostat is inactivated via glucuronidation by the enzyme UGT1A1.[55] Individuals who are UGT1A1 PMs have significantly decreased belinostat clearance.[56]

Consequence of Drug–Gene Interaction

Serious adverse reactions associated with belinostat administration include hematologic toxicity, hepatotoxicity, and gastrointestinal toxicity.[57] In phase 1 studies, individuals who were UGT1A1 PMs had increased incidence of hematologic toxicity, hepatotoxicity, and QT prolongation.[58,59]

Treatment Recommendation

No clinical pharmacogenetic guidelines currently exist for belinostat prescribing, although CPIC rates the evidence for the drug–gene interaction between belinostat and *UGT1A1* as a level B, which indicates the information is clinically actionable. The FDA package labeling recommends an initial 25% dose reduction in individuals who are known UGT1A1 PMs to minimize the risk of treatment toxicity.

Investigational Pharmacogenomic Relationships That Predict Medication Toxicity

Methotrexate and SLCO1B1

Methotrexate (MTX) is a dihydrofolate reductase inhibitor that prevents the formation of tetrahydrofolate required for de novo purine synthesis, subsequently preventing cellular replication. MTX is commonly used in the treatment of ALL and osteosarcoma.

Mechanism of Drug–Gene Interaction

After administration, MTX undergoes hepatic uptake via the organic anion transporter (OATP) 1B1, which is encoded by the gene *SLCO1B1*.[60] *SLCO1B1* has a common genetic variation (521 C>T) that results in decreased function of the transporter.[61] Individuals who carry one decreased-function variant have the SLCO1B1 decreased-function phenotype, while individuals with two decreased-function variants have the SLCO1B1 poor-function phenotype.[62] Decreased and poor function of the SLCO1B1 transporter results in higher exposure of MTX caused by less of the drug being transported into the liver for metabolic elimination.

Consequence of Drug–Gene Interaction

MTX can be administered via multiple dosing strategies, including high-dose MTX (>2 g/m^2). Both ALL and osteosarcoma utilize high-dose MTX in their treatment plans, although dosing can vary widely (2 to 12 g/m^2).[3,63] SLCO1B1 poor function decreases MTX clearance and increases MTX exposure approximately twofold to threefold compared with SLCO1B1 normal-function patients.[64–68] There is evidence the increase in MTX exposure due to SLCO1B1 poor function is associated with an increased rate of adverse events, including gastrointestinal toxicity outcomes.[65,69,70]

Treatment Recommendation

There are currently no clinical guidelines or other recommendations regarding MTX and *SLCO1B1* genotype. However, based on the currently available evidence, if a patient has known poor function of SLCO1B1, increased monitoring, especially post high-dose MTX treatment, may be warranted. Patients with SLCO1B1 poor function may require higher leucovorin rescue doses post high-dose MTX treatment, although specific recommendations for adjustment to the MTX and leucovorin doses have not been determined.[65]

Vincristine and CEP72

Vincristine is a microtubule-targeting chemotherapeutic agent that is commonly used in many leukemias, lymphomas, and several solid tumors, including kidney, liver, and lung cancer. Similar to other drugs that affect microtubules, one of the dose-limiting toxicities of vincristine is motor and sensory peripheral neuropathy that manifests as numbness, tingling, or burning pain in the hands and feet.[71] There are no effective ways to prevent or treat peripheral neuropathy, so patients who experience mild neuropathy typically require dose modifications to prevent progression to severe, sometimes irreversible, neuropathy.[51] Several studies have investigated genetic predictors of vincristine-induced neuropathy, particularly in pediatric patients with ALL.

Mechanism and Consequence of Drug-Gene Interaction

A genome-wide association study revealed that patients who are homozygous for the rs924607 *CEP72* promoter polymorphism have increased risk of peripheral neuropathy during long-term vincristine continuation treatment and cannot tolerate cumulative doses as large as those typically administered.[72] Unlike most other pharmacogenetic associations, this polymorphism does not affect vincristine pharmacokinetics. Instead, the promoter SNP decreases CEP72 expression, which increases the sensitivity of cells to the toxic effects of vincristine in vitro. Independent replication has been reported in a case-control study and a retrospective cohort study of patients with ALL receiving long-term treatment.[73] However, the association was not confirmed in several other attempted replication studies.[75–77]

Treatment Recommendation

Based on these inconsistent findings, this association likely has not been adequately validated for clinical translation and implementation, and there are currently no clinical practice guidelines for this drug–gene pair. However, there is an ongoing prospective clinical trial (NCT03117751) with an embedded *CEP72*-guided vincristine substudy that will attempt to determine whether patients with the high-risk homozygous variant genotype should be treated with lower vincristine doses or shorter overall regimens to reduce neuropathy while maintaining efficacy. These results may provide evidence of a clinical benefit for *CEP72*-guided vincristine treatment and could be the basis for future guidelines and implementation in clinical practice.

Clinically Actionable Pharmacogenomic Relationships Associated with Treatment Efficacy

Tamoxifen and CYP2D6

Tamoxifen is a selective estrogen receptor modulator (SERM) used in the treatment of hormone receptor–positive (HR+) breast cancer, particularly in premenopausal patients. Long-term tamoxifen treatment reduces tumor recurrence and improves overall survival.[78] Tamoxifen acts as an antagonist of the estrogen receptor on cancer cells, interfering with the estrogenic signaling that drives cellular replication and tumor growth. Tamoxifen itself is not a potent antiestrogen, but is metabolically bioactivated to endoxifen, the most potent and abundant metabolite that is thought to be responsible for tamoxifen's effectiveness.

Mechanism of Drug–Gene Interaction

Bioactivation of tamoxifen to endoxifen proceeds through two parallel pathways, both of which are rate limited by CYP2D6.[79] CYP2D6 is a highly polymorphic enzyme, with well over 100 recurrent haplotypes. These variants include gene deletions and duplications and polymorphisms in coding and regulatory regions that affect overall CYP2D6 activity.[80] It is well established that genotype-predicted CYP2D6 activity is the primary determinant of steady-state endoxifen concentrations in patients receiving tamoxifen.[81,82] CYP2D6 genotype-to-phenotype translation uses the CYP2D6 activity scoring system; each CYP2D6 allele is assigned an activity score relative to the functional activity of the allele (e.g., normal function is assigned an activity score of 1). The CYP2D6 phenotype is determined according to the sum of the patient's individual allele activity scores, and each phenotype has standard activity score ranges.[83,84] Other CYP450 enzyme families, including CYP2C and CYP3A; phase II enzymes such as SULTs and UGTs; and clinical variables, including concomitant CYP2D6 inhibitor intake, also contribute to the variability in steady-state endoxifen concentration.[85–87]

Consequence of Drug–Gene Interaction

While the direct effect of CYP2D6 genotype on endoxifen levels is well-established, the downstream effect of endoxifen concentration or CYP2D6 genotype on tamoxifen treatment efficacy has not been sufficiently validated. Several studies have reported that patients with low endoxifen concentrations have worse survival, though each reported a distinct endoxifen cutoff.[88–90] However, other studies, including several recent prospective trials, were not able to validate these thresholds or detect any association between low endoxifen concentrations and worse treatment outcome.[91–93] Similarly, several dozen retrospective pharmacogenetic studies have assessed the putative association between CYP2D6 genotype and tamoxifen treatment outcomes, which have reported highly inconsistent results.[94–98] This has led to differing opinions as to whether this association has been validated and has generally impeded the progress toward clinical translation of personalized treatment based on CYP2D6 genotype or measured endoxifen concentration.

Treatment Recommendation

Despite the unclear validation that genotype or endoxifen is predictive of tamoxifen treatment outcome, several studies have prospectively tested tamoxifen dose adjustment based on CYP2D6 genotype and/or endoxifen concentrations.[99–102] These studies have consistently found that personalized tamoxifen dosing can normalize endoxifen concentrations without affecting treatment safety or patient quality of life. However, none of these studies have reported that this strategy has any meaningful clinical benefit in terms of improved efficacy or safety. Given the lack of validation of endoxifen concentration as a surrogate of treatment efficacy, there is currently no rationale for testing CYP2D6 genetics or measuring endoxifen concentration to guide tamoxifen dosing. However, similar to many other pharmacogenetic associations, known CYP2D6 genetic information is worth considering when selecting an appropriate dose for a given patient. Based on CPIC guidelines, dose escalation from the standard 20 mg/day to 40 mg/day should be considered in patients with CYP2D6 PM or IM phenotype, as this has been demonstrated to normalize their endoxifen without increasing toxicity.[103]

ONCOLOGY SUPPORTIVE CARE MEDICATIONS WITH PHARMACOGENOMIC CONSIDERATIONS

Clinically Actionable Pharmacogenomic Relationships Associated with Toxicity

Rasburicase and G6PD

Rasburicase is a recombinant urate oxidase enzyme indicated for the treatment of tumor lysis syndrome.[104] Tumor lysis syndrome is characterized by a rise in uric acid concentrations and other laboratory abnormalities that can cause significant morbidity to patients.[105] Uric acid is formed via purine catabolism (Figure 7-2) and cannot be excreted from the body; high concentrations of uric acid can contribute to acute renal failure. Urate oxidase is able to convert uric acid into allantoin, which can be excreted from the body. Humans do not produce an endogenous

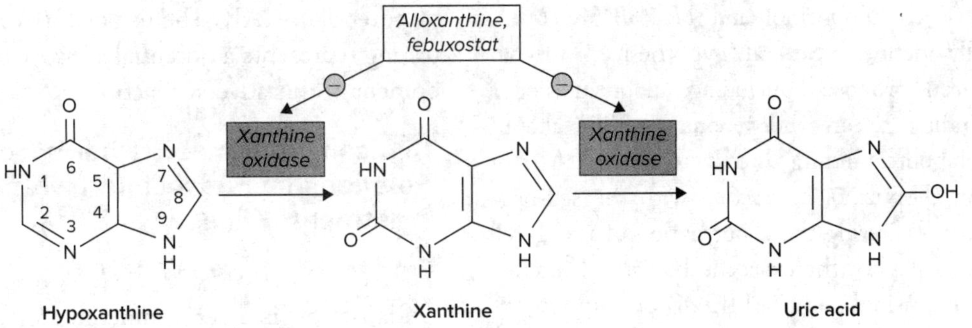

FIGURE 7-2 • **Purine catabolism pathway**. (Adapted from Meyers FH, Jawetz E, Goldfien A: Review of Medical Pharmacology, 7th ed. New York: McGraw-Hill, 1980.)

urate oxidase, so exogenous products are used to prevent the toxicities associated with acutely elevated uric acid concentrations. Hydrogen peroxide (H_2O_2) is a by-product of the uric acid conversion to allantoin.

Mechanism of Drug–Gene Interaction

Glucose-6-phosphate dehydrogenase (G6PD) is involved in maintaining cellular homeostasis, particularly in RBCs, through the production of nicotinamide adenine dinucleotide phosphate hydrogen (NADPH).[106] NADPH is a cofactor that plays an essential role in pathways that neutralize reactive oxygen species (ROS), such as H_2O_2. G6PD activity can be reduced to varying degrees due to many different genetic variants in the G6PD gene.[107] G6PD variant activity is classified according to the World Health Organization classification scheme, with class I variants conferring the most severe deficiency.[108]

The G6PD gene is located on the X chromosome, so all males are hemizygous (carry only one allele copy), and their phenotype will always correspond with the severity of the class of the G6PD variant they carry. Genotype may not be enough to determine the G6PD phenotype in females due to mosaicism.[106] Mosaicism is when one allele may be expressed at a higher percentage within a cell than another. For example, a female patient may carry one normal G6PD allele and one deficient G6PD allele (class II to III); however, she may have a normal phenotype because the normal G6PD allele is expressed at a higher percentage than the deficient allele.[106] Mosaicism is further complicated by the fact that this expression can change over time, so in the future the same female patient may have a deficient G6PD phenotype.[109] The only way to conclusively determine the G6PD phenotype in female patients is to perform a G6PD activity assay.

Consequence of Drug–Gene Interaction

ROS such as H_2O_2 formed as a by-product of rasburicase administration cause oxidative stress within the cell. Cells regulate oxidative stress by breaking down ROS through

pathways that require NADPH. Cells that are G6PD deficient have lower NADPH stores and therefore have an impaired ability to combat ROS. When a precipitating exposure, such as rasburicase administration, occurs in a G6PD-deficient cell, there is an inability to break down the increased ROS that can lead to cellular lysis. Because G6PD is particularly important for NADPH stores in erythrocytes, this drug–gene interaction causes hemolytic anemia.[110,111] This drug–gene interaction can also cause methemoglobinemia, which can be fatal.[112]

Treatment Recommendation

Due to the severity of the adverse drug reaction between rasburicase and G6PD, rasburicase is contraindicated per FDA drug labeling in patients who have known G6PD deficiency.[104] The FDA Black Box Warning also recommends testing G6PD activity prior to rasburicase administration in patients at high risk for being G6PD deficient (African or Mediterranean ancestry).[104] CPIC also recommends performing G6PD activity testing prior to drug administration in patients with known G6PD genotypes that could result in variable G6PD activity, or female patients with heterozygous or compound heterozygous G6PD class II to IV variants.[113]

Allopurinol and HLA-B

Allopurinol is a xanthine oxidase inhibitor that is used to prevent the formation of uric acid. Allopurinol is used as a prophylactic therapy in patients at risk for tumor lysis syndrome to decrease the formation of uric acid (Figure 7-2).

Mechanism of Drug–Gene Interaction

Human leukocyte antigen-B (HLA-B) is a major histocompatibility complex I (MHC-I) molecule that is part of the immune system. HLA-B is responsible for presenting peptides to T cells to mount immune responses. Genetic variation with HLA is common. The HLA-B*58:01 variant is associated with increased sensitivity to allopurinol and is most frequently found in patients of East Asian descent.[114,115] The mechanism of the drug–gene interaction between allopurinol and *HLA-B*58:01* has not been fully defined. Several hypothesized mechanisms have been proposed, including allopurinol or a metabolite binding to an endogenous peptide, allopurinol or a metabolite binding directly to the HLA-B or T-cell receptor, allopurinol interacting with the self-peptide, or allopurinol altering the confirmation of the T-cell receptor.[116] Regardless of the exact mechanism of interaction between allopurinol and the HLA-B or T-cell receptor, the drug–gene interaction can lead to an inappropriate immune activation.

Consequence of Drug–Gene Interaction

The inappropriate immune activation caused by the allopurinol–*HLA-B*58:01* drug–gene interaction causes the body to attack itself. This risk is the same for patients whether they are heterozygous or homozygous for the *HLA-B*58:01* variant. The most common manifestation for the allopurinol-*HLA-B*58:01* interaction is the development of severe cutaneous adverse reactions (SCARs) such as Steven-Johnson syndrome (SJS), toxic epidermal necrolysis (TEN), or drug reaction with eosinophilia and systemic symptoms (DRESS); these typically occur within the first few weeks to months of therapy with allopurinol.[117–120] Other patient characteristics, particularly decreased renal function, also increase the risk for the development of SCAR.[121,122] The estimated negative predictive value of *HLA-B*58:01* genotype for allopurinol adverse reactions is 100% for the high-risk populations. The positive predictive value is ~1.5%, meaning not all patients who carry *HLA-B*58:01* will develop SCAR if given allopurinol. Prospective studies of preemptive *HLA-B*58:01* genotyping demonstrated a significantly decreased rate of SCAR in the genotyped group compared to historical rates, demonstrating potential clinical utility for preemptive testing in at-risk populations.[123,124]

Treatment Recommendation

Although the positive predictive value of *HLA-B*58:01* testing is low, SCARs are associated with a significant risk for mortality, so CPIC states allopurinol should be contraindicated in all patients who carry *HLA-B*58:01*.[114] The American College of Rheumatology also recommends considering testing for *HLA-B*58:01* prior to initiating allopurinol in at-risk populations (e.g., Koreans with stage 3 or worse chronic kidney disease or those of Han Chinese and Thai descent).[125] *HLA-B*58:01* genotype is not included in the FDA drug labeling for allopurinol, but cutaneous adverse reactions are included in the warnings and precautions information, and it is recommended to discontinue the medication at the first sign

of potential SCAR. The use of *HLA-B*58:01* genotype testing represents a potential strategy to avoid the development of this adverse reaction.[126]

Clinically Actionable Pharmacogenomic Relationships Associated with Treatment Efficacy

Ondansetron and CYP2D6

Ondansetron is a serotonin receptor (5-HT3) antagonist that is recommended as a first-line antiemetic either alone or in combination for chemotherapy-induced nausea and vomiting (CINV) prophylaxis.[127] Many patients with cancer may also receive ondansetron as prophylaxis for postoperative nausea and vomiting (PONV).

Mechanism of Drug–Gene Interaction

Ondansetron undergoes extensive hepatic metabolism primarily to inactive hydroxylated metabolites via multiple cytochrome P450 enzymes, including CYP3A4, CYP1A2, and CYP2D6. CYP2D6 is estimated to facilitate metabolism for a minority of the ondansetron dose administered, primarily contributing to the metabolism of the S-enantiomer.[128,129]

As previously described in this chapter, *CYP2D6* is highly polymorphic. Changes in CYP2D6 activity have been associated with altered ondansetron pharmacokinetics. S-ondansetron enantiomer plasma concentrations have been shown to differ between CYP2D6 phenotypes, with CYP2D6 PMs having the highest concentrations and CYP2D6 UMs the lowest concentrations.[129]

Consequence of Drug–Gene Interaction

Although the number of studies investigating this relationship is limited, the CYP2D6 ultra-rapid metabolizer (UM) phenotype has been associated with increased rates of vomiting after treatment with ondansetron. In one large study of patients with cancer, CYP2D6 UMs had higher rates of vomiting within the first 24 hours after chemotherapy administration.[130] The same relationship was identified in a large PONV cohort, where 45% of CYP2D6 UMs experienced vomiting episodes after treatment with ondansetron.[131] A smaller study in PONV identified patients with higher CYP2D6 activity experienced more severe PONV. However, this study only had one CYP2D6 UM, and results have not been confirmed.[132] Although CYP2D6 PMs have higher ondansetron concentrations, it is currently unknown whether this correlates with an increased risk for experiencing adverse events associated with ondansetron, such as QT prolongation or headache.

Treatment Recommendation

Current evidence supports that patients who are CYP2D6 UMs are at an increased risk for treatment failure when ondansetron is selected as a prophylactic antiemetic. Therefore, CPIC recommends avoiding the use of ondansetron in patients who are known to be CYP2D6 UMs.[133] Prior pharmacokinetic evidence suggests ondansetron dose increases would not be effective at normalizing ondansetron concentrations in CYP2D6 UMs.[129] CPIC recommends selecting an alternative antiemetic that is not predominately metabolized via CYP2D6 in these patients. Alternative 5-HT3 receptor antagonists include dolasetron, palonosetron, and granisetron. Both dolasetron and palonosetron are metabolized via CYP2D6, while granisetron is metabolized via CYP3A4. Granisetron is therefore recommended as the alternative treatment.[134] Although it is well known that CYP2D6 contributes to dolasetron and palonosetron metabolism, there is currently no clinical evidence to demonstrate an association between CYP2D6 phenotype and dolasetron and palonosetron treatment efficacy.

GERMLINE PHARMACOGENOMICS IN FDA DRUG LABELING

The FDA maintains a list of all medications that contain genetic information within medication package inserts in the Table of Pharmacogenomic Biomarkers in Drug Labeling, which is freely available on the FDA web page. This table does not differentiate between germline and somatic genetics, so both types of drug–gene interactions are represented. There is not a standard location for genetic information within drug labeling information, but it is frequently found in the warnings and precautions or clinical pharmacology sections. Another important consideration for evaluating pharmacogenomic information in the drug labeling is that the lack of a drug–gene interaction may be represented within the drug label and included within this table. For example, rucaparib is a PARP inhibitor that is linked with CYP2D6 and CYP1A2 in the pharmacogenomic biomarkers table. However, the drug labeling information states that there was no significant difference in the drug pharmacokinetics among CYP2D6 or CYP1A2 genotype groups, suggesting pharmacogenomics should not be used to guide rucaparib therapy. Additionally, some drug–gene pairs with strong associations are not included in the drug labeling information, such as allopurinol and HLA-B*58:01. Because CPIC does not provide recommendations on whether to conduct pharmacogenomic testing, this table is the best resource to identify which drug–gene pairs have required or recommended testing.

GENETIC TESTING IN PATIENTS WITH CANCER

Genetic testing in patients with cancer is increasing due to both an increase in screening for germline genetic predisposition genes such as BRCA and an increase in the number of targeted therapies approved for the treatment of cancers with specific somatic mutations. Many laboratories are beginning to test both the somatic and germline genome of patients with cancer. This source of genetic information represents a resource that clinicians can leverage for obtaining relevant pharmacogenomic information for their patients.[135] Clinicians should evaluate the availability of pre-existing germline genetic information for patients to identify if any of the test results can be used to personalize either the chemotherapy or the supportive care treatment plan that is developed.

CASE SCENARIOS

Case 1

KR is a 62-year-old Caucasian male who was recently diagnosed with unresectable metastatic colon cancer. KR also has a history of type 2 diabetes, moderate diabetic peripheral neuropathy, hypertension, and Gilbert syndrome. Genetic testing for KR was ordered to determine KRAS mutation status, and the laboratory also performed germline genetic testing. The genetic results for KR were reported as follows: KRAS mutation positive, DPD intermediate metabolizer (activity score =1), CYP2D6 ultra-rapid metabolizer. Based on these genetic results and KR's clinical comorbidities, KR's physician plans for treatment with 5-FU 400 mg/m² bolus then 1200 mg/m²/day continuous infusion for 2 days, leucovorin 400 mg/m2 on day 1, and irinotecan 180 mg/m² on day 1 (FOLFIRI) every 14 days. KR's physician plans to prescribe dexamethasone 10 mg IV on day 1 and ondansetron 8 mg IV on day 1 and 8 mg PO BID on days 2 to 3 for CINV prophylaxis. You are reviewing the medication orders for KR's cycle 1, day 1 chemotherapy treatment.

1. According to current clinical evidence and CPIC recommendations, which of the following would be the most appropriate recommendation for KR's 5-FU dosing?

a. KR's 5-FU dose should be decreased by 75% to decrease the risk of myelosuppression

b. KR should not receive 5-FU due to the increased risk for myelosuppression

c. KR's 5-FU dose should be decreased by 50% to decrease the risk of myelosuppression

d. KR's 5-FU dose should not be adjusted unless KR experiences 5-FU toxicity

Answer: KR is a DPD intermediate metabolizer, indicating he will have impaired metabolism of 5-FU when administered at standard doses, which is associated with an increased risk for toxicity. Answer c is the correct response, as current CPIC guidelines recommend decreasing the 5-FU dose by 50% in patients who are DPD intermediate metabolizers to decrease the risk of toxicity due to the decreased DPD metabolism.

2. Based on current clinical evidence, which of the following would be the most appropriate recommendation for KR's irinotecan dosing?

a. KR's irinotecan dose should be increased, as KR has increased UGT1A1 activity

b. KR's irinotecan dose should be decreased by 25% because KR has decreased UGT1A1 activity

c. KR's irinotecan dose should not be adjusted because KR has normal UGT1A1 activity

d. KR's UGT1A1 genotype is unknown, and no recommendation can be provided

Answer: Although KR does not have a UGT1A1 genotype included in the pharmacogenetic testing that was returned, KR's diagnosis of Gilbert syndrome is synonymous with the UGT1A1 poor metabolizer phenotype. The current FDA labeling for irinotecan recommends a 25% dose reduction in patients who are UGT1A1 poor metabolizers; therefore, answer b would be correct.

3. Based on the current evidence and CPIC recommendations, which of the following modifications would be most appropriate for KR's supportive care therapy?

a. KR's ondansetron dose should be doubled to decrease the risk of CINV

b. KR's ondansetron dose should not be adjusted unless he experiences toxicity

c. KR's ondansetron should be switched to palonosetron

d. KR's ondansetron should be switched to granisetron

Answer: KR's testing identified he is a CYP2D6 ultra-rapid metabolizer. CYP2D6 is responsible for the inactivation of ondansetron, and use of ondansetron in CYP2D6 ultra-rapid metabolizers has been associated with reduced treatment efficacy. Current CPIC guidelines recommend selecting an alternative antiemetic therapy that is not metabolized via CYP2D6 in these patients. Palonosetron is also a CYP2D6 substrate, while granisetron is a CYP3A4 substrate; therefore, answer d, to switch to granisetron, is the correct answer.

Case 2

EM is a 15-year-old Asian male who is undergoing therapy for high-risk B-cell, Ph-negative, ALL. EM undergoes genetic testing for TPMT and is found to be a TPMT normal metabolizer (*1/*1 genotype). He begins maintenance therapy with daily oral mercaptopurine and weekly oral methotrexate. After two weeks of maintenance therapy EM experiences grade 3 neutropenia and is hospitalized for febrile neutropenia.

1. Which of the following additional pharmacogenetic tests would be most appropriate to recommend for EM to determine the cause of the neutropenia and guide further treatment decisions?

a. TPMT enzyme activity test

b. NUDT15 genotype test

c. SLCO1B1 genotype test

d. Confirm TPMT genotype test

Answer: TPMT and NUDT15 genotypes have both been associated with thiopurine toxicity. TPMT genetic variants are most common in Caucasian and African ethnicities, while NUDT15 genetic variants are more common in Asian ethnicities. Because of EM's ethnicity, the most appropriate test to guide further treatment decisions would be a NUDT15 genotype test, answer b.

2. EM's physician orders a panel pharmacogenetic test and the following pharmacogenetic results are returned: NUDT15 intermediate metabolizer (NUDT15 *1/*2), SLCO1B1 intermediate function (*1/*5), CEP72 normal function. Which of the following therapeutic recommendations would be most appropriate for EM's treatment based on his recent genetic results?

a. Decrease the methotrexate dose by 50%

b. Decrease the mercaptopurine dose by 50%

c. Neither a nor b

d. Both a and b

Answer: The NUDT15 genotype contributes to mercaptopurine toxicity. The SLCO1B1 genotype has been associated with methotrexate tolerability. However, only NUDT15 and mercaptopurine currently have clinical guideline recommendations for how to modify drug therapy based on the genotype result. Therefore, the only dose adjustment that can be confidently recommended is a decrease in the mercaptopurine dose, answer b.

Case 3

JM is a 42-year-old female diagnosed with early stage, ER+/PR+/HER2– breast cancer. The tumor has low recurrence risk, and you have decided to initiate tamoxifen treatment.

1. What pharmacogenetic testing would be appropriate to order at this time?
   a. CYP2D6 testing to inform tamoxifen dosing
   b. Pharmacogenetic panel testing to inform tamoxifen dosing
   c. Pharmacogenetic panel testing to inform dosing of tamoxifen and supportive care
   d. No testing is warranted at this time

Answer: The correct answer is d. While there are dosing guidelines for tamoxifen from CPIC and for other potentially relevant supportive care agents, there is no indication for preemptive pharmacogenetic testing.

2. Although you didn't order pharmacogenetic testing, your patient informs you that she was previously genotyped and is CYP2D6*5/*5. What is her activity score and metabolizer phenotype?

CYP2D6 Allele	Activity Score
*1	1
*2	1
*3	0
*4	0
*5	0

CYP2D6 Phenotype	Activity Score
Ultra-rapid metabolizer	>2.25
Normal metabolizer	1.25–2.25
Intermediate metabolizer	0.25–1
Poor metabolizer	0

   a. Activity score = 0, Poor metabolizer
   b. Activity score = 1.0, Intermediate metabolizer
   c. Activity score = 2.0, Normal metabolizer
   d. Activity score = 4.0, Ultra-rapid metabolizer

Answer: The correct answer is a. A CYP2D6*5 allele has an activity score of 0.0, so this patient would have a total activity score of 0.0, which makes them a CYP2D6 poor metabolizer.

3. Based on the patient's known genotype and CYP2D6 metabolizer activity, what would be her appropriate treatment regimen based on CPIC guidelines?
   a. CPIC guidelines recommend using tamoxifen 20 mg/day in patients, regardless of their genotype
   b. CPIC guidelines recommend a tamoxifen dose reduction to 10 mg/day in this patient due to their poor metabolizer phenotype
   c. CPIC guidelines recommend a tamoxifen dose escalation to 40 mg/day in this patient due to their poor metabolizer phenotype
   d. CPIC has not published guidelines for tamoxifen dosing based on CYP2D6 genotype

Answer: The correct answer is c. CPIC guidelines for tamoxifen dosing in patients with known CYP2D6 genotype recommend considering dose escalation to 40 mg/day in poor metabolizers. This is due to their limited ability to activate tamoxifen to endoxifen. Dose escalation to 40 mg/day in poor and intermediate metabolizers has been demonstrated to increase systemic endoxifen concentrations without increasing treatment-related toxicity. However, there is a lack of prospective evidence that increasing the dose or endoxifen concentration will improve treatment efficacy.

PHARMACOGENOMICS CLINICAL PEARLS

- Oncology pharmacogenomics has considerations for more than one genome: the tumor genome (somatic) and the inherited genome (germline).
- Genetics can be used to identify targeted therapies for patients whose cancer carries a specific somatic mutation or patients who carry a cancer predisposition variant.
- Germline pharmacogenomics can help to predict the efficacy and toxicity of anticancer and supportive care treatments.

- Patients who have variants in TPMT and NUDT15 are at an increased risk for potentially life-threatening myelosuppression when treated with thiopurines.
- Preemptively decreasing fluoropyrimidine doses in DPD intermediate metabolizers decreases the risk of toxicity during treatment.
- UGT1A1-guided dosing could decrease the risk of toxicity with irinotecan and belinostat therapy.

- Rasburicase and allopurinol, both used to treat tumor lysis syndrome, are affected by germline pharmacogenetics that can predict adverse events.
- CYP2D6 phenotype may help to explain ondansetron treatment failure.
- Clinicians should consider existing germline genetic data in treatment decisions when it is available from previous genetic testing.

KEY TERMS, ABBREVIATIONS AND ACRONYMS

Germline: Inherited DNA sequence

Somatic: Acquired genetic changes

CPIC: Clinical Pharmacogenetics Implementation Consortium

FDA: Food and Drug Administration

TPMT: Thiopurine methyltransferase

NUDT15: Nudix T hydrolase

DPYD: Dihydropyrimidine Dehydrogenase gene

DPD: Dihydropyrimidine Dehydrogenase enzyme

UGT1A1: Uridine diphosphate glucuronosyltransferase 1A1

SLCO1B1: Solute carrier organic anion transporter 1B1

CEP72: Centrosomal protein 72

CYP2D6: Cytochrome P450 2D6

G6PD: Glucose-6-phosphate dehydrogenase

HLA-B: Human leukocyte antigen-B

UM: Ultra-rapid metabolizer

NM: Normal metabolizer

IM: Intermediate metabolizer

PM: Poor metabolizer

REFERENCES

1. Ettinger DS, W.D., Aisner DL, et al. *NCCN Clinical Practice Guidelines in Oncology: Non-Small Cell Lung Cancer. Version 2.2020.* Accessed May 5, 2020.

2. VITRAKVI (larotrectinib) [package insert]. Stamford, CT: Loxo Oncology, Inc.; 2018.

3. Brown P, I.H., Annesley C, et al. *NCCN Clinical Practice Guidelines in Oncology: Pediatric Acute Lymphoblastic Leukemia. Version 1.2020.* 2019. Available at https://www.nccn.org/professionals/physician_gls/default.aspx. Accessed May 5, 2020.

4. Brown P, Wieduwilt M, Logan A, et al. *NCCN Clinical Practice Guidelines in Oncology: Acute Lymphoblastic Leukemia. Version 1.2019.* 2019. Available at nccn.org. Accessed May 5, 2020.

5. Remy CN. Metabolism of thiopyrimidines and thiopurines. S-Methylation with S-adenosylmethionine transmethylase and catabolism in mammalian tissues. *J Biol Chem.* 1963;238:1078–1084.

6. Zaza G, Cheok M, Krynetskaia N, et al. Thiopurine pathway. *Pharmacogenet Genomics.* 2010;20(9):573–574.

7. CPIC. CPIC Guideline for Thiopurines and TPMT and NUDT15. TPMT frequency table. 2018. Available at https://cpicpgx.org/guidelines/guideline-for-thiopurines-and-tpmt/. Accessed May 5, 2020.

8. PharmGKB. Gene-Specific Information Tables for TPMT.

9. Wiwattanakul S, et al. Development and validation of a reliable method for thiopurine methyltransferase (TPMT) enzyme activity in human whole blood by LC-MS/MS: An application for phenotypic and genotypic correlations. *J Pharm Biomed Anal.* 2017;145:758–764.

10. Cheung ST, Allan RN. Mistaken identity: Misclassification of TPMT phenotype following blood transfusion. *Eur J Gastroenterol Hepatol.* 2003;15(11):1245–1247.

11. Moriyama T, et al. NUDT15 polymorphisms alter thiopurine metabolism and hematopoietic toxicity. *Nat Genet.* 2016;48(4):367–373.

12. Yang SK, et al. A common missense variant in NUDT15 confers susceptibility to thiopurine-induced leukopenia. *Nat Genet.* 2014;46(9):1017–1020.

13. CPIC. CPIC Guideline for Thiopurines and TPMT and NUDT15. NUDT15 Frequency Table. 2018. Available at https://cpicpgx.org/guidelines/guideline-for-thiopurines-and-tpmt/. Accessed May 5, 2020..

14. Yang JJ, et al. Inherited NUDT15 variant is a genetic determinant of mercaptopurine intolerance in children with acute lymphoblastic leukemia. *J Clin Oncol.* 2015;33(11):1235–1242.

15. PharmGKB. Gene-Specific Information Tables for NUDT15.

16. Schaeffeler E, et al. Impact of NUDT15 genetics on severe thio-purine-related hematotoxicity in patients with European ancestry. *Genet Med.* 2019;21(9):2145–2150.

17. Zhu Y, et al. Combination of common and novel rare NUDT15 variants improves predictive sensitivity of thiopurine-induced leuko-penia in children with acute lymphoblastic leukemia. *Haematologica.* 2018;103(7):e293–e295.

18. Relling MV, et al. Mercaptopurine therapy intolerance and hetero-zygosity at the thiopurine S-methyltransferase gene locus. *J Natl Cancer Inst.* 1999; 91(23):2001–2008.

19. Lennard L, et al. Thiopurine pharmacogenetics in leukemia: cor-relation of erythrocyte thiopurine methyltransferase activity and 6-thioguanine nucleotide concentrations. *Clin Pharmacol Ther.* 1987;41(1):18–25.

20. Moriyama T, et al. The effects of inherited NUDT15 polymorphisms on thiopurine active metabolites in Japanese children with acute lym-phoblastic leukemia. *Pharmacogenet Genomics.* 2017;27(6):236–239.

21. Relling MV, et al. Prognostic importance of 6-mercaptopu-rine dose intensity in acute lymphoblastic leukemia. *Blood.* 1999;93(9):2817–2823.

22. Relling MV, et al. Clinical Pharmacogenetics Implementation Consortium guideline for thiopurine dosing based on TPMT and NUDT15 genotypes: 2018 update. *Clin Pharmacol Ther.* 2019;105(5):1095–1105.

23. Mercaptopurine [package insert]. Coral Springs, FL: Quinn Pharmaceuticals, LLC; 2018.

24. Relling MV, et al. Thiopurine methyltransferase in acute lympho-blastic leukemia. *Blood.* 2006;107(2): 843–8444.

25. Conroy T, et al. FOLFIRINOX versus gemcitabine for metastatic pancreatic cancer. *N Engl J Med.* 2011;364(19):1817–1825.

26. Andre T, et al. Oxaliplatin, fluorouracil, and leucovorin as adjuvant treatment for colon cancer. *N Engl J Med.* 2004;350(23):2343–2351.

27. Gelmon K, Chan A, Harbeck N. The role of capecitabine in first-line treatment for patients with metastatic breast cancer. *Oncologist.* 2006;11(Suppl 1): 42–51.

28. Masuda N, et al. Adjuvant capecitabine for breast cancer after preop-erative chemotherapy. *N Engl J Med.* 2017;376(22):2147–2159.

29. Ison G, et al. FDA approval: Uridine triacetate for the treatment of patients following fluorouracil or capecitabine overdose or exhibiting early-onset severe toxicities following administration of these drugs. *Clin Cancer Res.* 2016;22(18):4545–4549.

30. Maring JG, et al. Reduced 5-FU clearance in a patient with low DPD activity due to heterozygosity for a mutant allele of the DPYD gene. *Br J Cancer.* 2002;86(7):1028–1033.

31. Meulendijks D, et al. Clinical relevance of DPYD variants c.1679T>G, c.1236G>A/HapB3, and c.1601G>A as predic-tors of severe fluoropyrimidine-associated toxicity: A systematic review and meta-analysis of individual patient data. *Lancet Oncol.* 2015;16(16):1639–1650.

32. PharmGKB. Gene-Specific Information Tables for DPYD. Available at https://www.pharmgkb.org/page/dpydRefMaterials.

33. Rai K, Batukbhai BDO, Brooks GA. Risk of treatment-related death in carriers of pathogenic DPYD polymorphisms treated with fluoropyrimidine chemotherapy: A systematic review and patient-level analysis. *J Clin Oncol.* 2019;37(Suppl 15):e15132.

34. Amstutz U, et al. Clinical Pharmacogenetics Implementation Consortium (CPIC) guideline for dihydropyrimidine dehydro-genase genotype and fluoropyrimidine dosing: 2017 update. *Clin Pharmacol Ther.* 2018;103(2):210–216.

35. Deenen MJ, Cats A, Sechterberger MK, et al. Safety, pharmacokinet-ics (PK), and cost-effectiveness of upfront genotyping of DPYD in fluoropyrimidine therapy. *ASCO Meeting Abstracts.* 2011;29:3606.

36. Henricks LM, et al. DPYD genotype-guided dose individualisation of fluoropyrimidine therapy: Who and how?—Authors' reply. *Lancet Oncol.* 2019;20(2):e67.

37. Henricks LM, et al. Capecitabine-based treatment of a patient with a novel DPYD genotype and complete dihydropyrimidine dehydro-genase deficiency. *Int J Cancer.* 2018;142(2):424–430.

38. Paoluzzi L, et al. Influence of genetic variants in UGT1A1 and UGT1A9 on the in vivo glucuronidation of SN-38. *J Clin Pharmacol.* 2004;44(8):854–860.

39. Stewart CF, et al. UGT1A1 promoter genotype correlates with SN-38 pharmacokinetics, but not severe toxicity in patients receiv-ing low-dose irinotecan. *J Clin Oncol.* 2007;25(18):2594–2600.

40. Toffoli G, et al. The role of UGT1A1*28 polymorphism in the phar-macodynamics and pharmacokinetics of irinotecan in patients with metastatic colorectal cancer. *J Clin Oncol.* 2006;24(19):3061–3068.

41. Innocenti F, et al. Genetic variants in the UDP-glucuronosy-ltransferase 1A1 gene predict the risk of severe neutropenia of irinotecan. *J Clin Oncol.* 2004;22(8):1382–1388.

42. Iyer L, et al. UGT1A1*28 polymorphism as a determinant of irinote-can disposition and toxicity. *Pharmacogenomics J.* 2002;2(1):43–47.

43. Hazama S, et al. Phase I study of irinotecan and doxifluridine for metastatic colorectal cancer focusing on the UGT1A1*28 polymor-phism. *Cancer Sci.* 2010;101(3):722–727.

44. Satoh T, et al. Genotype-directed, dose-finding study of irinotecan in cancer patients with UGT1A1*28 and/or UGT1A1*6 polymor-phisms. *Cancer Sci.* 2011;102(10):1868–1873.

45. Sharma MR, et al. A UGT1A1 genotype-guided dosing study of modified FOLFIRINOX in previously untreated patients with advanced gastrointestinal malignancies. *Cancer.* 2019;125(10): 1629–1636.

46. Paez D, et al. Pharmacogenetic clinical randomised phase II trial to evaluate the efficacy and safety of FOLFIRI with high-dose irinote-can (HD-FOLFIRI) in metastatic colorectal cancer patients accord-ing to their UGT1A 1 genotype. *Br J Cancer.* 2019;120(2):190–195.

47. McWilliams RR, et al. North Central Cancer Treatment Group N0543 (Alliance): A phase 2 trial of pharmacogenetic-based dos-ing of irinotecan, oxaliplatin, and capecitabine as first-line therapy for patients with advanced small bowel adenocarcinoma. *Cancer.* 2017;123(18):3494–3501.

48. Boisdron-Celle M, et al. A multicenter phase II study of personal-ized FOLFIRI-cetuximab for safe dose intensification. *Semin Oncol.* 2017;44(1):24–33.

49. Fujii H, et al. Dose adjustment of irinotecan based on UGT1A1 polymorphisms in patients with colorectal cancer. *Cancer Chemother Pharmacol.* 2019;83(1):123–129.

50. Swen JJ, et al. Pharmacogenetics: From bench to byte—An update of guidelines. *Clin Pharmacol Ther.* 2011;89(5):662–673.

51. Hershman DL, et al. Prevention and management of chemotherapy-induced peripheral neuropathy in survivors of adult cancers:

American Society of Clinical Oncology clinical practice guideline. *J Clin Oncol.* 2014;32(18):1941–1967.

52. Singer JB, et al. UGT1A1 promoter polymorphism increases risk of nilotinib-induced hyperbilirubinemia. *Leukemia.* 2007;21(11): 2311–2315.

53. Motzer RJ, et al. Hyperbilirubinemia in pazopanib- or sunitinib-treated patients in COMPARZ is associated with UGT1A1 polymorphisms. *Ann Oncol.* 2013;24(11):2927–2928.

54. Xu CF, et al. Pazopanib-induced hyperbilirubinemia is associated with Gilbert's syndrome UGT1A1 polymorphism. *Br J Cancer.* 2010;102(9):1371–1377.

55. Wang LZ, et al. Glucuronidation by UGT1A1 is the dominant pathway of the metabolic disposition of belinostat in liver cancer patients. *PLoS One.* 2013;8(1):e54522.

56. Peer CJ, et al. UGT1A1 genotype-dependent dose adjustment of belinostat in patients with advanced cancers using population pharmacokinetic modeling and simulation. *J Clin Pharmacol.* 2016;56(4):450–460.

57. Beleodaq (belinostat) [package insert]. Irvine, CA: Spectrum Pharmaceuticals, Inc.; 2014.

58. Goey AK, et al. Effects of UGT1A1 genotype on the pharmacokinetics, pharmacodynamics, and toxicities of belinostat administered by 48-hour continuous infusion in patients with cancer. *J Clin Pharmacol.* 2016;56(4):461–473.

59. Balasubramaniam S, et al. Phase I trial of belinostat with cisplatin and etoposide in advanced solid tumors, with a focus on neuroendocrine and small cell cancers of the lung. *Anticancer Drugs.* 2018;29(5):457–465.

60. van de Steeg E, et al. Methotrexate pharmacokinetics in transgenic mice with liver-specific expression of human organic anion-transporting polypeptide 1B1 (SLCO1B1). *Drug Metab Dispos.* 2009;37(2):277–281.

61. Kameyama Y, et al. Functional characterization of SLCO1B1 (OATP-C) variants, SLCO1B1*5, SLCO1B1*15 and SLCO1B1*15+C1007G, by using transient expression systems of HeLa and HEK293 cells. *Pharmacogenet Genomics.* 2005;15(7):513–522.

62. Ramsey LB, et al. The clinical pharmacogenetics implementation consortium guideline for SLCO1B1 and simvastatin-induced myopathy: 2014 update. *Clin Pharmacol Ther.* 2014;96(4):423–428.

63. Biermann JS, Chow W, Adkins DR, et al. NCCN *Clinical Practice Guidelines in Oncology: Bone Cancer.* Version 1.2020. 2019. Accessed May 5, 2020.

64. Liu SG, et al. Polymorphisms in methotrexate transporters and their relationship to plasma methotrexate levels, toxicity of high-dose methotrexate, and outcome of pediatric acute lymphoblastic leukemia. *Oncotarget.* 2017;8(23):37761–37772.

65. Zhang HN, et al. Impact of SLCO1B1 521T > C variant on leucovorin rescue and risk of relapse in childhood acute lymphoblastic leukemia treated with high-dose methotrexate. *Pediatr Blood Cancer.* 2014;61(12):2203–2207.

66. Ramsey LB, et al. Genome-wide study of methotrexate clearance replicates SLCO1B1. *Blood.* 2013;121(6):898–904.

67. Goricar K, et al. Influence of the folate pathway and transporter polymorphisms on methotrexate treatment outcome in osteosarcoma. *Pharmacogenet Genomics.* 2014;24(10):514–521.

68. Radtke S, et al. Germline genetic variations in methotrexate candidate genes are associated with pharmacokinetics, toxicity, and outcome in childhood acute lymphoblastic leukemia. *Blood.* 2013;121(26):5145–5153.

69. Trevino LR, et al. Germline genetic variation in an organic anion transporter polypeptide associated with methotrexate pharmacokinetics and clinical effects. *J Clin Oncol.* 2009;27(35):5972–5978.

70. Yang L, et al. SLCO1B1 rs4149056 genetic polymorphism predicting methotrexate toxicity in Chinese patients with non-Hodgkin lymphoma. *Pharmacogenomics.* 2017;18(17):1557–1562.

71. Mora E, et al. Vincristine-induced peripheral neuropathy in pediatric cancer patients. *Am J Cancer Res.* 2016;6(11):2416–2430.

72. Diouf B, et al. Association of an inherited genetic variant with vincristine-related peripheral neuropathy in children with acute lymphoblastic leukemia. *JAMA.* 2015;313(8):815–823.

73. Stock W, et al. An inherited genetic variant in CEP72 promoter predisposes to vincristine-induced peripheral neuropathy in adults with acute lymphoblastic leukemia. *Clin Pharmacol Ther.* 2017;101(3):391–395.

74. Wright GEB, et al. Pharmacogenomics of vincristine-induced peripheral neuropathy implicates pharmacokinetic and inherited neuropathy genes. *Clin Pharmacol Ther.* 2019;105(2):402–410.

75. Gutierrez-Camino A, et al. Lack of association of the CEP72 rs924607 TT genotype with vincristine-related peripheral neuropathy during the early phase of pediatric acute lymphoblastic leukemia treatment in a Spanish population. *Pharmacogenet Genomics.* 2016;26(2):100–102.

76. Zgheib NK, et al. Genetic polymorphisms in candidate genes are not associated with increased vincristine-related peripheral neuropathy in Arab children treated for acute childhood leukemia: A single institution study. *Pharmacogenet Genomics.* 2018;28(8):189–195.

77. Li L, et al. Genetic variants associated with vincristine-induced peripheral neuropathy in two populations of children with acute lymphoblastic leukemia. *Clin Pharmacol Ther.* 2019;105(6):1421–1428.

78. Early Breast Cancer Trialists' Collaborative Group, et al. Relevance of breast cancer hormone receptors and other factors to the efficacy of adjuvant tamoxifen: Patient-level meta-analysis of randomised trials. *Lancet.* 2011;378(9793):771–784.

79. Murdter TE, et al. Activity levels of tamoxifen metabolites at the estrogen receptor and the impact of genetic polymorphisms of phase I and II enzymes on their concentration levels in plasma. *Clin Pharmacol Ther.* 2011;89(5):708–717.

80. Ingelman-Sundberg M. Genetic polymorphisms of cytochrome P450 2D6 (CYP2D6): Clinical consequences, evolutionary aspects and functional diversity. *Pharmacogenomics J.* 2005;5(1):6–13.

81. Jin Y, et al. CYP2D6 genotype, antidepressant use, and tamoxifen metabolism during adjuvant breast cancer treatment. *J Natl Cancer Inst.* 2005;97(1):30–39.

82. Hertz DL, et al. In vivo assessment of the metabolic activity of CYP2D6 diplotypes and alleles. *Br J Clin Pharmacol.* 2015;80(5):1122–1130.

83. Caudle KE, et al. Standardizing CYP2D6 genotype to phenotype translation: consensus recommendations from the Clinical Pharmacogenetics Implementation Consortium and Dutch Pharmacogenetics Working Group. *Clin Transl Sci.* 2020;13(1):116–124.

84. Gaedigk A, et al. The CYP2D6 activity score: Translating genotype information into a qualitative measure of phenotype. *Clin Pharmacol Ther.* 2008;83(2):234–242.

85. Marcath LA, et al. Comprehensive assessment of cytochromes P450 and transporter genetics with endoxifen concentration during tamoxifen treatment. *Pharmacogenet Genomics*. 2017;27(11):402–409.

86. Teft WA, et al. CYP3A4 and seasonal variation in vitamin D status in addition to CYP2D6 contribute to therapeutic endoxifen level during tamoxifen therapy. *Breast Cancer Res Treat*. 2013;139(1):95–105.

87. Powers JL, et al. Multigene and drug interaction approach for tamoxifen metabolite patterns reveals possible involvement of CYP2C9, CYP2C19, and ABCB1. *J Clin Pharmacol*. 2016;56(12):1570–1581.

88. Madlensky L, et al. Tamoxifen metabolite concentrations, CYP2D6 genotype, and breast cancer outcomes. *Clin Pharmacol Ther*. 2011;89(5):718–725.

89. Saladores P, et al. Tamoxifen metabolism predicts drug concentrations and outcome in premenopausal patients with early breast cancer. *Pharmacogenomics J*. 2015;15(1):84–94.

90. Helland T, et al. Serum concentrations of active tamoxifen metabolites predict long-term survival in adjuvantly treated breast cancer patients. *Breast Cancer Res*. 2017;19(1):125.

91. Lintermans A, V.A.K., Jongen L, et al. Prospective study evaluating the effect of impaired tamoxifen metabolisation on efficacy in breast cancer patients receiving tamoxifen in the neo-adjuvant or metastatic setting. ASCO Meeting Abstracts. 2016;34:523.

92. Love RR, et al. CYP2D6 genotypes, endoxifen levels, and disease recurrence in 224 Filipino and Vietnamese women receiving adjuvant tamoxifen for operable breast cancer. *Springerplus*. 2013;2(1):52.

93. Sanchez-Spitman A, et al. Tamoxifen pharmacogenetics and metabolism: Results from the prospective CYPTAM study. *J Clin Oncol*. 2019;37(8):636–646.

94. Hertz DL, McLeod HL, Irvin WJ Jr. Tamoxifen and CYP2D6: A contradiction of data. *Oncologist*. 2012;17(5):620–630.

95. Hertz DL, Rae JM. One step at a time: CYP2D6 guided tamoxifen treatment awaits convincing evidence of clinical validity. *Pharmacogenomics*. 2016;17(8):823–826.

96. Province MA, et al. CYP2D6 genotype and adjuvant tamoxifen: Meta-analysis of heterogeneous study populations. *Clin Pharmacol Ther*. 2014;95(2):216–227.

97. Berry DA. CYP2D6 genotype and adjuvant tamoxifen. *Clin Pharmacol Ther*. 2014;96(2):138–140.

98. Kiyotani K, et al. Important and critical scientific aspects in pharmacogenomics analysis: Lessons from controversial results of tamoxifen and CYP2D6 studies. *J Hum Genet*. 2013;58(6):327–333.

99. Hertz DL, et al. Tamoxifen dose escalation in patients with diminished CYP2D6 activity normalizes endoxifen concentrations without increasing toxicity. *Oncologist*. 2016;21(7):795–803.

100. Irvin WJ Jr. et al. Genotype-guided tamoxifen dosing increases active metabolite exposure in women with reduced CYP2D6 metabolism: A multicenter study. *J Clin Oncol*. 2011;29(24):3232–3239.

101. Fox P, et al. Dose escalation of tamoxifen in patients with low endoxifen level: Evidence for therapeutic drug monitoring—The TADE study. *Clin Cancer Res*. 2016;22(13):3164–3171.

102. Kiyotani K, et al. Dose-adjustment study of tamoxifen based on CYP2D6 genotypes in Japanese breast cancer patients. *Breast Cancer Res Treat*. 2012;131(1):137–145.

103. Goetz MP, et al. Clinical Pharmacogenetics Implementation Consortium (CPIC) guideline for CYP2D6 and tamoxifen therapy. *Clin Pharmacol Ther*. 2018;103(5):770–777.

104. Elitek (rasburicase) [package insert]. New York, NY: Sanofi-Aventis U.S. LLC; 2017.

105. Coiffier B, et al. Guidelines for the management of pediatric and adult tumor lysis syndrome: An evidence-based review. *J Clin Oncol*. 2008;26(16):2767–2778.

106. Cappellini MD, Fiorelli G. Glucose-6-phosphate dehydrogenase deficiency. *Lancet*. 2008;371(9606):64–74.

107. McDonagh EM, et al. PharmGKB summary: Very important pharmacogene information for G6PD. *Pharmacogenet Genomics*. 2012;22(3):219–228.

108. WHO Working Group. Glucose-6-phosphate dehydrogenase deficiency. *Bull World Health Organ*. 1989;67(6):601–611.

109. Lim F, Vulliamy T, Abdalla SH. An Ashkenazi Jewish woman presenting with favism. *J Clin Pathol*. 2005;58(3):317–319.

110. Akande M, Audino AN, Tobias JD. Rasburicase-induced hemolytic anemia in an adolescent with unknown glucose-6-phosphate dehydrogenase deficiency. *J Pediatr Pharmacol Ther*. 2017;22(6):471–475.

111. Ferguson D, Kovach AE. Rasburicase-induced hemolytic anemia in previously undiagnosed G6PD deficiency. *Blood*. 2018;132(6):673.

112. Sherwood GB, Paschal RD, Adamski J. Rasburicase-induced methemoglobinemia: Case report, literature review, and proposed treatment algorithm. *Clin Case Rep*. 2016;4(4):315–319.

113. Relling MV, et al. Clinical Pharmacogenetics Implementation Consortium (CPIC) guidelines for rasburicase therapy in the context of G6PD deficiency genotype. *Clin Pharmacol Ther*. 2014;96(2):169–174.

114. Saito Y, et al. Clinical Pharmacogenetics Implementation Consortium (CPIC) guidelines for human leukocyte antigen B (HLA-B) genotype and allopurinol dosing: 2015 update. *Clin Pharmacol Ther*. 2016;99(1):36–37.

115. CPIC. Frequencies of HLA-B and HLA-A variants in major race/ethnic groups. 2017. Available at https://cpicpgx.org/guidelines/guideline-for-carbamazepine-and-hla-b/. Accessed May 5, 2020.

116. Fan WL, Shiao MS, Hui RC, et al. HLA association with drug-induced adverse reactions. *J Immunol Res*. 2017;2017:3186328.

117. Cao ZH, et al. HLA-B*58:01 allele is associated with augmented risk for both mild and severe cutaneous adverse reactions induced by allopurinol in Han Chinese. *Pharmacogenomics*. 2012;13(10):1193–1201.

118. Chiu ML, et al. Association between HLA-B*58:01 allele and severe cutaneous adverse reactions with allopurinol in Han Chinese in Hong Kong. *Br J Dermatol*. 2012;167(1):44–49.

119. Hung SI, et al. HLA-B*5801 allele as a genetic marker for severe cutaneous adverse reactions caused by allopurinol. *Proc Natl Acad Sci U S A*. 2005;102(11):4134–4139.

120. Tassaneeyakul W, et al. Strong association between HLA-B*5801 and allopurinol-induced Stevens-Johnson syndrome and toxic epidermal necrolysis in a Thai population. *Pharmacogenet Genomics*. 2009;19(9):704–709.

121. Stamp LK, et al. Starting dose is a risk factor for allopurinol hypersensitivity syndrome: A proposed safe starting dose of allopurinol. *Arthritis Rheum*. 2012;64(8):2529–2536.

122. Chung WH, et al. Insights into the poor prognosis of allopurinol-induced severe cutaneous adverse reactions: The impact of renal insufficiency, high plasma levels of oxypurinol and granulysin. *Ann Rheum Dis.* 2015;74(12):2157–2164.

123. Park HW, et al. Efficacy of the HLA-B(*)58:01 screening test in preventing allopurinol-induced severe cutaneous adverse reactions in patients with chronic renal insufficiency—A prospective study. *J Allergy Clin Immunol Pract.* 2019;7(4):1271–1276.

124. Ko TM, et al. Use of HLA-B*58:01 genotyping to prevent allopurinol induced severe cutaneous adverse reactions in Taiwan: National prospective cohort study. *BMJ.* 2015;351:h4848.

125. Khanna D, et al. 2012 American College of Rheumatology guidelines for management of gout. Part 1: Systematic nonpharmacologic and pharmacologic therapeutic approaches to hyperuricemia. *Arthritis Care Res (Hoboken).* 2012;64(10):1431–1446.

126. Ponzo MG, et al. HLA-B*58:01 genotyping to prevent cases of DRESS and SJS/TEN in East Asians treated with allopurinol—A Canadian missed opportunity. *J Cutan Med Surg.* 2019:1203475419867599.

127. Berger MJ, et al. NCCN Guidelines insights: Antiemesis, Version 2.2017. *J Natl Compr Canc Netw.* 2017;15(7):883–893.

128. Fischer V, et al. The polymorphic cytochrome P-4502D6 is involved in the metabolism of both 5-hydroxytryptamine antagonists, tropisetron and ondansetron. *Drug Metab Dispos.* 1994;22(2):269–274.

129. Stamer UM, et al. CYP2D6- and CYP3A-dependent enantioselective plasma concentrations of ondansetron in postanesthesia care. *Anesth Analg.* 2011;113(1):48–54.

130. Kaiser R, et al. Patient-tailored antiemetic treatment with 5-hydroxytryptamine type 3 receptor antagonists according to cytochrome P-450 2D6 genotypes. *J Clin Oncol.* 2002;20(12):2805–2811.

131. Candiotti KA, et al. The impact of pharmacogenomics on postoperative nausea and vomiting: Do CYP2D6 allele copy number and polymorphisms affect the success or failure of ondansetron prophylaxis? *Anesthesiology.* 2005;102(3):543–549.

132. Niewinski PA, et al. CYP2D6 basic genotyping as a potential tool to improve the antiemetic efficacy of ondansetron in prophylaxis of postoperative nausea and vomiting. *Adv Clin Exp Med.* 2018;27(11):1499–1503.

133. Bell GC, et al. Clinical Pharmacogenetics Implementation Consortium (CPIC) guideline for CYP2D6 genotype and use of ondansetron and tropisetron. *Clin Pharmacol Ther.* 2017;102(2):213–218.

134. Janicki PK. Cytochrome P450 2D6 metabolism and 5-hydroxytryptamine type 3 receptor antagonists for postoperative nausea and vomiting. *Med Sci Monit.* 2005;11(10):RA322–RA328.

135. Hertz DL, McLeod HL. Integrated patient and tumor genetic testing for individualized cancer therapy. *Clin Pharmacol Ther.* 2016;99(2):143–146.

CHAPTER 8

PSYCHIATRY AND NEUROLOGY PHARMACOGENOMICS

Kimberly Hamann, Rachel A. Daut, and Mary A. Gutierrez

LEARNING OBJECTIVES

1. Recognize and interpret common pharmacogenomic relationships that affect adverse events or efficacy of medications used to treat psychiatric and neurological conditions.

2. Utilize the available information of pharmacogenomics for the treatment of psychiatric and neurological disorders.

ANTIDEPRESSANTS AND ANTIPSYCHOTICS

Selective serotonin reuptake inhibitors (SSRIs) are first-line pharmacotherapy options for depression.[1] The six traditional SSRIs (citalopram, escitalopram, fluoxetine, fluvoxamine, paroxetine, and sertraline) function by blocking the serotonin transporter, preventing reuptake of serotonin into the presynaptic neuron. This is thought to lead to elevated serotonin levels in the synapse and therefore increase the amount of serotonin available to bind to postsynaptic receptors.

SSRIs and *CYP2D6* and *CYP2C19*

Many CYP450 genes are involved in the metabolism of SSRIs, and the Clinical Pharmacogenetics Implementation Consortium (CPIC) has issued guidelines on prescribing SSRIs in the presence of genetic variation in two important pathways: *CYP2D6* and

CYP2C19. The clinical impact of genetic variation in these pathways on SSRI metabolism is addressed next.

Mechanism of Drug–Gene Interaction

In addition to the potential biological activity of the resulting metabolite, the impact of genetic variation on a drug's metabolism depends on the overall contribution of the enzymatic pathway. Because *CYP2D6* and *CYP2C19* genes are involved in the metabolism of SSRIs, variation in these pathways can have significant effects on drug efficacy and safety.

Consequence of Drug–Gene Interaction

Paroxetine and fluoxetine rely heavily on *CYP2D6* for biotransformation. Fluvoxamine is metabolized by both *CYP2D6* and *CYP1A2*. For this reason, *CYP2D6* variation may greatly affect the activity of these SSRIs. *CYP2D6* ultrarapid metabolizers (UMs) have been shown to have low or undetectable paroxetine plasma concentrations compared to extensive metabolizers (EMs), putting individuals with this phenotype at risk of therapeutic failure.[2–5] However, while one might reasonably expect to see a decrease in plasma concentrations of fluvoxamine in *CYP2D6* UMs, data are currently lacking. For both paroxetine and fluvoxamine, *CYP2D6* poor metabolizers (PMs) have significantly greater drug exposure.[2,6–8]

On the other hand, *CYP2C19* is a major pathway for the biotransformation of citalopram, escitalopram, and sertraline, and thus variations in this gene may alter drug exposure. For citalopram and escitalopram, studies have shown that *CYP2C19* UMs have significantly lower drug exposure and therefore increased risk of therapeutic failure.[9–11] It would be reasonable to expect a similar trend for *CYP2C19* UMs taking sertraline; however, limited published data for these individuals show only slightly increased metabolism.[12] The *CYP2C19* PM phenotype results in elevated concentrations of all three drugs, putting individuals with this phenotype at risk for adverse events.[11,13–15]

Treatment Recommendation

CPIC has made recommendations for paroxetine and fluvoxamine based on *CYP2D6* phenotype.[16] For paroxetine, they advise considering a 50% reduction of the recommended starting dose or selecting a drug that uses a different primary metabolism pathway for *CYP2D6* PMs. For UMs, CPIC recommends selecting a drug that uses a primary pathway other than *CYP2D6*. In the case of fluvoxamine, they recommend considering a 25% to 50% reduction of the recommended starting dose or selecting a drug that uses a different primary metabolism pathway for *CYP2D6* PMs (Table 8-1).

CPIC has also made recommendations for sertraline and citalopram/escitalopram based on *CYP2C19*

phenotype.[16] For *CYP2C19* PMs, they advise considering a 50% reduction of the recommended starting dose for all three drugs or selecting a drug that uses a primary metabolism pathway other than *CYP2C19*. For *CYP2C19* UMs, they recommend initiating sertraline therapy at the recommended starting dose and if the patient does not respond to the recommended maintenance dosing, consider an alternative drug that is not primarily metabolized through *CYP2C19*. For citalopram/escitalopram, they advise considering an alternative drug that is not primarily metabolized through *CYP2C19* for UMs (Table 8-2). Note that it is helpful to refer directly to CPIC guidelines, as recommendations are classified as strong, moderate, or optional, and information about clinical implications is provided.

In addition to guideline recommendations, some SSRIs have pharmacogenomic language in their Food and Drug Administration (FDA)–approved package inserts. See Table 8-3 for the list of FDA-approved psychiatry drugs with pharmacogenomic biomarker/gene information in the labeling. For example, the package insert of Celexa (citalopram) states that the maximum dose should be limited to 20 mg per day for *CYP2C19* PMs due to the fact that the drug was found to be associated with a dose-dependent increase in the QTc interval.[17] The package insert for Luvox CR (fluvoxamine) encourages caution in using this drug for patients with reduced *CYP2D6* activity.[18]

SSRIs and *SLC6A4*

Mechanism of Drug–Gene Interaction

The serotonin transporter gene, *SLC6A4*, has been researched extensively regarding its ability to predict efficacy and adverse events with SSRI treatment. Several

TABLE 8-1 SSRIs and CYP2D6

Medication	CYP2D6 Phenotype	Recommendations	Classification of Recommendations
Paroxetine	Ultra-rapid Metabolizer (UM)	Use a medication that is metabolized by another pathway other than CYP2D6	Strong
	Poor Metabolizer (PM)	Reduce the starting dose by 50% or select a medication that uses a different metabolism pathway	Optional
Fluvoxamine	Poor Metabolizer (PM)	Reduce the starting dose by 25%–50%, or select a medication that uses a different metabolism pathway	Optional

Source: Reproduced, with permission, from Hicks JK, Bishop JR, Sangkuhl K, et al. Clinical Pharmacogenetics Implementation Consortium (CPIC) Guideline for CYP2D6 and CYP2C19 Genotypes and Dosing of Selective Serotonin Reuptake Inhibitors. Clin Pharmacol Ther. 2015;98(2):127–134.

TABLE 8-2 SSRIs and CYP2C19

Medication	CYP2C19 Phenotype	Recommendations	Classification of Recommendations
Citalopram, escitalopram, sertraline	Ultra-rapid Metabolizer (UM)	*Sertraline*: Initiate at the recommended starting dose; consider an alternative medication not primarily metabolized by CYP2C19 if patient does not respond to the recommended maintenance dose.	Optional
		Citalopram/escitalopram: Use an alternative medication that is not primarily metabolized by CYP2C19.	Moderate
	Poor Metabolizer (PM)	*Sertraline*: Reduce the starting dose by 50% or select a medication that uses a different metabolism pathway.	Optional
		Citalopram†/escitalopram: Reduce the starting dose by 50% or select a medication that uses a different metabolism pathway.	Moderate

†*Citalopram maximum recommended dose should be 20 mg/day in CYP2C19 poor metabolizers due to the risk of QT prolongation. FDA product labeling additionally cautions that citalopram dose should be limited to 20 mg/day in patients with hepatic impairment, those taking a CYP2C19 inhibitor, and patients >60 years old.*

Reprinted with permission, from Hicks JK, Bishop JR, Sangkuhl K, et al. Clinical Pharmacogenetics Implementation Consortium (CPIC) Guideline for CYP2D6 and CYP2C19 Genotypes and Dosing of Selective Serotonin Reuptake Inhibitors. Clin Pharmacol Ther. 2015;98(2):127–134.

polymorphisms have been identified for this gene, including two variants in the serotonin transporter–linked polymorphic region (5-HTTLPR). 5-HTTLPR is a 44 base pair insertion/deletion polymorphism in the promoter region of the *SLC6A4* and may have either short or long (S or L) alleles, with the S allele resulting in reduced transcriptional activity.

A second variant, the single nucleotide polymorphism (SNP) rs25531, is present within the L allele of 5-HTTLPR. Depending on whether a G or an A is present in the gene sequence, rs25531 alleles are denoted as L_A or L_G. These variants have been proposed to stratify the L allele into high/normal transcription (L_A) or impaired transcription (L_G), similar to the function of the S allele.

Consequence of Drug–Gene Interaction

5-HTTLPR. Multiple meta-analyses have shown the S allele to be associated with reduced response to SSRIs.[19] This association appears to be strongest in Caucasians, with mixed results in patient populations of other ethnicities. The effect size is moderate. For example, one analysis assessing nine studies of Caucasians taking SSRIs found S/S individuals to be 1.71-fold less likely to respond to SSRIs than L/L genotype individuals.[20]

The 5-HTTLPR variant has also been assessed in other medication classes. The predictive value of this variant for outcomes with serotonin and norepinephrine reuptake inhibitors (SNRIs) has been studied with several compounds, including venlafaxine, desvenlafaxine, milnacipran, and duloxetine. Further research is warranted, but current publications indicate mixed results, with the plurality of studies for SNRIs and *SLC6A4* having no significant association.[21–26] Other compounds studied with *SLC6A4* include mirtazapine (with little affinity for serotonin transporter) and nortriptyline, both of which have a mixture of studies showing no association or favoring clinical outcomes when the S allele is present (opposite of the effect seen with SSRIs).[27–32]

rs25531. Outcomes studies where the rs25531 SNP was assessed in conjunction with 5-HTTLPR have produced mixed outcomes, with some studies indicating L_A is predictive of improved response to SSRIs[27,33–35] and others showing no significant association.[36–39] All published studies evaluating whether rs25531 alone predicts outcomes to antidepressants have shown no significant association.[40–43]

Treatment Recommendation

There are currently no clinical guidelines regarding *SLC6A4* genotype and medication selection or dosing. However, CPIC does note in a 2015 publication that "[t]here is increasing evidence that variations in the genes encoding the serotonin transporter (*5-HTT, SLC6A4*) and the serotonin 2A receptor (*HTR2A*) are associated with SSRI response and adverse effects. As additional studies are published, gene-based dosing recommendations for *SLC6A4* and/or *HTR2A* may be warranted."[16]

TABLE 8-3 List of FDA-Approved Psychiatry Drugs with Pharmacogenomic Biomarker/Gene Information in Labeling

Drug	Therapeutic Area	Gene	FDA Labeling Section(s)	CPIC Level	CPIC Guidelines PubMed ID	PharmGKB Level
Amitriptyline	Psychiatry	*CYP2D6*	Actionable PGx Precautions	A	23486447 27997040	1A
FDA summary:		UM, IM, or PM status "may alter systemic concentrations."				
Amoxapine	Psychiatry	*CYP2D6*	Actionable PGx Precautions	A	None	1A
FDA summary:		UM, IM, or PM status "may alter systemic concentrations."				
Amphetamine	Psychiatry	*CYP2D6*	Informative PGx Clinical Pharmacology	None	None	None
FDA summary:		PM status "may affect systemic concentrations and adverse reaction risk. Consider lower starting dosage or use an alternative agent."				
Aripiprazole	Psychiatry	*CYP2D6*	Actionable PGx Dosage and Administration, Use in Specific Populations, Clinical Pharmacology	B	None	3
FDA summary:		PM status "results in higher systemic concentrations and higher adverse reaction risk. Dosage adjustment is recommended. Refer to FDA labeling for specific dosing recommendations."				
Aripiprazole lauroxil	Psychiatry	*CYP2D6*	Actionable PGx Dosage and Administration, Use in Specific Populations, Clinical Pharmacology	None	None	None
FDA summary:		PM status "results in higher systemic concentrations. Dosage adjustment is recommended. Refer to FDA labeling for specific dosing recommendations."				
Atomoxetine	Psychiatry	*CYP2D6*	Actionable PGx Dosage and Administration, Warnings and Precautions, Adverse Reactions, Drug Interactions, Use in Specific Populations, Clinical Pharmacology	A	30801677	1A
FDA summary:		PM status "results in higher systemic concentrations and higher adverse reaction risk. Adjust titration interval and increase dosage if tolerated. Refer to FDA labeling for specific dosing recommendations."				
Brexpiprazole	Psychiatry	*CYP2D6*	Actionable PGx Dosage and Administration, Use in Specific Populations, Clinical Pharmacology	B	None	None
FDA summary:		PM status "results in higher systemic concentrations. Dosage adjustment is recommended. Refer to FDA labeling for specific dosing recommendations."				
Cariprazine	Psychiatry	*CYP2D6*	Informative PGx Clinical Pharmacology	None	None	None
Citalopram	Psychiatry	*CYP2C19*	Actionable PGx Dosage and Administration, Warnings, Clinical Pharmacology	A	25974703	1A
Citalopram	Psychiatry	*CYP2D6*	Actionable PGx Clinical Pharmacology	None	None	None
Clomipramine	Psychiatry	*CYP2D6*	Actionable PGx Precautions	B	23486447 27997040	1A

TABLE 8-3   List of FDA-Approved Psychiatry Drugs with Pharmacogenomic Biomarker/Gene Information in Labeling (*Continued*)

Drug	Therapeutic Area	Gene	FDA Labeling Section(s)	CPIC Level	CPIC Guidelines PubMed ID	PharmGKB Level
Clozapine	Psychiatry	CYP2D6	Actionable PGx Dosage and Administration, Use in Specific Populations, Clinical Pharmacology	C	None	None
FDA summary:	PM status "results in higher systemic concentrations. Dosage reductions may be necessary."					
Desipramine	Psychiatry	CYP2D6	Actionable PGx Precautions	B	23486447 27997040	1A
FDA summary:	UM, IM, or PM status "may alter systemic concentrations."					
Desvenlafaxine	Psychiatry	CYP2D6	Informative PGx Clinical Pharmacology	None	None	None
Doxepin	Psychiatry	CYP2D6	Actionable PGx Clinical Pharmacology	B	23486447 27997040	1A
FDA summary:	UM, IM, or PM status "may alter systemic concentrations."					
Doxepin	Psychiatry	CYP2C19	Actionable PGx Clinical Pharmacology	B	23486447 27997040	3
FDA summary:	IM or PM status "results in higher systemic concentrations."					
Duloxetine	Psychiatry	CYP2D6	Actionable PGx Drug Interactions	C	None	None
Escitalopram	Psychiatry	CYP2D6	Actionable PGx Drug Interactions	None	None	None
Escitalopram	Psychiatry	CYP2C19	Actionable PGx Adverse Reactions	A	25974703	1A
FDA summary:	PM status "may result in higher systemic concentrations."					
Fluoxetine	Psychiatry	CYP2D6	Informative PGx Precautions, Clinical Pharmacology	C	None	3
Fluvoxamine	Psychiatry	CYP2D6	Actionable PGx Drug Interactions	A	25974703	1A
FDA summary:	PM status "results in higher systemic concentrations. Use with caution."					
Iloperidone	Psychiatry	CYP2D6	Actionable PGx Dosage and Administration, Warnings and Precautions, Drug Interactions, Clinical Pharmacology	B/C	None	3
FDA summary:	PM status "results in higher systemic concentrations and higher adverse reaction risk (QT prolongation). Reduce dosage by 50%."					
Imipramine	Psychiatry	CYP2D6	Actionable PGx Precautions	B	23486447 27997040	1A
FDA summary:	UM, IM, or PM status "may alter systemic concentrations."					
Modafinil	Psychiatry	CYP2D6	Actionable PGx Clinical Pharmacology	C	None	None

(Continued)

TABLE 8-3 List of FDA-Approved Psychiatry Drugs with Pharmacogenomic Biomarker/Gene Information in Labeling (*Continued*)

Drug	Therapeutic Area	Gene	FDA Labeling Section(s)	CPIC Level	CPIC Guidelines PubMed ID	PharmGKB Level
Nefazodone	Psychiatry	CYP2D6	Informative PGx Precautions	None	None	None
Nortriptyline	Psychiatry	CYP2D6	Actionable PGx Precautions	A	23486447 27997040	1A
FDA summary:	UM, IM, or PM status "may alter systemic concentrations."					
Paliperidone	Psychiatry	CYP2D6	Informative PGx Clinical Pharmacology	None	None	None
Paroxetine	Psychiatry	CYP2D6	Informative PGx Drug Interactions	A	25974703	1A
FDA summary:	UM, IM, or PM status "may alter systemic concentrations."					
Perphenazine	Psychiatry	CYP2D6	Actionable PGx Precautions, Clinical Pharmacology	B/C	None	None
FDA summary:	PM status "results in higher systemic concentrations and higher adverse reaction risk."					
Pimozide	Psychiatry	CYP2D6	Testing Required Dosage and Administration, Precautions	B	None	4
FDA summary:	PM status "results in higher systemic concentrations. Dosages should not exceed 0.05 mg/kg in children or 4 mg/day in adults who are poor metabolizers and dosages should not be increased earlier than 14 days."					
Protriptyline	Psychiatry	CYP2D6	Actionable PGx Precautions	B	None	None
FDA summary:	PM status "results in higher systemic concentrations."					
Risperidone	Psychiatry	CYP2D6	Informative PGx Clinical Pharmacology	B	None	2A
FDA summary:	PM status "alters systemic parent drug and metabolite concentrations."					
Thioridazine	Psychiatry	CYP2D6	Actionable PGx Contraindications, Warnings, Precautions	C	None	3
FDA summary:	PM status "results in higher systemic concentrations and higher adverse reaction risk (QT prolongation). Predicted effect based on experience with CYP2D6 inhibitors. Contraindicated in poor metabolizers."					
Trimipramine	Psychiatry	CYP2D6	Actionable PGx Precautions	B	23486447 27997040	1A
FDA summary:	UM, IM, or PM status "may alter systemic concentrations."					
Venlafaxine	Psychiatry	CYP2D6	Actionable PGx Drug Interactions, Use in Specific Populations, Clinical Pharmacology	B	None	2A
FDA summary:	PM status "alters systemic parent drug and metabolite concentrations. Consider dosage reductions."					
Vortioxetine	Psychiatry	CYP2D6	Actionable PGx Dosage and Administration, Clinical Pharmacology	B	None	3
FDA summary:	PM status "results in higher systemic concentrations. The maximum recommended dose is 10 mg."					

Source: Data from Table of Pharmacogenetic Associations. FDA U.S. Food & Drug Adminstration. February 25, 2020. (https://www.fda.gov/medical-devices/precision-medicine/table-pharmacogenetic-associations). For specific pharmacogenetic verbiage please refer to the FDA package insert.

PharmGKB denotes the level of evidence for citalopram/escitalopram and *SLC6A4* as 2B. Clinically, *5-HTTLPR* is among the most frequently tested pharmacodynamic gene in neuropsychiatry, and rs25531, while utilized less often, can certainly be found in commercial markets.

SSRIs and *HTR2A*

Mechanism of Drug–Gene Interaction

The serotonin 2A receptor, encoded by *HTR2A*, is responsible for postsynaptic serotonin signaling. Three *HTR2A* SNPs have been evaluated for potential pharmacogenomic associations. Two of these, rs6311 (-1438G>A) and rs6313 (102C>T), are in strong linkage disequilibrium. This means that when a variation is observed at one SNP, it is nearly always observed at the other, and thus research studies for either may be used interchangeably. It has been proposed that variation in these SNPs may be associated with reduced messenger RNA (mRNA) levels and thus reduced receptor density; however, ribonucleic acid (RNA) expression studies and receptor density studies have failed to demonstrate consistent associations, leaving the functional effect of these polymorphisms unclear.[44–55] A third SNP, rs7997012, has also been evaluated. This SNP is located in the intronic region of *HTR2A* and its function is unknown.[56]

Consequence of Drug–Gene Interaction

Adverse Events. For paroxetine, some data suggest an increased risk of adverse events when the -1438GG (102CC) genotype is present.[57–59] The impact of this SNP is fairly robust, with a weighted average of several studies indicating side effect risk may be increased by 15% for carriers and 42% for homozygotes. However, two studies evaluating paroxetine and this SNP found no association.[60,61]

Efficacy. There does not appear to be an association between *HTR2A* genotype and antidepressant efficacy in studies evaluating -1438G>A/102C>T variation.[56,62] One publication of the STAR*D (Sequenced Treatment Alternatives to Relieve Depression) study identified rs7997012 to be predictive of citalopram response, but this has not been replicated, with several studies finding no association and others finding an opposite association.[56,62–66]

Treatment Recommendation

There are currently no clinical guidelines regarding *HTR2A* genotype and pharmacogenomics. However, CPIC does note in a 2015 publication that "[t]here is increasing evidence that variations in the genes encoding the serotonin transporter (5-HTT, SLC6A4) and the serotonin 2A receptor (HTR2A) are associated with SSRI response and adverse effects. As additional studies are published, gene-based dosing recommendations for *SLC6A4* and/or *HTR2A* may be warranted."[16] PharmGKB denotes an evidence level of 2B for citalopram and *HTR2A*. For antidepressants (as a medication class) and *HTR2A*, they assigned a lower evidence level of 3.

Tricyclic Antidepressants and CYPs

Tricyclic antidepressants (TCAs) are mixed SNRIs that were originally used to treat depression, but are also effective for other neuropsychiatric disorders (e.g., obsessive-compulsive disease [OCD]), chronic pain, and migraine prophylaxis. TCAs are divided into two groups based on their chemical structure (i.e., number of substitutions of side chain amines) and are so named: tertiary amines and secondary amines. Pharmacological properties also vary by TCA group. Tertiary amines have a greater impact on the serotonin system, whereas secondary amines have a greater influence on the norepinephrine system. Side effects are common with TCAs because they also block a variety of receptors (e.g., H_1 histamine, α1-adrenergic, and muscarinic receptors). As a result, more selective antidepressants (e.g., SSRIs), which are better tolerated, have widely replaced the use of TCAs in treating depression.

Mechanism of Drug–Gene Interaction

The tertiary amines (e.g., amitriptyline, imipramine, doxepin) are primarily metabolized by *CYP2C19* into desmethyl metabolites, referred to as secondary amines (e.g., nortriptyline, desipramine). Note that some secondary amines also serve as effective antidepressants with clinical features distinct from that of their parent compounds. Both the tertiary and secondary amines are also metabolized via *CYP2D6* into less active hydroxy metabolites.

Consequence of Drug–Gene Interaction

CYP2C19. CYP2C19 PMs are predicted to have a higher ratio of amitriptyline to nortriptyline, resulting in a greater risk of side effects compared to EMs.[67] CYP2C19 intermediate metabolizers (IMs) and, to a greater extent, PMs exhibit reduced TCA metabolism, leading to an increased risk of side effects.

CYP2D6. CYP2D6 UMs exhibit increased metabolism of TCAs to less active metabolites compared to CYP2D6 EMs. Therefore, CYP2D6 UMs have decreased plasma concentrations of the parent compound leading to greater likelihood of therapeutic failure. CYP2D6 gene duplication was examined in 108 patients with persistent mood disorders; 75% of patients did not respond to antidepressants metabolized by *CYP2D6*, and *CYP2D6* UMs were more common in the nonresponder vs. responder group. *CYP2D6* gene duplication was also predictive of depression severity.[68] Furthermore, one retrospective population-based study in Dutch patients taking TCAs showed that the probability of switching to another antidepressant was greater in *CYP2D6* PMs than EMs and the average TCA dose was significantly lower in PMs.[69] *CYP2D6* IMs and, to a greater extent, PMs exhibit reduced metabolism of TCAs to less active metabolites compared to EMs. Therefore, *CYP2D6* IMs and PMs can have increased plasma concentrations of TCA parent compounds, leading to increased risk of adverse events.[70]

Treatment Recommendation

Language regarding the pharmacokinetic effects of PM status for *CYP2D6* and *CYP2C19* is included in the FDA package labeling for several TCAs. CPIC guidelines are specific to amitriptyline and nortriptyline, but can likely be generalized to other TCAs because they share similar pharmacokinetic properties. CPIC recommends that TCAs should be avoided in *CYP2D6* UMs due to potential lack of efficacy, and to consider administering an alternative drug not metabolized by *CYP2D6*. If a TCA is deemed necessary, then an increased dose should be considered in conjunction with therapeutic drug monitoring to guide appropriate dosing. For *CYP2D6* EMs, therapy should be initiated with standard dosing. For *CYP2D6* IMs, a dose reduction of 25% should be considered. For *CYP2D6* PMs, TCAs should be avoided due to the potential for side effects, and alternative drug not metabolized by *CYP2D6* should be considered. CPIC also acknowledges there may be an additive effect of *CYP2D6* and *CYP2C19* genotype on TCA response. A combinatorial dosing algorithm can be found on the PharmGKB website (see https://www.pharmgkb.org/guidelineAnnotation/PA166105006).

L-methylfolate and *MTHFR*

L-methylfolate, the active form of folic acid, has been shown to be a beneficial treatment option for patients with depression, both alone[71–74] and as an augmentation to an antidepressant.[74–76] L-methylfolate crosses the blood–brain barrier and is believed to stimulate the production of monoamine neurotransmitters.

Mechanism of Drug–Gene Interaction

Methylenetetrahydrofolate reductase (*MTHFR*) encodes an enzyme that helps convert folic acid into its active form, L-methylfolate. Carriers of the *MTHFR* C677T (rs1801133) polymorphism have reduced enzyme activity, with C/C, C/T, and T/T genotypes exhibiting approximately 100%, 65%, and 30% enzyme activity, respectively.[77,78] Studies of another variant, the A1298C (rs1801131) polymorphism, have shown mixed results. Some studies of this polymorphism showed reduced *MTHFR* enzyme levels when the C variant is present, though to a lesser extent than the variation in C677T.[79–81] Theoretically, individuals with variation in *MTHFR* would be ideal candidates for L-methylfolate supplementation, which could bypass the reduced enzymatic conversion of folic acid and promote normal levels of monoamine neurotransmitter production.

Consequence of Drug–Gene Interaction

The relationship between *MTHFR* genotype and L-methylfolate response is not well studied; however, one study evaluated the *MTHFR* A1298C and C677T genotypes in depressed patients taking L-methylfolate supplementation.[82] This study found no significant improvement for either polymorphism using the 28-item Hamilton Depression Rating Scale (HDRS-28), though they noted a trend for *MTHFR* C677T CT/TT patients benefiting more from L-methylfolate supplementation, which is consistent with the proposed hypothesis. The *MTHFR* C677T CT/TT cohort did significantly outperform in other scales, including the Clinical Global Impressions-Severity of Illness (CGI-S) scale and the Cognitive and Physical Functioning Questionnaire (CPFQ), but not the seven-item Hamilton Depression Rating Scale (HDRS-7). The *MTHFR* A1298C genotype did not significantly affect outcome on any scale.

Treatment Recommendation

There are currently no guidelines regarding L-methylfolate supplementation in general or pertaining to *MTHFR* genotype. It is worth noting that L-methylfolate is classified as a medical food and thus is not regulated as a drug by the FDA.

Antidepressants/Antipsychotics and *CACNA1C*

Mechanism of Drug–Gene Interaction

CACNA1C encodes the α-1C subunit of the voltage-gated L-type Ca^{2+} channel, which plays a critical role in calcium signaling. This gene has been identified as a risk marker for bipolar disorder and schizophrenia, conferring a small increased risk. It has also been studied as a pharmacogenomic marker. Several *CACNA1C* SNPs have been evaluated for their impacts on medication response, with the most studied being rs1006737, which is discussed next.

Consequence of Drug–Gene Interaction

Multiple studies have evaluated the impact of the *CACNA1C* rs1006737 SNP on treatment outcomes, with mixed findings. One study evaluating Caucasians taking citalopram found rs1006737 to have no association with response or remission.[83] Another study evaluating antidepressant response had mixed results, showing rs1006737 to be associated with better treatment response and remission rates in one European group, with increased rates of treatment-resistant depression in a second European group, and to have no significant associations in a third group with Italian ancestry.[84] A third study evaluating response to olanzapine in a Korean population reported no association with rs1006737 and treatment response for schizophrenia.[85]

Treatment Recommendation

No guidelines exist for *CACNA1C* use in pharmacogenomics.

Antipsychotics and *DRD2*

Mechanism of Drug–Gene Interaction

DRD2 encodes the dopamine receptor D2 subtype, the site of action for antipsychotics. The -141C Ins/Del polymorphism is a well-studied SNP of *DRD2* that has been proposed to alter D2 receptor density and consequently modulate antipsychotic efficacy and side effect burden.

Consequence of Drug–Gene Interaction

Efficacy. The majority of publications evaluating the effect of the *DRD2* -141C Ins/Del variant on antipsychotic efficacy have resulted in no significant association.[86–97] Several publications found the Ins allele to be associated with improved response to antipsychotics,[98–101] but one study found the Del allele to have the better outcome.[102]

Adverse Effects. An overwhelming majority of studies evaluating the -141C Ins/Del polymorphism on antipsychotic side effect risk have found no significant association.[93,103–115] One study found the -141 Ins/Del allele to be associated with rigidity caused by antipsychotics in males, but not in females.[116] Similarly, most publications evaluating risk of weight gain with antipsychotics found the -141C Ins/Del variant to have no significant predictive power.[115,117,118] One study found Del carriers to have increased weight gain.[119]

Treatment Recommendation

No clinical guidelines currently exist regarding *DRD2* genotype and medication selection or dosing.

MOOD STABILIZERS AND ANTIEPILEPTICS

The three main classes of mood stabilizers include lithium, antiepileptics, and antipsychotics. Mood stabilizers were originally designed to treat manic episodes and are the most common drug class for the treatment of bipolar disorder, but their mechanism of action is not well understood. For example, the FDA package insert for lithium carbonate simply states "[t]he mechanism of action of lithium as a mood stabilizing agent is unknown."[120] See Table 8-4 for the list of FDA-approved neurology drugs with pharmacogenomic biomarker/gene information in labeling.

Mood Stabilizers and HLAs

Mechanism of Drug–Gene Interaction

The human leukocyte antigen (HLA) complex helps the immune system differentiate between its own proteins and foreign proteins, like viral and bacterial peptides. HLA proteins function by presenting foreign peptides to the immune system so that infected cells can be destroyed. Genetic variation in the immune system is thought to increase population survival odds; therefore, genes related to the HLA complex are highly polymorphic. Two well-studied variants, *HLA-B*15:02* and *HLA-A*31:01*, are predictive of severe cutaneous adverse drug reactions, like Stevens-Johnson syndrome (SJS) and toxic epidermal necrolysis (TEN).

Consequence of Drug–Gene Interaction

Variations in *HLA-B*15:02* have been shown to be predictive of SJS/TEN in patients taking carbamazepine, lamotrigine, oxcarbazepine, and phenytoin, with respective odds ratios of 80.7, 2.4, 26.4, and 5.65.[121–124] These odds ratios reflect how many times more likely a person with the *HLA-B*15:02* variant is to develop SJS/TEN while taking a medication compared to someone in the general population.

Variation in *HLA-A*31:01* has also been shown to be predictive of SJS/TEN, as well as drug reaction with eosinophilia and systemic symptoms (DRESS) and maculopapular exanthema (MPE) for patients taking carbamazepine, with an odds ratio of 5.65.[121]

Treatment Recommendation

Treatment recommendations regarding HLA variants exist for carbamazepine and oxcarbazepine. A Black Box Warning on the package insert of Tegretol (carbamazepine) warns against use of this drug for *HLA-B*15:02*-positive individuals, stating that "patients testing positive

TABLE 8-4 List of FDA-Approved Neurology Drugs with Pharmacogenomic Biomarker/Gene Information in Labeling

Drug	Therapeutic Area	Gene	FDA Labeling Section(s)	CPIC Level	CPIC Guidelines PubMed ID	PharmGKB Level
Amifampridine	Neurology	NAT2	Actionable PGx Dosage and Administration, Adverse Reactions, Use in Specific Populations, Clinical Pharmacology	None	None	None
FDA summary:			PM status "results in higher systemic concentrations and higher adverse reaction risk. Use lowest recommended starting dosage and monitor for adverse reactions. Refer to FDA labeling for specific dosing recommendations."			
Amifampridine phosphate	Neurology	NAT2	Actionable PGx Dosage and Administration, Use in Specific Populations, Clinical Pharmacology	None	None	None
FDA summary:			PM status "results in higher systemic concentrations. Use lowest recommended starting dosage (15 mg/day) and monitor for adverse reactions."			
Brivaracetam	Neurology	CYP2C19	Actionable PGx Clinical Pharmacology	B/C	None	4
FDA summary:			IM or PM status "results in higher systemic concentrations and higher adverse reaction risk. Consider dosage reductions in poor metabolizers."			
Carbamazepine	Neurology/ Psychiatry	HLA-A (HLA-A*31:01)	Actionable PGx Warnings	A	23695185 29392710	1A
Carbamazepine	Neurology/ Psychiatry	HLA-B (HLA-B*15:02)	Testing Required Boxed Warning, Warnings, Precautions	A	23695185 29392710	1A
FDA summary:			HLA-B*15:02 positive "results in higher adverse reaction risk (severe skin reactions). Avoid use unless potential benefits outweigh risks and consider risks of alternative therapies. Patients positive for HLA-B*15:02 may be at increased risk of severe skin reactions with other drugs that are associated with a risk of Stevens Johnson Syndrome/Toxic Epidermal Necrolysis (SJS/TEN). Genotyping is not a substitute for clinical vigilance."			
Clobazam	Neurology	CYP2C19	Actionable PGx Dosage and Administration, Use in Specific Populations, Clinical Pharmacology	C	None	2A
FDA summary:			IM or PM status "results in higher systemic active metabolite concentrations. Poor metabolism results in higher adverse reaction risk. Dosage adjustment is recommended. Refer to FDA labeling for specific dosing recommendations."			
Deutetrabenazine	Neurology	CYP2D6	Actionable PGx Dosage and Administration, Warnings and Precautions, Use in Specific Populations, Clinical Pharmacology	None	None	None
FDA summary:			PM status "results in higher systemic concentrations and adverse reaction risk (QT prolongation). The maximum recommended dosage should not exceed 36 mg (maximum single dose of 18 mg)."			
Dextromethorphan	Neurology	CYP2D6	Testing Recommended Warnings and Precautions, Clinical Pharmacology	B	None	3

TABLE 8-4 List of FDA-Approved Neurology Drugs with Pharmacogenomic Biomarker/Gene Information in Labeling (*Continued*)

Drug	Therapeutic Area	Gene	FDA Labeling Section(s)	CPIC Level	CPIC Guidelines PubMed ID	PharmGKB Level
Quinidine	Neurology	CYP2D6	Informative PGx Warnings and Precautions, Clinical Pharmacology	B	None	None
Diazepam	Neurology	CYP2C19	Actionable PGx Clinical Pharmacology	C	None	3
FDA summary:	PM status "may affect systemic concentrations."					
Donepezil	Neurology	CYP2D6	Actionable PGx Clinical Pharmacology	B/C	None	3
FDA summary:	UM or PM status "alters systemic concentrations."					
Eteplirsen	Neurology	DMD	Testing Required Indications and Usage, Adverse Reactions, Use in Specific Populations, Clinical Studies	None	None	None
Fosphenytoin	Neurology	HLA-B	Actionable PGx Warnings and Precautions	None	None	None
Galantamine	Neurology	CYP2D6	Informative PGx Clinical Pharmacology	D	None	3
FDA summary:	PM status "results in higher systemic concentrations. Titrate dosage based on tolerability."					
Inotersen	Neurology	TTR	Informative PGx Adverse Reactions, Clinical Pharmacology	None	None	None
Lacosamide	Neurology	CYP2C19	Informative PGx Clinical Pharmacology	None	None	None
Meclizine	Neurology	CYP2D6	Actionable PGx Warnings and Precautions	None	None	None
Nusinersen	Neurology	SMN2	Informative PGx Clinical Pharmacology, Clinical Studies	None	None	None
Oxcarbazepine	Neurology/Psychiatry	HLA-B	Testing Recommended Warnings and Precautions	A	29392710	1A
Patisiran	Neurology	TTR	Adverse Reactions, Clinical Pharmacology, Clinical Studies	C	None	None
Phenytoin	Neurology	CYP2C9	Actionable PGx Clinical Pharmacology	A	32779747	1A
Phenytoin	Neurology	CYP2C19	Actionable PGx Clinical Pharmacology	None	None	None
Phenytoin	Neurology	HLA-B (HLA-B*15:02)	Actionable PGx Warnings	A	32779747	1A

(*Continued*)

TABLE 8-4 List of FDA-Approved Neurology Drugs with Pharmacogenomic Biomarker/Gene Information in Labeling (*Continued*)

Drug	Therapeutic Area	Gene	FDA Labeling Section(s)	CPIC Level	CPIC Guidelines PubMed ID	PharmGKB Level
Siponimod	Neurology	*CYP2C9*	Testing Required Dosage and Administration, Contraindications, Drug Interactions, Use in Specific Populations, Clinical Pharmacology	A	None	None
Tetrabenazine	Neurology	*CYP2D6*	Testing Required Dosage and Administration, Warnings and Precautions, Use in Specific Populations, Clinical Pharmacology	C	none	None
Valbenazine	Neurology	*CYP2D6*	Actionable PGx Dosage and Administration, Warnings and Precautions, Use in Specific Populations, Clinical Pharmacology	None	None	None
Valproic acid	Neurology	*POLG*	Testing Required Boxed Warning, Contraindications, Warnings and Precautions	B	None	3
Valproic acid	Neurology	Nonspecific	Actionable PGx Contraindications, Warnings and Precautions	n/a	None	n/a

Source: Data from Table of Pharmacogenetic Associations. FDA U.S. Food & Drug Adminstration. February 25, 2020. (https://www.fda.gov/medical-devices/precision-medicine/table-pharmacogenetic-associations). For specific pharmacogenetic verbiage please refer to the FDA package insert.

for the allele should not be treated with Tegretol unless the benefit clearly outweighs the risk." It also cautions to evaluate the risks and benefits of using Tegretol in *HLA-A*31:01*–positive patients. The package insert for Trileptal (oxcarbazepine) states that "[p]atients carrying the HLA-B*1502 allele may be at increased risk for SJS/TEN with Trileptal treatment."[125]

CPIC's guideline cautions against the use of carbamazepine if a patient is *HLA-B*15:02* or *HLA-A*31:01* positive and against the use of oxcarbazepine if the patient is *HLA-B*15:02* positive. These recommendations are for treatment-naive patients, as SJS/TEN are unlikely to develop if a patient has been taking carbamazepine or oxcarbazepine consistently for at least three months.[126] CPIC and PharmGKB assign their highest levels of evidence, A and 1A, respectively, to the drug–gene pairs mentioned earlier. For *HLA-A*31:01* and oxcarbazepine, CPIC assigns a level C, while PharmGKB has not designated a level.

Phenytoin and *CYP2C9*

Mechanism of Drug–Gene Interaction

Phenytoin is one of the most utilized antiepileptic medications in the U.S., accounting for approximately 52% of all antiepileptic prescriptions next to valproic acid (19%), carbamazepine (11%), and phenobarbital (7%).[127] The pharmacokinetic properties of phenytoin are highly complex. Phenytoin is metabolized by CYP450 enzymes primarily into two distinct isomers of its inactive metabolite, 5-(p-hydroxyphenyl-),5-phenylhydantoin (HPPH). When the reaction is catalyzed by *CYP2C19*, the ratio of S and R isomers is nearly equivalent.[128] However, when the reaction is instead catalyzed by *CYP2C9*, the reaction favors the S isomer by a ratio of 40 to 1.[128,129] There are two types of phenytoin-induced adverse drug reactions: dose-dependent (e.g., sedation, ataxia, dizziness, nystagmus, nausea, and cognitive impairment) and more severe, life-threatening hypersensitivity reactions (e.g., SJS and TEN).

Consequence of Drug–Gene Interaction

Higher plasma concentrations of phenytoin in *CYP2C9* IMs and PMs increase the probability of toxicity. One study demonstrated that the average phenytoin dose required to achieve a steady-state concentration (i.e., 10 to 20 µg/mL) in patients with one or two reduced-metabolism alleles (*CYP2C9*2 or *3*) was 37% lower than that in NMs.[130] This finding is further supported by a case study in which a 41-year-old woman was admitted to the hospital and treated for seizures with a 15 mg/kg dose of phenytoin administered over 30 minutes. Following treatment, the patient exhibited reduced respiration and became unresponsive. Subsequent investigation revealed that she had a phenytoin serum concentration of 79 µg/mL, and genotyping confirmed that she was a *CYP2C9* PM (*1*3 diplotype*). Interestingly, there are racial/ethnic differences in *CYP2C9* allelic frequencies; the *2 allele is more prevalent in Caucasian (10% to 20%) than Asian (1% to 3%) or African (0% to 6%) populations, whereas the *3 allele is less common in most populations (<10%) and is extremely rare in African populations.[131]

Treatment Recommendation

The FDA-approved drug label for Dilantin (phenytoin) states that consideration should be given to avoiding phenytoin as an alternative for carbamazepine in patients positive for *HLA-B*15:02*.[132] CPIC guidelines state that *HLA-B*15:02*-positive individuals who are phenytoin-naïve should not be administered phenytoin due to an increased risk of SJS/TEN, and an alternative antiepileptic medication should be considered (except for carbamazepine and oxcarbazepine).[130] For phenytoin-naïve and *HLA-B*15:02*-negative individuals, *CYP2C9* genotype should be used to guide dosing. *CYP2C9* NMs and IMs [Activity Score (AS) >1.5] should be administered the standard starting and maintenance doses. *HLA-B*15:02* recommendations apply regardless of an individual's *CYP2C9* genotype, age, race, or ancestry. There are multiple reports that *CYP2C9* PMs exhibit an increased risk of phenytoin-induced toxicities, and the *3 allele is strongly linked to the occurrence of SJS/TEN. For IMs (AS of 1.0), consider using a standard starting dose and then a maintenance dose that is reduced by 25%. For PMs, consider using a standard starting dose and then a maintenance dose that is reduced by 50%. Because phenytoin has a very narrow therapeutic window, maintenance dosing for IMs and PMs should be determined by therapeutic drug monitoring.

ALZHEIMER DISEASE MEDICATIONS

Alzheimer disease (AD) pathology is characterized by a loss of cholinergic neurons, accumulation of amyloid beta peptide (plaques), and formation of tau protein (neurofibrillary tangles). One mainstay treatment for AD is second-generation acetylcholinesterase (AChE) inhibitors (donepezil, galantamine, and rivastigmine), which prevent degradation of acetylcholine into choline and acetate, thereby increasing the amount of acetylcholine available at the synapse. Notably, only 10% to 20% of AD patients exhibit a moderate response to conventional AD medications.[133]

Acetylcholinesterase Inhibitors and *CYP2D6*

Mechanism of Drug–Gene Interaction

AChE inhibitors donepezil and galantamine are primarily metabolized in the liver by *CYP2D6*, *CYP3A4*, and to a lesser extent, *CYP1A2*.[134] There are differences in clearance values among *CYP2D6* phenotypes, with PMs exhibiting a 31.5% slower clearance and UMs exhibiting a 24% faster clearance rate compared to EMs.[135] The two most well-studied *CYP2D6* variants in response to AChE inhibitors are the rs1080985 SNP (-1584C>G) and *CYP2D6*10* allele.

Consequence of Drug–Gene Interaction

Efficacy. The rs1080985 SNP (-1584C>G) in the promoter region of the *CYP2D6* gene is linked to higher gene expression and enzymatic activity in vivo.[136] Two studies reported a higher frequency of AD patients carrying the G allele in responders compared to nonresponders to donepezil;[137,138] however, two other studies found no association between the polymorphism and drug response.[139,140] In addition, AD patients carrying at least one *CYP2D6*10* (i.e., reduced function) allele show greater cognitive improvement compared to *CYP2D6*1* (i.e., normal function) carriers treated with donepezil or galantamine,[141–144] likely due to higher steady-state plasma drug concentrations.[141,145] These findings may be particularly relevant for AD patients with Asian ancestry because the *CYP2D6*10* haplotype is common in this population.[146]

Adverse Effects. One study reported that the *CYP2D6*10* allele is also associated with fewer adverse effects in AD patients treated with donepezil or galantamine.[144]

Treatment Recommendation

Additional studies are required to determine the impact of the CYP450 family of enzymes on AD medications.

There are currently no clinical guidelines for *CYP2D6* and AChE inhibitors. CPIC and PharmGKB rate the evidence supporting the relationship between *CYP2D6* and donepezil as levels B/C and 3, respectively. However, it is important to consider that geriatric patients may have impaired production of CYP450 enzymes. For example, when compared to 65-year-old subjects, 90-year-old subjects had a 17% decrease in clearance, whereas 40-year-old subjects exhibited 33% increase in clearance of donepezil. However, it is unknown whether the impact of age on donepezil clearance is clinically meaningful.[147]

Acetylcholinesterase Inhibitors and APOE

Mechanism of Drug–Gene Interaction

In the brain, apolipoprotein E (APOE) is synthesized by a type of glial cell called an astrocyte and regulates lipid homeostasis by transporting cholesterol to neurons. There are three common alleles of the APOE gene: ε2, ε3, and ε4, which have a global incidence of 8.4%, 77.9%, and 13.7%, respectively.[148] APOE isoforms are characterized by a single amino acid substitution (cystine or arginine) at positions 112 and 158. Carriers of the APOE ε4 allele have a greater risk of developing AD, as well as earlier age of onset.[149] Individuals with one copy of the allele exhibit 2 to 3 times greater risk, whereas those with two copies are at 12 times greater risk of developing AD.[149] A recent meta-analysis of genome-wide association studies on longevity-related genes found that the APOE ε4 allele was associated with the lowest odds of surviving to the 90th and 99th percentile age.[150] The APOE ε4 copy number is negatively correlated with brain choline acetyltransferase activity in AD patients,[151] suggesting that APOE may play a role in cholinergic function.

Consequence of Drug–Gene Interaction

APOE ε4 is associated with a reduced response to AChE inhibitors. One study reported that APOE ε4 carriers had considerably poorer cognitive outcomes than APOE ε4 noncarriers in response to treatment with donepezil.[152] Another study found that 80% of APOE ε4–negative AD patients exhibited marked cognitive improvement as assessed via the AD scores on the Alzheimer's Disease Assessment Scale (ADAS) following 30 weeks maintained on the AChE inhibitor tacrine, whereas 60% of APOE ε4 carriers had lower ADAS scores compared to baseline.[151] However, results are inconsistent, as two other studies reported no impact of APOE ε4 genotype and AChE inhibitor efficacy.[141,153]

Treatment Recommendation

Additional studies are warranted to determine whether APOE variants affect response to AChE inhibitors. Currently, there are no clinical guidelines for this drug–gene pair.

ANTIPARKINSONIAN MEDICATIONS

Parkinson disease (PD) is a neurological disorder that causes progressive death of dopamine neurons in the substantia nigra pathway, resulting in impaired motor function. The hallmark features of PD include resting tremor, bradykinesia, postural instability, rigidity, and albeit less frequently, mild cognitive impairment. Gold-standard treatment for PD is levodopa (L-dopa), the immediate precursor to dopamine, which is co-administered with carbidopa, a noncompetitive L-amino acid decarboxylase, that prevents the conversion of L-dopa to dopamine in the periphery because it does not cross the blood–brain barrier. Thus, when taken together, these drugs selectively increase dopamine synthesis in the central nervous system.

Levodopa and *DRD3*

Mechanism of Drug–Gene Interaction

The rs6280 SNP (Ser9Gly) is a functional missense mutation in the *DRD3* gene, which encodes for the dopamine receptor D3 subtype. A positron emission tomography (PET) scan of dopamine 2/3 receptor agonist activity showed that the C allele (Gly) in the rs6280 SNP was associated with enhanced D3 receptor–binding affinity in the striatum of healthy subjects.[154]

Consequence of Drug–Gene Interaction

Efficacy. In one study, PD patients with the rs6280 CC genotype (Gly/Gly) required higher doses of dopamine agonists to manage symptoms of PD compared to other genotypes.[155]

Adverse Effects. There are several studies linking the rs6280 SNP with L-dopa–induced central and peripheral side effects. Approximately 15% of PD patients report gastrointestinal issues (i.e., nausea and vomiting) with L-dopa therapy.[156] The rs6280 TT genotype (Ser/Ser) was predictive of gastrointestinal symptoms associated with L-dopa therapy.[157] In addition, approximately 25% to 40% of PD patients experience visual hallucinations with L-dopa therapy; duration of illness and cognitive impairment are also risk factors for this adverse event.[156] Carriers of at least one rs6280 C allele (Gly) and

CC homozygotes had a greater likelihood of experiencing visual hallucinations with L-dopa therapy, with odds ratios of 1.88 and 3.31, respectively.[156] This polymorphism was also a risk factor for younger age of PD onset in one Caucasian cohort.[158]

Treatment Recommendation

To date, there are no clinical guidelines for L-dopa and *DRD3*. PharmGKB rates the evidence supporting the relationship between the drug–gene pair as level 3.

ANALGESICS AND ADDICTION MEDICATIONS

Nonsteroidal Anti-Inflammatory Drugs

Nonsteroidal anti-inflammatory drugs (NSAIDs) are a group of nonopioid drugs that are commonly used to treat acute and chronic pain. The principal analgesic effect of NSAIDs occurs via inhibition of prostaglandin biosynthesis from arachidonic acid by the prostaglandin G/H synthases 1 and 2, also known as cyclooxygenases (COX). Most NSAIDs are reversible inhibitors of both the COX-1 and COX-2 isoforms; however, some NSAIDs are selective COX-2 inhibitors.

Mechanism of Drug–Gene Interaction

CYP2C9 is involved in the metabolism and clearance of several NSAIDs although their pharmacokinetic properties are unique. The two most well-studied variants are *CYP2C9*2* and *CYP2C9*3*. *CYP2C9* PMs (AS of 0) are predicted to have extended NSAID half-life and increased plasma levels. For example, a meta-analysis of seven small studies evaluating the impact of *CYP2C9* genotype on celecoxib exposure found that *3/*3 carriers have nearly a 400% increase in area under the curve (AUC) compared to NMs (*1/*1 diplotype).[159] A separate meta-analysis of four studies evaluating the impact of *CYP2C9* genotype on meloxicam exposure found that *1/*3 carriers have approximately an 80% increase in AUC compared to *1/*1 (wild type).[159]

Consequence of Drug–Gene Interaction

CYP2C9 PMs have higher plasma levels of NSAIDs, which can increase the likelihood and/or severity of adverse events. Even though some NSAIDs are available over-the-counter, they can produce serious side effects such as gastrointestinal bleeding, hypertension, myocardial infarction, heart failure, and renal damage, especially with long-term use. For example, *CYP2C9* PMs have an increased risk of developing NSAID-induced gastrointestinal distress and bleeding, with respective odds ratios of 1.86 and 1.90.[160] In addition, the *CYP2C9*3* allele is a strong predictor of NSAID-related adverse events and so genotyping may help reduce their risk.

Treatment Recommendation

CPIC guidelines are organized according to the plasma elimination half-life of NSAIDs in *CYP2C9* NMs. Furthermore, the phenotypes are categorized by activity scores: 2.0 (EM or NM: an individual carrying two normal-function alleles), 1.5 to 1.0 (IM: an individual carrying one normal-function allele plus one decreased-function allele, or one normal-function allele plus one nonfunction allele, or two decreased-function alleles), and 0.5 to 0 (PM: an individual carrying one no-function allele plus one decreased-function allele, or two no-function alleles)

Celecoxib, Flurbiprofen, and Ibuprofen. For celecoxib, flurbiprofen, and ibuprofen, *CYP2C9* NMs and IMs (AS of 1.5) should use the recommended starting dose. However, *CYP2C9* IMs (AS of 1.0) should begin NSAID therapy with the lowest recommended starting dose and titrate to therapeutic effect. *CYP2C9* PMs should begin NSAID therapy with 25% to 50% of the maximum recommended starting dose. Upward dose titration should not be initiated until after steady state has been achieved (within five to eight days depending on the drug), or consider using an alternative drug not affected by *CYP2C9*. Both IMs and PMs should be monitored for side effects such as elevated blood pressure and kidney dysfunction.

Meloxicam. For meloxicam, *CYP2C9* EMs and IMs (AS of 1.5) should use the recommended starting dose. *CYP2C9* IMs (AS of 1.0) should begin NSAID therapy with 50% of the maximum recommended starting dose. Upward dose titration should not be initiated until after steady state has been achieved (at least seven days). Both IMs (AS of 1.0) and PMs should consider using an alternative drug not affected by *CYP2C9* or an NSAID with a shorter half-life than meloxicam.

Piroxicam. For piroxicam, *CYP2C9* EMs and IMs (AS of 1.5) should use the recommended starting dose. *CYP2C9* IMs (AS of 1.5) and PMs should consider using an alternative drug not affected by *CYP2C9* or an NSAID with a shorter half-life than piroxicam.

Topiramate and *GRIK1*

Topiramate is an antiepileptic agent indicated for treatment of epilepsy and migraine prevention. It has also been shown to reduce heavy drinking in patients with alcoholism.[161–163] This drug has several proposed mechanisms of action, including the antagonism of the AMPA/kainate subtype of glutamate receptors.

Mechanism of Drug–Gene Interaction

The glutamate ionotropic receptor kainate type subunit 1 (GRIK1) gene encodes a subunit of certain ionotropic glutamate receptors and is involved in excitatory neurotransmission. The rs2832407 variant is an SNP located in a noncoding intronic region of GRIK1. While its functional effects are not well understood, it has been postulated that this SNP or one linked to it may reduce the density of GluK1-containing kainate receptors and thereby lower the effect of topiramate. As evidence for this, one study showed that the GRIK1 rs2832407 variant was predictive of the effects of topiramate on heavy alcohol drinking days.[164]

Consequence of Drug–Gene Interaction

In one European American subsample (N = 122), CC homozygotes of rs2832407, but not A carriers, experienced significantly fewer heavy drinking days when taking topiramate compared to placebo.[164]

Treatment Recommendation

No guidelines exist for topiramate treatment and GRIK1.

Naltrexone and OPRM1

Naltrexone is an opioid receptor antagonist with high affinity for the mu-opioid receptor. Its mechanism of action allows it to displace drugs from opioid receptors, making it able to reverse their effects. Naltrexone is FDA approved in the U.S. for the treatment of opioid and alcohol use disorders.

Mechanism of Drug–Gene Interaction

The opioid receptor μ 1 (OPRM1) gene encodes the mu-opioid receptor, which is the site of action for many endogenous and exogenous opioids. One OPRM1 SNP, rs1799971 (also referred to as A118G and Asn40Asp), is believed to reduce receptor expression when the G allele is present.[165,166] Because naltrexone is an OPRM1 antagonist, the reduction in binding targets caused by rs1799971 variation may explain improved responses to naltrexone observed in clinical studies (discussed next).

Consequence of Drug–Gene Interaction

Patients with one or more copies of the G allele may be more likely to respond to naltrexone treatment for alcohol use disorder compared with A/A genotype individuals. Some studies suggest that G carriers have an increased percentage of days abstinent, decreased heavy drinking days, decreased chance of relapse, and reduced self-reported alcohol intoxication intensity.[166-169] One meta-analysis calculated that G carriers treated with naltrexone had lower relapse rates than those of A/A genotype with an odds ratio of 2.02.[169] Another more recent meta-analysis assessed treatment outcomes for patients with alcohol use disorder treated with naltrexone, but presence of the G allele was associated only with a statistically significant reduction in number of drinks per day.[170]

Treatment Recommendation

No guidelines currently exist for OPRM1 testing in pharmacogenomics.

OPIOID ANALGESIC MEDICATIONS

Opioids are natural and synthetic derivatives of opium and are some of the most commonly prescribed drugs for pain management. There is significant individual variability in dosing required to achieve sufficient pain relief, and this could be due, in part, to pharmacogenomic factors. Most opioids are metabolized by CYP450 enzymes. Opioids have significant abuse potential and can cause fatal overdose through respiratory depression, especially when combined with other sedatives (e.g., alcohol and benzodiazepines).

Codeine and CYP2D6

Mechanism of Drug–Gene Interaction

Codeine is a prodrug and is primarily metabolized by the CYP2D6 enzyme into its active metabolite, morphine. Codeine is also directly inactivated by the CYP3A4 enzyme into norcodeine and codeine-6-glucuronide. Roughly 5% to 10% of the administered dose of codeine is converted to morphine,[171,172] which has a 200-fold greater affinity for the μ-opioid receptor than its parent compound.[173] Morphine is further metabolized via glucuronidation into morphine-3-glucuronide and morphine-6-glucuronide, but these metabolites exhibit little to no analgesic properties.

Consequence of Drug–Gene Interaction

Because CYP2D6 PMs slowly metabolize codeine into morphine, they have decreased plasma concentrations of morphine and may experience inadequate pain relief. For example, following administration of a 170 mg oral dose of codeine CYP2D6 PMs exhibited approximately 95% lower morphine AUC (plasma exposure) and Cmax (maximum concentration) compared to CYP2D6 EMs.[174] One study found a decrease in peripheral side effects (e.g., constipation) in PMs compared to EMs.[174] However, another study found no difference in the incidence of codeine-related central side effects (e.g., sedation, nausea, and dry mouth) between PMs and EMs.[174] On the other hand, following administration of a 30 mg oral dose of codeine CYP2D6 UMs exhibited approximately 45% higher morphine AUC and 24% greater Cmax compared to CYP2D6 EMs.[175] CYP2D6 UMs rapidly convert codeine into morphine, which can lead to opioid intoxication even with small doses.[176]

Treatment Recommendation

The FDA package insert for codeine warns that "life-threatening respiratory depression and death have occurred in children who received codeine; most cases followed tonsillectomy and/or adenoidectomy and many of the children had evidence of being an ultra-rapid metabolizer of codeine due to a CYP2D6 polymorphism." As a result, codeine is contraindicated in children <12 years old and children <18 years of age following tonsillectomy and/or adenoidectomy.[177]

Individuals who are CYP2D6 UMs with activity score of greater than 2.0 may have a higher risk of toxicity/side effects (e.g., respiratory depression, cardiotoxicity, or nausea) as compared to individuals with *1/*1 (wild type) genotype who are CYP2D6 NMs. For CYP2D6 UMs, reduce the codeine dose or choose an alternative medication (e.g., acetaminophen, NSAID, morphine) due to potential for toxicity and monitor the patient for adverse drug events.

CPIC guidelines for codeine state that UMs can undergo increased formation of morphine following codeine administration, leading to a higher risk of toxicity. In contrast, PMs can experience greatly reduced morphine formation following codeine administration, leading to insufficient pain relief. As a result, CPIC strongly recommends avoiding the use of codeine in both phenotypes and to use alternative analgesics. Furthermore, IMs should be closely monitored to determine whether they respond to codeine.[178] One nonrandomized, prospective open-label trial comparing CYP2D6 genotype–guided treatment vs. treatment as usual for management of chronic pain over a period of months found that there was greater improvement in pain control among IMs/PMs that were prescribed codeine or tramadol at baseline.[179] These data support CYP2D6 genotype–guided treatment for pain.

Tramadol and CYP2D6

Tramadol is a synthetic opioid that exerts its analgesic effects primarily through the OPRM1. Like codeine, tramadol is also a prodrug; tramadol is metabolized, in part, by CYP2D6 into the O-desmethyltramadol (ODMT) metabolite, which has a 200-fold greater affinity for OPRM1 than its parent compound.[180] Tramadol is a racemic mixture; both isomers weakly inhibit serotonin and norepinephrine reuptake[181] and inhibit pain transmission in the spinal cord.

Consequence of Drug–Gene Interaction

CYP2D6 PMs have lower ODMT plasma concentrations and decreased analgesic effects to tramadol compared to CYP2D6 EMs. For example, one prospective study of patients with postoperative pain found that tramadol nonresponders were almost two times more likely to be CYP2D6 PMs than EMs (46.7% vs. 21.6 %, respectively).[182] Furthermore, CYP2D6 PMs required approximately 30% higher doses of tramadol than EMs to achieve adequate pain relief.[182] CYP2D6 UMs exhibit higher plasma ODMT concentrations and increased analgesia and adverse events following tramadol administration compared to CYP2D6 NMs.[183]

Treatment Recommendation

DPWG guidelines state that CYP2D6 UMs are advised to select an alternative medication for pain management, but if an alternative is not possible, use 40% of the standard tramadol dose and monitor patient-reported side effects (e.g., drowsiness, confusion, constipation, nausea and vomiting, respiratory distress, urine retention). A specific dose adjustment is not provided for CYP2D6 IMs or PMs, but clinicians are advised to monitor the patient for reduced efficacy. If inadequate analgesia is reported, consider increasing the dose or using an alternative analgesic that is not metabolized by CYP2D6.

In 2017, the FDA issued a safety announcement to restrict the use of codeine and tramadol in children and also advised against the use of these medications in breastfeeding mothers due to potential harm to their infants. The American Academy for Pediatrics echoed this concern, but acknowledged the need for additional pharmacogenetic studies and safety data on alternative analgesics in pediatric populations.[184] Importantly, the relative abundance of drug-metabolizing enzymes in the liver changes during child development. Therefore, pharmacogenetic data in adults might not be applicable to children.

ADHD MEDICATIONS

Atomoxetine and CYP2D6

Mechanism of Drug–Gene Interaction

Atomoxetine is an SNRI indicated for the treatment of attention deficit hyperactivity disorder (ADHD). Unlike stimulants, this medication typically takes two to four weeks for its clinical effect to be observed.[185] Atomoxetine is metabolized through two enzyme pathways, CYP2D6 and CYP2C19, with CYP2D6 being the major pathway.[186,187]

Consequence of Drug–Gene Interaction

On average, atomoxetine exposure (when assessed by AUC) is tenfold higher in CYP2D6 PMs than individuals with other CYP2D6 phenotypes.[186–190] CYP2D6 PMs are reported to have both higher treatment response rates and greater risk of adverse effects, likely due to increased serum levels of the parent compound.[188,190,191] It has been postulated that CYP2D6 UMs could likely have atomoxetine serum levels below the therapeutic window, but this has not yet been validated.[192]

Treatment Recommendation

CPIC has issued a guideline on atomoxetine and CYP2D6, with specific recommendations for adults and children.[193] In children, for ultrarapid, extensive, and extensive/intermediate metabolizers" to "UM, EM, and EM/IMs *without* the *10 allele, CPIC recommends initiating a dose of 0.5 mg/kg, increasing to 1.2 mg/kg after three days, and, in the absence of both clinical response and adverse events after two weeks, to consider obtaining a peak plasma concentration. If levels are under 200 ng/mL, a dose increase may be appropriate to approach 400 ng/mL. For children who are poor, intermediate, or extensive/intermediate metabolizers" to "PM, IM, and EM/IMs *with* the *10 allele, CPIC recommends initiating a dose of 0.5 mg/kg and, in the absence of both clinical response and adverse events after two weeks, to consider obtaining a peak plasma concentration prior to increasing the dose. If levels are under 200 ng/mL, a dose increase may be appropriate to approach 400 ng/mL.

For adults who are ultrarapid, extensive, and extensive/intermediate metabolizers" to "UM, EM, and EM/IMs *without* the *10 allele, CPIC recommends initiating a dose of 40 mg, increasing to 80 mg after three days, and, in the absence of both clinical response and adverse events after two weeks, increasing to 100 mg. If still no clinical response is observed after two weeks, CPIC advises to consider obtaining a peak plasma concentration. If levels are under 200 ng/mL, a dose increase may be appropriate to approach 400 ng/mL. For adults who are poor, intermediate, or extensive/intermediate metabolizers *with* the *10 allele, CPIC recommends initiating a dose of 40 mg and, in the absence of both clinical response and adverse events after two weeks, increasing to 80 mg. If still no clinical response is observed after two weeks, CPIC advises to consider obtaining a peak plasma concentration. If levels are under 200 ng/mL, a dose increase may be appropriate to approach 400 ng/mL.

The FDA-approved prescribing information for Strattera (atomoxetine) recommends dosing adjustments for patients who are CYP2D6 PMs or taking a strong CYP2D6 inhibitor concomitantly. For such children and adolescents up to 70 kg body weight, they advise initiating Strattera at 0.5 mg/kg/day and only increasing to the usual target dose of 1.2 mg/kg/day if symptoms do not improve after four weeks and the initial dose is tolerated. For individuals over 70 kg body weight who are taking strong CYP2D6 inhibitors, they recommend initiating Strattera at 40 mg/day and only increasing to the target dose of 80 mg/day if symptoms do not improve after four weeks and the initial dose is tolerated. Additionally, the prescribing information advises that CYP2D6 poor metabolism results in a tenfold AUC increase, fivefold higher peak plasma concentrations, and slower elimination.[194] It also cautions that CYP2D6 inhibitors increase the AUC of atomoxetine approximately sixfold to eightfold.

Stimulants and COMT

Mechanism of Drug–Gene Interaction

The catechol-O-methyltransferase (COMT) encodes an enzyme that degrades catecholamines such as dopamine and norepinephrine. The best-studied polymorphism of COMT, Val158Met (rs4680), results in a threefold to fourfold decrease in enzymatic activity.[195] Patients with this variation are expected to degrade catecholamines more slowly and have higher baseline levels of catecholamines in the prefrontal cortex. It has been postulated that these individuals may be less likely to respond to stimulant medications, which could cause catecholamine levels to be increased beyond the range of optimal biological function.[196]

Consequence of Drug–Gene Interaction

Amphetamine Salts. There have been multiple studies evaluating the modulating effect of COMT genotype on healthy adults completing cognitive tasks. These studies have been largely negative, with some suggesting Val carriers have improved response. Two studies showed no significant association.[197,198] Furthermore, two studies showed Val carriers had improved performance over Met carriers,[196,199] and while another study replicated this result, it was only in one scale of 13 evaluated (the remaining 12 scales showed no association).[200]

Methylphenidates. Most studies evaluating the predictive value of COMT on methylphenidate response have shown no significant association.[201–206] Those showing positive associations had mixed results, with three studies and one meta-analysis showing better outcomes associated with the Val allele[207–210] and two studies showing better outcomes associated with the Met allele.[211,212]

Treatment Recommendation

No guidelines exist for prescribing stimulant medications using COMT genotype.

Stimulants/α-2A Agonists and *ADRA2A*

The adrenoceptor alpha 2A (*ADRA2A*) gene encodes the α-2A adrenergic receptor, a direct site of action for the two α-2A agonists used to treat ADHD: guanfacine[213] and clonidine.[214] These drugs stimulate postsynaptic α-2 receptors and thereby increase norepinephrine signaling. Stimulant medications, as discussed earlier, block norepinephrine and dopamine transporters and increase the levels of these neurotransmitters. Thus, both stimulants and α-2 agonists affect norepinephrine function at α-2A adrenergic receptors. Since ADHD symptoms are attributed to low concentrations of norepinephrine in the prefrontal cortex, increasing norepinephrine signaling is hypothesized to decrease hyperactive-impulsive and inattentive symptoms.

Mechanism of Drug–Gene Interaction

The most-studied pharmacogenomic variant in *ADRA2A* is rs1800544, also known as -1291C>G. The mechanism of this variant is not well understood, but is thought to reduce binding affinity.[215]

Consequence of Drug–Gene Interaction

Initial studies evaluating the effect of -1291C>G on methylphenidate response in individuals with ADHD concluded the G polymorphism to be associated with improved response to methylphenidate treatment.[216–218] Endpoints associated with the G allele in these studies included improved inattentive symptoms and greater improvement of inattentive and total ADHD symptoms. Other studies exhibited mixed results where most endpoints evaluated showed no association, but one endpoint or subgroup analysis was significant for the G allele and improved outcomes on a scale or subscale, respectively.[219–221] In contrast, few studies found no significant association between the *ADRA2A* genotype and methylphenidate response.[222–224] Others—generally more recent publications—found an opposite effect of the

original hypothesis, reporting the G variant to be associated with reduced response to methylphenidates.[204,225,226]

The effect of *ADRA2A* on response to amphetamine salts and the α-2A agonists has not been studied in subjects with ADHD. However, two studies have analyzed the effect of this variant on clonidine efficacy in other disease states. One found subjects with the C/C genotype to have decreased response to clonidine used to treat irritable bowel syndrome[227]; the other failed to find an association between this variant and clonidine response in patients with cirrhosis with refractory ascites.[228] One study evaluated this SNP's effect on atomoxetine response in children with ADHD, but no associations were found.[229]

Treatment Recommendation

No treatment guidelines exist for using *ADRA2A* as a pharmacogenomic maker.

Methylphenidates and *DRD4*

Mechanism of Drug–Gene Interaction

The *DRD4* gene encodes the dopamine receptor D4 subset. Two relatively common variants, 4R and 7R, have been evaluated for their effects on methylphenidate response.

Consequence of Drug–Gene Interaction

A majority of studies on the 7R allele have shown no significant predictive ability of this variant on methylphenidate response.[205,208,230–235] However, two studies show this variant to reduce response to methylphenidates,[236,237] and one shows an improved response.[238] Data on the 4R allele, while also mixed, seem more positive than those of the 7R allele, with some studies showing this variant to increase the effects of methylphenidate (for at least some symptoms or scales evaluated, but not necessarily all)[203,204,239] and others showing no significant association.[223,230,234,240]

Treatment Recommendation

No treatment guidelines exist for using *DRD4* as a pharmacogenomic maker.

CASE SCENARIOS

Case 1

CW is a 48-year-old Caucasian woman with recurrent major depressive disorder on the maximum dose of escitalopram at 20 mg/day. She was recently switched to

escitalopram from paroxetine due to a potential interaction with her metoprolol. For the last 15 years, her dose of paroxetine was maintained at a low dose of 10 mg/day with good efficacy for her major depression. She had intolerable adverse drug reactions when her paroxetine dose was at 20 mg/day. Her prescriber ordered a pharmacogenomic test for CW before making any further changes to her antidepressant therapy.

CW's pertinent PGx test results:

CYP2C9	*1/*1	Extensive metabolizer
CYP2C19	*1/*17	Rapid metabolizer
CYP2D6	*4/*41	Poor metabolizer
CYP3A4	*1B/*1B	Intermediate metabolizer
SLC6A4	L/L	Good activity

Questions:

1. Based on her PGx test results, which of the following would you recommend?
   A. Increase escitalopram to beyond the recommended maximum dose of 20 mg/day.
   B. Discontinue escitalopram and initiate sertraline to be titrated to a maximum dose of 200 mg/day.
   C. Discontinue escitalopram and restart paroxetine at a low dose of 10 mg/day.
   D. Discontinue escitalopram and initiate an antidepressant with no need for serotonin transporters for its mechanism of action.

Answer: C

CYP2C19 ultrarapid metabolizers have significantly lower drug exposure and therefore increased risk of therapeutic failure with escitalopram. It would be reasonable to expect a similar trend for CYP2C19 ultrarapid metabolizers taking sertraline.

2. Explain why paroxetine at below the recommended daily dose of 10 mg/day worked well for this patient with major depression.
   A. With the L/L allele of the *SCL6A4* gene, Caucasians with European descent can use a lower therapeutic dose of SSRIs for optimal antidepressant responses.
   B. As a poor metabolizer of the CYP2D6 enzyme, the patient achieves therapeutic levels at lower paroxetine daily doses.
   C. As a rapid metabolizer of CYP2C19, the patient achieves therapeutic levels at lower paroxetine daily doses.
   D. A and B

Answer: B

CPIC's recommendations for paroxetine is a 50% reduction of the recommended starting dose or selecting a drug that uses a different primary metabolism pathway for CYP2D6 poor metabolizers. CW did well for years on low-dose paroxetine as a CYP2D6 PM and has the SLC6A4 L/L allele.

3. What is the recommendation for other CYP2D6-metabolized medications (e.g., metoprolol) if CW was maintained on paroxetine?
   A. Accommodate for the poor metabolism of CYP2D6 medications by utilizing a low daily dose and monitor blood pressure and heart rate.
   B. Accommodate for the potential drug interactions between CYP2D6 medications by utilizing a low daily dose and monitor blood pressure.
   C. Consider another beta blocker that is not metabolized by the CYP2D6 enzyme.
   D. All of the above.

Answer: D

4. Which of the following SSRIs may not be effective for a CYP2C19 rapid metabolizer at the recommended maximum therapeutic daily dose?
   A. Citalopram
   B. Escitalopram
   C. Sertraline
   D. All of the above

Answer: D

5. As a poor metabolizer for CYP2D6, which pain medications may not work optimally for CW?
   A. Tramadol
   B. Codeine
   C. Hydrocodone
   D. All of the above

Answer: D

Case 2

LB is a 20-year-old female presenting with major depressive disorder. She had a history of good grades in school but began failing classes and lost all motivation to study. LB dropped out of school on medical leave. She had a partial response to escitalopram; however, motivation issues remained. While on escitalopram 10 mg/day, LB stated she "can't imagine anything except sleeping." Her prescriber ordered a pharmacogenomic test to help support the "next steps" in treatment.

LB's pertinent PGx test results:

CYP1A2	163C>A – C/A, 5347C>T – C/T	Ultrarapid metabolizer
CYP2C9	*1/*1	Extensive metabolizer
CYP2C19	*1/*2	Intermediate metabolizer
CYP2D6	*1/*1	Extensive metabolizer
CYP3A4	*1/*1	Extensive metabolizer
SLC6A4	L/S	Intermediate activity
HTR2A	G/A	Reduced activity

Reference: https://genesight.com/20-year-old-with-major-depressive-disorder/

Questions:

1. Which of the following is the most appropriate recommendation for LB based on her PGx results?

   A. Increase escitalopram to 20 mg/day
   B. Decrease escitalopram to 5 mg/day
   C. Discontinue escitalopram and start sertraline 50 mg/day
   D. Taper off escitalopram and switch to another class of antidepressant

Answer: D

2. Based on her PGx results, which antidepressant would you switch LB to?

   A. Bupropion
   B. Duloxetine
   C. Fluoxetine
   D. Paroxetine

Answer: A

3. Which psychotropic medication will be less effective at the recommended therapeutic doses for this patient?

   A. Clozapine
   B. Duloxetine
   C. Olanzapine
   D. All of the above

Answer: D

Case 3

A 5-year-old boy had undergone surgery to remove his tonsils and adenoids to treat obstructive sleep apnea syndrome. The surgery was successful, and he was sent home that same evening. At about 11 pm that night, he complained of increasing pain and was given 20 mg of tramadol. The next morning, his parents found him lethargic and took him back to the hospital. By the time they arrived in the emergency room, the boy was comatose. He received ventilation therapy and naloxone, a medication used to counter the effects of opioid overdose. He was able to return home the next day with discontinuation of tramadol. Genotype testing revealed that he is an ultrarapid metabolizer for the CYP2D6 enzyme, which metabolizes tramadol.[241]

Questions:

1. Explain why an ultrarapid metabolizer of CYP2D6 can increase the toxicity of tramadol at low doses.

Answer: Tramadol is a prodrug that needs the CYP2D6 enzyme to convert to the active metabolite that has 200 times more affinity to the opioid mu receptor.

2. Based on this patient's PGx results, which opioid medication can convert to excessive morphine and opioid toxicity?

Answer: Codeine

Case 4

LP is a 20-year-old Chinese male who is admitted to the emergency department for intermittent high-grade fever and sore throat for a week. He complains of non-itchy skin eruptions on his body and yellowish eye discoloration five days after the onset of fever. LP was started on carbamazepine for the treatment of epilepsy one week prior to his admission to the emergency department. He does not take any other medications and has no known drug allergies. The emergency department physician discontinues carbamazepine and plans to initiate him on phenytoin for seizure management.

1. What could be the possible cause of LP's symptoms upon his ED admission?

Answer: Drug-induced hypersensitivity reaction associated with carbamazepine

2. Would you recommend pharmacogenomic testing for LP prior to starting him on phenytoin? Explain why or why not.

Answer: Yes, because LP is of Asian ethnicity. There is a high prevalence of the expression of a hypersensitivity allele in Asians, especially those of Han Chinese and Southeastern Asian descent.

3. If a pharmacogenomic test is requested, what specific test should be ordered?

*Answer: HLA-B*1502 allele*

4. LP's pharmacogenomic test result shows that he is positive for the HLA-B*1502 allele (he is a carrier for this allele). Do you agree or disagree with initiating LP on phenytoin?

*Answer: Disagree to initiate LP on phenytoin. Both carbamazepine and phenytoin are associated with drug-induced hypersensitivity reactions because of the HLA-B*1502 allele.*

5. What would be your treatment recommendation for LP?

*Answer: An alternative anticonvulsant that is not structurally related to carbamazepine and phenytoin and is not linked to HLA-B*1502. One option is valproic acid.*

PHARMACOGENOMICS CLINICAL PEARLS

- The *CYP2D6* and *CYP2C19* genes are involved in the metabolism of SSRIs, and variation in these pathways can have significant effects on drug efficacy and safety. *CYP2D6* UMs have been shown to have low or undetectable paroxetine plasma concentrations compared to extensive metabolizers, putting individuals with this phenotype at risk of therapeutic failure, while for citalopram and escitalopram, studies have shown that *CYP2C19* UMs have significantly lower drug exposure and therefore increased risk of therapeutic failure.

- For paroxetine, CPIC advises considering a 50% reduction of the recommended starting dose or selecting a drug that uses a different primary metabolism pathway for *CYP2D6* PMs. For UMs, CPIC recommends selecting a drug that uses a primary pathway other than *CYP2D6*.

- For *CYP2C19* PMs, CPIC advises considering a 50% reduction of the recommended starting dose for citalopram, escitalopram, and sertraline or selecting a drug that uses a primary metabolism pathway other than *CYP2C19*. For *CYP2C19* UMs, CPIC recommends initiating sertraline therapy at the recommended starting dose and if the patient does not respond to the recommended maintenance dosing, to then consider an alternative drug that is not primarily metabolized through *CYP2C19*. For citalopram/escitalopram, CPIC advises considering an alternative drug that is not primarily metabolized through *CYP2C19* for UMs.

- *CYP2C19* PMs are predicted to have a higher ratio of amitriptyline to nortriptyline, resulting in a greater risk of side effects compared to EMs. *CYP2C19* IMs and, to a greater extent, PMs exhibit greatly reduced TCA metabolism, leading to an increased risk of side effects.

- CPIC recommends that *CYP2D6* UMs avoid TCA use due to potential lack of efficacy and to consider administering an alternative drug not metabolized by CYP2D6. If a TCA is necessary, an increased dose should be considered in conjunction with therapeutic drug monitoring to guide appropriate dosing. *CYP2D6* IMs should consider a dose reduction of 25%. For *CYP2D6* PMs, avoid TCAs due to the potential for side effects and consider administering an alternative drug not metabolized by CYP2D6.

- On average, atomoxetine exposure is tenfold higher in *CYP2D6* PMs than in individuals with other *CYP2D6* phenotypes. CPIC has specific recommendations for atomoxetine dosing in adults and children who are ultrarapid, extensive, and extensive/intermediate metabolizers without the *10* allele.

- The serotonin transporter gene, *SLC6A4*, has been researched extensively regarding its ability to predict efficacy and adverse events with SSRI treatment. Several polymorphisms have been identified for this gene, including two variants in the serotonin transporter–linked polymorphic region (5-HTTLPR). 5-HTTLPR is a base pair insertion/deletion polymorphism in the promoter region of *SLC6A4* and may have either short or long (S or L) alleles, with the S allele resulting in reduced transcriptional activity. Multiple meta-analyses have shown the S allele to be associated with reduced response to SSRIs. This association appears to be strongest in Caucasians, with mixed results in patient populations of other ethnicities. There are currently no clinical guidelines regarding *SLC6A4* genotype and medication selection or dosing.

- Variations in *HLA-B*15:02* have been shown to be predictive of SJS and TEN in patients taking carbamazepine, lamotrigine, oxcarbazepine, and phenytoin, with respective odds ratios of 80.7, 2.4, 26.4, and 5.65. CPIC's guideline cautions against the use of carbamazepine if a patient is *HLA-B*15:02* or *HLA-A*31:01* positive and against the use of oxcarbazepine if the patient is *HLA-B*15:02* positive.

- CPIC guidelines state that *HLA-B*15:02–*positive individuals should not be administered phenytoin/fosphenytoin regardless of *CYP2C9* phenotype, ethnicity, or age. However, if the patient is *HLA-B*15:02* negative, follow *CYP2C9* phenotype–specific recommendations. *CYP2C9* EMs should initiate therapy based on standard dosing for phenytoin. *CYP2C9* IMs should consider a 25% reduction in dose, whereas *CYP2C9* PMs should consider a 50% dose reduction. Phenytoin has a very narrow therapeutic window, and so maintenance doses for *CYP2C9* IMs and PMs should be determined with therapeutic drug monitoring.

- *CYP2C9* PMs have an increased risk of developing NSAID-induced gastrointestinal distress and bleeding, with respective odds ratios of 1.86, and 1.90. *CYP2C9* PMs should begin NSAID therapy with 25% to 50% of the maximum recommended starting dose. Upward dose titration should not be initiated until after steady state has been achieved, or consider using an alternative drug not affected by *CYP2C9*.

- CPIC guidelines for codeine state that UMs can undergo increased formation of morphine following codeine administration, leading to a higher risk of toxicity. In contrast, PMs can experience greatly reduced morphine formation following codeine administration, leading to insufficient pain relief. CPIC strongly recommends avoiding the use of codeine in both phenotypes and to use alternative analgesics.

- For tramadol, *CYP2D6* UMs are advised to select an alternative medication for pain management. If an alternative is not possible, use 40% of the standard dose and monitor patient-reported side effects. A specific dose adjustment is not provided for *CYP2D6* IMs or PMs, but clinicians are advised to monitor the patient for reduced efficacy. If inadequate analgesia is reported, consider increasing the dose or using an alternative analgesic that is not metabolized by *CYP2D6*.

ABBREVIATIONS AND ACRONYMS

AChE: acetylcholinesterase

ADRA2A: adrenoceptor alpha 2A

APOE: apolipoprotein E

CACNA1C: calcium voltage-gated channel subunit α-1C

COMT: catechol-O-methyltransferase

COX: cyclooxygenases

CYP450: cytochrome P450

CPIC: Clinical Pharmacogenetics Implementation Consortium

DPWG: Dutch Pharmacogenetics Working Group

DRD2: dopamine receptor D2

DRD3: dopamine receptor D3

DRD4: dopamine receptor D4

GRIK1: glutamate ionotropic receptor kainate type subunit 1

HLA: human leukocyte antigen

HTR2A: 5-hydroxytryptamine receptor 2A or serotonin 2A receptor

MTHFR: methylenetetrahydrofolate reductase

OPRM1: opioid receptor μ 1

SJS: Stevens Johnson syndrome

SLC6A4: serotonin transporter gene

SNP: single nucleotide polymorphism

SNRIs: serotonin and norepinephrine reuptake inhibitors

SSRIs: selective serotonin reuptake inhibitors

5-HTTLPR: serotonin transporter linked polymorphic region

TEN: toxic epidermal necrolysis

REFERENCES

1. Practice guideline for the treatment of patients with major depressive disorder (revision). American Psychiatric Association. *The American Journal of Psychiatry.* 2000;157(4 suppl):1-45.

2. Charlier C, Broly F, Lhermitte M, et al. Polymorphisms in the CYP 2D6 gene: association with plasma concentrations of fluoxetine and paroxetine. *Ther Drug Monit.* 2003;25(6):738-742.

3. Gex-Fabry M, Eap CB, Oneda B, et al. CYP2D6 and ABCB1 genetic variability: influence on paroxetine plasma level and therapeutic response. *Ther Drug Monit.* 2008;30(4):474-482.

4. Güzey C, Spigset O. Low serum concentrations of paroxetine in CYP2D6 ultrarapid metabolizers. *J Clin Psychopharmacol.* 2006;26(2):211-212.

5. Lam YW, Gaedigk A, Ereshefsky L, et al. CYP2D6 inhibition by selective serotonin reuptake inhibitors: analysis of achievable steady-state plasma concentrations and the effect of ultrarapid metabolism at CYP2D6. *Pharmacotherapy.* 2002;22(8):1001-1006.

6. Carrillo JA, Dahl ML, Svensson JO, et al. Disposition of fluvoxamine in humans is determined by the polymorphic CYP2D6 and also by the CYP1A2 activity. *Clin Pharmacol Ther.* 1996;60(2):183-190.

7. Sawamura K, Suzuki Y, Someya T. Effects of dosage and CYP2D6-mutated allele on plasma concentration of paroxetine. *Eur J Clin Pharmacol.* 2004;60(8):553-557.

8. Spigset O, Granberg K, Hägg S, et al. Relationship between fluvoxamine pharmacokinetics and CYP2D6/CYP2C19 phenotype polymorphisms. *Eur J Clin Pharmacol.* 1997;52(2):129-133.

9. Huezo-Diaz P, Perroud N, Spencer EP, et al. CYP2C19 genotype predicts steady state escitalopram concentration in GENDEP. *J Psychopharmacol.* 2012;26(3):398-407.

10. Hodgson K, Tansey K, Dernovsek MZ, et al. Genetic differences in cytochrome P450 enzymes and antidepressant treatment response. *J Psychopharmacol.* 2014;28(2):133-141.

11. Rudberg I, Mohebi B, Hermann M, et al. Impact of the ultrarapid CYP2C19*17 allele on serum concentration of escitalopram in psychiatric patients. *Clin Pharmacol Ther.* 2008;83(2):322-327.

12. Rudberg I, Hermann M, Refsum H, et al. Serum concentrations of sertraline and N-desmethyl sertraline in relation to CYP2C19 genotype in psychiatric patients. *Eur J Clin Pharmacol.* 2008;64(12):1181-1188.

13. Chen B, Xu Y, Jiang T, et al. Estimation of CYP2D6*10 genotypes on citalopram disposition in Chinese subjects by population pharmacokinetic assay. *J Clin Pharm Ther.* 2013;38(6):504-511.

14. Fudio S, Borobia AM, Piñana E, et al. Evaluation of the influence of sex and CYP2C19 and CYP2D6 polymorphisms in the disposition of citalopram. *Eur J Pharmacol.* 2010;626(2-3):200-204.

15. Noehr-Jensen L, Zwisler ST, Larsen F, et al. Impact of CYP2C19 phenotypes on escitalopram metabolism and an evaluation of pupillometry as a serotonergic biomarker. *Eur J Clin Pharmacol.* 2009;65(9):887-894.

16. Hicks JK, Bishop JR, Sangkuhl K, et al. Clinical Pharmacogenetics Implementation Consortium (CPIC) Guideline for CYP2D6 and CYP2C19 Genotypes and Dosing of Selective Serotonin Reuptake Inhibitors. *Clin Pharmacol Ther.* 2015;98(2):127-134.

17. PI C. Celexa (citalopram hydrobromide) [package insert]. St. Louis, MO: Forest Pharmaceuticals; 2013.

18. PI LE. Luvox ER (fluvoxamine maleate) [package insert]. Palo, Alto, CA: Jazz Pharmaceuticals; 2014.

19. Karlović D, Karlović D. Serotonin transporter gene (5-HTTLPR) polymorphism and efficacy of selective serotonin reuptake inhibitors--do we have sufficient evidence for clinical practice. *Acta Clin Croat.* 2013;52(3):353-362.

20. Porcelli S, Fabbri C, Serretti A. Meta-analysis of serotonin transporter gene promoter polymorphism (5-HTTLPR) association with antidepressant efficacy. *Eur Neuropsychopharmacol.* 2012;22(4):239-258.

21. Ng C, Sarris J, Singh A, et al. Pharmacogenetic polymorphisms and response to escitalopram and venlafaxine over 8 weeks in major depression. *Hum Psychopharmacol.* 2013;28(5):516-522.

22. Lee SH, Choi TK, Lee E, et al. Serotonin transporter gene polymorphism associated with short-term treatment response to venlafaxine. *Neuropsychobiology.* 2010;62(3):198-206.

23. Proft F, Kopf J, Olmes D, et al. SLC6A2 and SLC6A4 variants interact with venlafaxine serum concentrations to influence therapy outcome. *Pharmacopsychiatry.* 2014;47(7):245-250.

24. Ng CH, Bousman C, Smith DJ, et al. A Prospective study of serotonin and norepinephrine transporter genes and the response to desvenlafaxine over 8 weeks in major depressive disorder. *Pharmacopsychiatry.* 2016;49(5):210-212.

25. Yoshida K, Takahashi H, Higuchi H, et al. Prediction of antidepressant response to milnacipran by norepinephrine transporter gene polymorphisms. *Am J Psychiatry.* 2004;161(9):1575-1580.

26. Perlis RH, Fijal B, Dharia S, et al. Failure to replicate genetic associations with antidepressant treatment response in duloxetine-treated patients. *Biol Psychiatry.* 2010;67(11):1110-1113.

27. Staeker J, Leucht S, Laika B, et al. Polymorphisms in serotonergic pathways influence the outcome of antidepressant therapy in psychiatric inpatients. *Genet Test Mol Biomarkers.* 2014;18(1):20-31.

28. Murphy GM,Jr., Hollander SB, Rodrigues HE, et al. Effects of the serotonin transporter gene promoter polymorphism on mirtazapine and paroxetine efficacy and adverse events in geriatric major depression. *Arch Gen Psychiatry.* 2004;61(11):1163-1169.

29. Kang RH, Wong ML, Choi MJ, et al. Association study of the serotonin transporter promoter polymorphism and mirtazapine antidepressant response in major depressive disorder. *Prog Neuropsychopharmacol Biol Psychiatry.* 2007;31(6):1317-1321.

30. Chang HS, Lee HY, Cha JH, et al. Interaction of 5-HTT and HTR1A gene polymorphisms in treatment responses to mirtazapine in patients with major depressive disorder. *J Clin Psychopharmacol.* 2014;34(4):446-454.

31. Kim H, Lim SW, Kim S, et al. Monoamine transporter gene polymorphisms and antidepressant response in koreans with late-life depression. *JAMA.* 2006;296(13):1609-1618.

32. Pollock BG, Ferrell RE, Mulsant BH, et al. Allelic variation in the serotonin transporter promoter affects onset of paroxetine treatment response in late-life depression. *Neuropsychopharmacology.* 2000;23(5):587-590.

33. Baffa A, Hohoff C, Baune BT, et al. Norepinephrine and serotonin transporter genes: impact on treatment response in depression. *Neuropsychobiology.* 2010;62(2):121-131.

34. Gudayol-Ferré E, Herrera-Guzmán I, Camarena B, et al. Prediction of remission of depression with clinical variables, neuropsychological performance, and serotonergic/dopaminergic gene polymorphisms. *Hum Psychopharmacol.* 2012;27(6):577-586.

35. Manoharan A, Shewade DG, Rajkumar RP, et al. Serotonin transporter gene (SLC6A4) polymorphisms are associated with response

to fluoxetine in south Indian major depressive disorder patients. *Eur J Clin Pharmacol.* 2016;72(10):1215-1220.

36. Domschke K, Tidow N, Schwarte K, et al. Serotonin transporter gene hypomethylation predicts impaired antidepressant treatment response. *Int J Neuropsychopharmacol.* 2014;17(8):1167-1176.

37. Gudayol-Ferré E, Herrera-Guzmán I, Camarena B, et al. The role of clinical variables, neuropsychological performance and SLC6A4 and COMT gene polymorphisms on the prediction of early response to fluoxetine in major depressive disorder. *J Affect Disord.* 2010;127(1-3):343-351.

38. Dreimüller N, Tadić A, Dragicevic A, et al. The serotonin transporter promoter polymorphism (5-HTTLPR) affects the relation between antidepressant serum concentrations and effectiveness in major depression. *Pharmacopsychiatry.* 2012;45(3):108-113.

39. Maron E, Tammiste A, Kallassalu K, et al. Serotonin transporter promoter region polymorphisms do not influence treatment response to escitalopram in patients with major depression. *Eur Neuropsychopharmacol.* 2009;19(6):451-456.

40. Kraft JB, Slager SL, McGrath PJ, et al. Sequence analysis of the serotonin transporter and associations with antidepressant response. *Biol Psychiatry.* 2005;58(5):374-381.

41. Kraft JB, Peters EJ, Slager SL, et al. Analysis of association between the serotonin transporter and antidepressant response in a large clinical sample. *Biol Psychiatry.* 2007;61(6):734-742.

42. Shiroma PR, Drews MS, Geske JR, et al. SLC6A4 polymorphisms and age of onset in late-life depression on treatment outcomes with citalopram: a Sequenced Treatment Alternatives to Relieve Depression (STAR*D) report. *Am J Geriatr Psychiatry.* 2014;22(11):1140-1148.

43. Mrazek DA, Rush AJ, Biernacka JM, et al. SLC6A4 variation and citalopram response. *Am J Med Genet B Neuropsychiatr Genet.* 2009;150b(3):341-351.

44. Smith RM, Papp AC, Webb A, et al. Multiple regulatory variants modulate expression of 5-hydroxytryptamine 2A receptors in human cortex. *Biol Psychiatry.* 2013;73(6):546-554.

45. Marinova Z, Monoranu CM, Fetz S, et al. Region-specific regulation of the serotonin 2A receptor expression in development and ageing in post mortem human brain. *Neuropathol Appl Neurobiol.* 2015;41(4):520-532.

46. Falkenberg VR, Gurbaxani BM, Unger ER, et al. Functional genomics of serotonin receptor 2A (HTR2A): interaction of polymorphism, methylation, expression and disease association. *Neuromolecular Med.* 2011;13(1):66-76.

47. Myers RL, Airey DC, Manier DH, Shelton RC, Sanders-Bush E. Polymorphisms in the regulatory region of the human serotonin 5-HT2A receptor gene (HTR2A) influence gene expression. *Biol Psychiatry.* 2007;61(2):167-173.

48. Polesskaya OO, Sokolov BP. Differential expression of the "C" and "T" alleles of the 5-HT2A receptor gene in the temporal cortex of normal individuals and schizophrenics. *J Neurosci Res.* 2002;67(6):812-822.

49. Smith RM, Banks W, Hansen E, et al. Family-based clinical associations and functional characterization of the serotonin 2A receptor gene (HTR2A) in autism spectrum disorder. *Autism Res.* 2014;7(4):459-467.

50. Kouzmenko AP, Scaffidi A, Pereira AM, et al. No correlation between A(-1438)G polymorphism in 5-HT2A receptor gene promoter and the density of frontal cortical 5-HT2A receptors in schizophrenia. *Hum Hered.* 1999;49(2):103-105.

51. Ono H, Shirakawa O, Kitamura N, et al. Tryptophan hydroxylase immunoreactivity is altered by the genetic variation in postmortem brain samples of both suicide victims and controls. *Mol Psychiatry.* 2002;7(10):1127-1132.

52. Hrdina PD, Du L. Levels of serotonin receptor 2A higher in suicide victims? *Am J Psychiatry.* 2001;158(1):147-148.

53. Du L, Faludi G, Palkovits M, et al. Frequency of long allele in serotonin transporter gene is increased in depressed suicide victims. *Biol Psychiatry.* 1999;46(2):196-201.

54. Turecki G, Brière R, Dewar K, et al. Prediction of level of serotonin 2A receptor binding by serotonin receptor 2A genetic variation in postmortem brain samples from subjects who did or did not commit suicide. *Am J Psychiatry.* 1999;156(9):1456-1458.

55. Khait VD, Huang YY, Zalsman G, et al. Association of serotonin 5-HT2A receptor binding and the T102C polymorphism in depressed and healthy Caucasian subjects. *Neuropsychopharmacology.* 2005;30(1):166-172.

56. Noro M, Antonijevic I, Forray C, et al. 5HT1A and 5HT2A receptor genes in treatment response phenotypes in major depressive disorder. *Int Clin Psychopharmacol.* 2010;25(4):228-231.

57. Wilkie MJ, Smith G, Day RK, et al. Polymorphisms in the SLC6A4 and HTR2A genes influence treatment outcome following antidepressant therapy. *Pharmacogenomics J.* 2009;9(1):61-70.

58. Murphy GM,Jr., Kremer C, Rodrigues HE, et al. Pharmacogenetics of antidepressant medication intolerance. *Am J Psychiatry.* 2003;160(10):1830-1835.

59. Kato M, Fukuda T, Wakeno M, et al. Effects of the serotonin type 2A, 3A and 3B receptor and the serotonin transporter genes on paroxetine and fluvoxamine efficacy and adverse drug reactions in depressed Japanese patients. *Neuropsychobiology.* 2006;53(4):186-195.

60. Tanaka M, Kobayashi D, Murakami Y, et al. Genetic polymorphisms in the 5-hydroxytryptamine type 3B receptor gene and paroxetine-induced nausea. *Int J Neuropsychopharmacol.* 2008;11(2):261-267.

61. Murata Y, Kobayashi D, Imuta N, et al. Effects of the serotonin 1A, 2A, 2C, 3A, and 3B and serotonin transporter gene polymorphisms on the occurrence of paroxetine discontinuation syndrome. *J Clin Psychopharmacol.* 2010;30(1):11-17.

62. Illi A, Setälä-Soikkeli E, Viikki M, et al. 5-HTR1A, 5-HTR2A, 5-HTR6, TPH1 and TPH2 polymorphisms and major depression. *Neuroreport.* 2009;20(12):1125-1128.

63. Perlis RH, Fijal B, Adams DH, et al. Variation in catechol-O-methyltransferase is associated with duloxetine response in a clinical trial for major depressive disorder. *Biol Psychiatry.* 2009;65(9):785-791.

64. Horstmann S, Lucae S, Menke A, et al. Polymorphisms in GRIK4, HTR2A, and FKBP5 show interactive effects in predicting remission to antidepressant treatment. *Neuropsychopharmacology.* 2010;35(3):727-740.

65. Lucae S, Ising M, Horstmann S, et al. HTR2A gene variation is involved in antidepressant treatment response. *Eur Neuropsychopharmacol.* 2010;20(1):65-68.

66. Niitsu T, Fabbri C, Bentini F, et al. Pharmacogenetics in major depression: a comprehensive meta-analysis. *Prog Neuropsychopharmacol Biol Psychiatry.* 2013;45:183-194.

67. Shimoda K, Someya T, Yokono A, et al. The impact of CYP2C19 and CYP2D6 genotypes on metabolism of amitriptyline in Japanese psychiatric patients. *J Clin Psychopharmacol.* 2002;22(4):371-378.

68. Kawanishi C, Lundgren S, Agren H, et al. Increased incidence of CYP2D6 gene duplication in patients with persistent mood disorders: ultrarapid metabolism of antidepressants as a cause of nonresponse. A pilot study. *Eur J Clin Pharmacol.* 2004;59(11):803-807.

69. Bijl MJ, Visser LE, Hofman A, et al. Influence of the CYP2D6*4 polymorphism on dose, switching and discontinuation of antidepressants. *Br J Clin Pharmacol.* 2008;65(4):558-564.

70. Bertilsson L, Mellström B, Sjökvist F, et al. Slow hydroxylation of nortriptyline and concomitant poor debrisoquine hydroxylation: clinical implications. *Lancet (London, England).* 1981;1(8219):560-561.

71. Di Palma C, Urani R, Agricola R, et al. Is methylfolate effective in relieving major depression in chronic alcoholics? A hypothesis of treatment. *Current Therapeutic Research.* 1994;55(5):559-568.

72. Guaraldi GP, Fava M, Mazzi F, et al. An open trial of methyltetrahydrofolate in elderly depressed patients. *Ann Clin Psychiatry.* 1993;5(2):101-105.

73. Passeri M, Cucinotta D, Abate G, et al. Oral 5′-methyltetrahydrofolic acid in senile organic mental disorders with depression: results of a double-blind multicenter study. *Aging (Milano).* 1993;5(1):63-71.

74. Shelton RC, Sloan Manning J, Barrentine LW, et al. Assessing Effects of l-Methylfolate in Depression Management: Results of a Real-World Patient Experience Trial. *Prim Care Companion CNS Disord.* 2013;15(4):PCC.13m01520.

75. Godfrey PS, Toone BK, Carney MW, et al. Enhancement of recovery from psychiatric illness by methylfolate. *Lancet (London, England).* 1990;336(8712):392-395.

76. Papakostas GI, Shelton RC, Zajecka JM, et al. L-methylfolate as adjunctive therapy for SSRI-resistant major depression: results of two randomized, double-blind, parallel-sequential trials. *Am J Psychiatry.* 2012;169(12):1267-1274.

77. Frosst P, Blom HJ, Milos R, et al. A candidate genetic risk factor for vascular disease: a common mutation in methylenetetrahydrofolate reductase. *Nat Genet.* 1995;10(1):111-113.

78. Chango A, Potier De Courcy G, Boisson F, et al. 5,10-methylenetetrahydrofolate reductase common mutations, folate status and plasma homocysteine in healthy French adults of the Supplementation en Vitamines et Mineraux Antioxydants (SU.VI.MAX) cohort. *Br J Nutr.* 2000;84(6):891-896.

79. Chango A, Boisson F, Barbé F, et al. The effect of 677C-->T and 1298A-->C mutations on plasma homocysteine and 5,10-methylenetetrahydrofolate reductase activity in healthy subjects. *Br J Nutr.* 2000;83(6):593-596.

80. van der Put NM, Gabreëls F, Stevens EM, et al. A second common mutation in the methylenetetrahydrofolate reductase gene: an additional risk factor for neural-tube defects? *Am J Hum Genet.* 1998;62(5):1044-1051.

81. Weisberg I, Tran P, Christensen B, et al. A second genetic polymorphism in methylenetetrahydrofolate reductase (MTHFR) associated with decreased enzyme activity. *Mol Genet Metab.* 1998;64(3):169-172.

82. Papakostas GI, Shelton RC, Zajecka JM, et al. Effect of adjunctive L-methylfolate 15 mg among inadequate responders to SSRIs in depressed patients who were stratified by biomarker levels and genotype: results from a randomized clinical trial. *J Clin Psychiatry.* 2014;75(8):855-863.

83. Casamassima F, Huang J, Fava M, et al. Phenotypic effects of a bipolar liability gene among individuals with major depressive disorder. *Am J Med Genet B Neuropsychiatr Genet.* 2010;153B(1):303-309.

84. Fabbri C, Corponi F, Albani D, et al. Pleiotropic genes in psychiatry: Calcium channels and the stress-related FKBP5 gene in antidepressant resistance. *Prog Neuropsychopharmacol Biol Psychiatry.* 2018;81:203-210.

85. Yu H, Yan H, Wang L, et al. Five novel loci associated with antipsychotic treatment response in patients with schizophrenia: a genome-wide association study. *Lancet Psychiatry.* 2018;5(4):327-338.

86. Shen YC, Chen SF, Chen CH, et al. Effects of DRD2/ANKK1 gene variations and clinical factors on aripiprazole efficacy in schizophrenic patients. *J Psychiatr Res.* 2009;43(6):600-606.

87. Arranz MJ, Li T, Munro J, et al. Lack of association between a polymorphism in the promoter region of the dopamine-2 receptor gene and clozapine response. *Pharmacogenetics.* 1998;8(6):481-484.

88. Hwang R, Shinkai T, Deluca V, et al. Dopamine D2 receptor gene variants and quantitative measures of positive and negative symptom response following clozapine treatment. *Eur Neuropsychopharmacol.* 2006;16(4):248-259.

89. Ikeda M, Yamanouchi Y, Kinoshita Y, et al. Variants of dopamine and serotonin candidate genes as predictors of response to risperidone treatment in first-episode schizophrenia. *Pharmacogenomics.* 2008;9(10):1437-1443.

90. Xing Q, Qian X, Li H, et al. The relationship between the therapeutic response to risperidone and the dopamine D2 receptor polymorphism in Chinese schizophrenia patients. *Int J Neuropsychopharmacol.* 2007;10(5):631-637.

91. Vehof J, Burger H, Wilffert B, et al. Clinical response to antipsychotic drug treatment: association study of polymorphisms in six candidate genes. *Eur Neuropsychopharmacol.* 2012;22(9):625-631.

92. Alenius M, Wadelius M, Dahl ML, et al. Gene polymorphism influencing treatment response in psychotic patients in a naturalistic setting. *J Psychiatr Res.* 2008;42(11):884-893.

93. Gunes A, Scordo MG, Jaanson P, et al. Serotonin and dopamine receptor gene polymorphisms and the risk of extrapyramidal side effects in perphenazine-treated schizophrenic patients. *Psychopharmacology.* 2007;190(4):479-484.

94. Zahari Z, Teh LK, Ismail R, et al. Influence of DRD2 polymorphisms on the clinical outcomes of patients with schizophrenia. *Psychiatr Genet.* 2011;21(4):183-189.

95. Tybura P, Samochowiec A, Beszlej A, et al. Some dopaminergic genes polymorphisms are not associated with response to antipsychotic drugs in schizophrenic patients. *Pharmacol Rep.* 2012;64(3):528-535.

96. Miura I, Kanno-Nozaki K, Hino M, et al. Influence of -141C Ins/Del Polymorphism in DRD2 Gene on Clinical Symptoms and Plasma Homovanillic Acid Levels in the Treatment of Schizophrenia With Aripiprazole. *J Clin Psychopharmacol.* 2015;35(3):333-334.

97. Bishop JR, Reilly JL, Harris MS, et al. Pharmacogenetic associations of the type-3 metabotropic glutamate receptor (GRM3) gene with working memory and clinical symptom response to antipsychotics in first-episode schizophrenia. *Psychopharmacology.* 2015;232(1):145-154.

98. Suzuki A, Kondo T, Mihara K, et al. The -141C Ins/Del polymorphism in the dopamine D2 receptor gene promoter region is associated with anxiolytic and antidepressive effects during treatment with dopamine antagonists in schizophrenic patients. *Pharmacogenetics.* 2001;11(6):545-550.

99. Yasui-Furukori N, Tsuchimine S, Saito M, et al. Comparing the influence of dopamine D_2 polymorphisms and plasma drug concentrations on the clinical response to risperidone. *J Clin Psychopharmacol.* 2011;31(5):633-637.

100. Lencz T, Robinson DG, Xu K, et al. DRD2 promoter region variation as a predictor of sustained response to antipsychotic medication in first-episode schizophrenia patients. *Am J Psychiatry.* 2006;163(3):529-531.

101. Wu S, Xing Q, Gao R, et al. Response to chlorpromazine treatment may be associated with polymorphisms of the DRD2 gene in Chinese schizophrenic patients. *Neurosci Lett.* 2005;376(1):1-4.

102. Lencer R, Bishop JR, Harris MS, et al. Association of variants in DRD2 and GRM3 with motor and cognitive function in first-episode psychosis. *Eur Arch Psychiatry Clin Neurosci.* 2014;264(4):345-355.

103. Dolzan V, Plesnicar BK, Serretti A, et al. Polymorphisms in dopamine receptor DRD1 and DRD2 genes and psychopathological and extrapyramidal symptoms in patients on long-term antipsychotic treatment. *Am J Med Genet B Neuropsychiatr Genet.* 2007;144B(6):809-815.

104. Hori H, Ohmori O, Shinkai T, et al. Association between three functional polymorphisms of dopamine D2 receptor gene and tardive dyskinesia in schizophrenia. *Am J Med Genet.* 2001;105(8):774-778.

105. Kaiser R, Tremblay PB, Klufmöller F, et al. Relationship between adverse effects of antipsychotic treatment and dopamine D(2) receptor polymorphisms in patients with schizophrenia. *Mol Psychiatry.* 2002;7(7):695-705.

106. Lafuente A, Bernardo M, Mas S, et al. Polymorphism of dopamine D2 receptor (TaqIA, TaqIB, and -141C Ins/Del) and dopamine degradation enzyme (COMT G158A, A-278G) genes and extrapyramidal symptoms in patients with schizophrenia and bipolar disorders. *Psychiatry Res.* 2008;161(2):131-141.

107. Liou YJ, Lai IC, Liao DL, et al. The human dopamine receptor D2 (DRD2) gene is associated with tardive dyskinesia in patients with schizophrenia. *Schizophr Res.* 2006;86(1-3):323-325.

108. Mihara K, Kondo T, Suzuki A, et al. No relationship between -141C Ins/Del polymorphism in the promoter region of dopamine D2 receptor and extrapyramidal adverse effects of selective dopamine D2 antagonists in schizophrenic patients: a preliminary study. *Psychiatry Res.* 2001;101(1):33-38.

109. Segman RH, Goltser T, Heresco-Levy U, et al. Association of dopaminergic and serotonergic genes with tardive dyskinesia in patients with chronic schizophrenia. *Pharmacogenomics J.* 2003;3(5):277-283.

110. Zai CC, Hwang RW, De Luca V, et al. Association study of tardive dyskinesia and twelve DRD2 polymorphisms in schizophrenia patients. *Int J Neuropsychopharmacol.* 2007;10(5):639-651.

111. de Leon J, Susce MT, Pan RM, et al. Polymorphic variations in GSTM1, GSTT1, PgP, CYP2D6, CYP3A5, and dopamine D2 and D3 receptors and their association with tardive dyskinesia in severe mental illness. *J Clin Psychopharmacol.* 2005;25(5):448-456.

112. Inada T, Arinami T, Yagi G. Association between a polymorphism in the promoter region of the dopamine D2 receptor gene and schizophrenia in Japanese subjects: replication and evaluation for antipsychotic-related features. *Int J Neuropsychopharmacol.* 1999;2(3):181-186.

113. Srivastava V, Varma PG, Prasad S, et al. Genetic susceptibility to tardive dyskinesia among schizophrenia subjects: IV. Role of dopaminergic pathway gene polymorphisms. *Pharmacogenet Genomics.* 2006;16(2):111-117.

114. Wu SN, Gao R, Xing QH, et al. Association of DRD2 polymorphisms and chlorpromazine-induced extrapyramidal syndrome in Chinese schizophrenic patients. *Acta Pharmacol Sin.* 2006;27(8):966-970.

115. Tybura P, Trześniowska-Drukała B, Bienkowski P, et al. Pharmacogenetics of adverse events in schizophrenia treatment: comparison study of ziprasidone, olanzapine and perazine. *Psychiatry Res.* 2014;219(2):261-267.

116. Al Hadithy AF, Wilffert B, Stewart RE, et al. Pharmacogenetics of parkinsonism, rigidity, rest tremor, and bradykinesia in African-Caribbean inpatients: differences in association with dopamine and serotonin receptors. *Am J Med Genet B Neuropsychiatr Genet.* 2008;147B(6):890-897.

117. Lane HY, Liu YC, Huang CL, et al. Risperidone-related weight gain: genetic and nongenetic predictors. *J Clin Psychopharmacol.* 2006;26(2):128-134.

118. Müller DJ, Zai CC, Sicard M, et al. Systematic analysis of dopamine receptor genes (DRD1-DRD5) in antipsychotic-induced weight gain. *Pharmacogenomics J.* 2012;12(2):156-164.

119. Lencz T, Robinson DG, Napolitano B, et al. DRD2 promoter region variation predicts antipsychotic-induced weight gain in first episode schizophrenia. *Pharmacogenet Genomics.* 2010;20(9):569-572.

120. PI L. Lithium (lithium carbonate) [package insert]. Columbus, Ohio: Roxane Laboratories; 2011.

121. Grover S, Kukreti R. HLA alleles and hypersensitivity to carbamazepine: an updated systematic review with meta-analysis. *Pharmacogenet Genomics.* 2014;24(2):94-112.

122. Deng Y, Li S, Zhang L, et al. Association between HLA alleles and lamotrigine-induced cutaneous adverse drug reactions in Asian populations: A meta-analysis. *Seizure.* 2018;60:163-171.

123. Tangamornsuksan W, Scholfield N, Lohitnavy M. Association between HLA genotypes and oxcarbazepine-induced cutaneous adverse drug reactions: A systematic review and meta-analysis. *J Pharm Pharm Sci.* 2018;21(1):1-18.

124. Li X, Yu K, Mei S, et al. HLA-B*1502 increases the risk of phenytoin or lamotrigine induced Stevens-Johnson Syndrome/toxic epidermal necrolysis: evidence from a meta-analysis of nine case-control studies. *Drug Res (Stuttg).* 2015;65(2):107-111.

125. PI T. Trileptal (oxcarbazepine) [package insert]. East Hanover, NJ: Novartis Pharmaceuticals Corportaion; 2013.

126. Phillips EJ, Sukasem C, Whirl-Carrillo M, et al. Clinical Pharmacogenetics Implementation Consortium Guideline for HLA Genotype and Use of Carbamazepine and Oxcarbazepine: 2017 Update. *Clin Pharmacol Ther.* 2018;103(4):574-581.

127. Chaudhry AS, Urban TJ, Lamba JK, et al. CYP2C9*1B promoter polymorphisms, in linkage with CYP2C19*2, affect phenytoin autoinduction of clearance and maintenance dose. *J Pharmacol Exp Ther.* 2010;332(2):599-611.

128. Bajpai M, Roskos LK, Shen DD, et al. Roles of cytochrome P4502C9 and cytochrome P4502C19 in the stereoselective metabolism of phenytoin to its major metabolite. *Drug Metab Dispos.* 1996;24(12):1401-1403.

129. Argikar UA, Cloyd JC, Birnbaum AK, et al. Paradoxical urinary phenytoin metabolite (S)/(R) ratios in CYP2C19*1/*2 patients. *Epilepsy Res.* 2006;71(1):54-63.

130. Karnes JH, Rettie AE, Somogyi AA, et al. Clinical Pharmacogenetics Implementation Consortium (CPIC) Guideline

for CYP2C9 and HLA-B Genotypes and Phenytoin Dosing: 2020 Update. *Clin Pharmacol Ther.* Aug 2020; doi: 10.1002/cpt.2008.

131. van der Weide J, Steijns LS, van Weelden MJ, et al. The effect of genetic polymorphism of cytochrome P450 CYP2C9 on phenytoin dose requirement. *Pharmacogenetics.* 2001;11(4):287-291.

132. PI D. Dilantin (phenytoin sodium) [package insert]. New York, NY: Pfizer; 2009.

133. Cacabelos R. Pharmacogenomics in Alzheimer's disease. *Methods Mol Biol.* 2008;448:213-357.

134. Cacabelos R, Llovo R, Fraile C, et al. Pharmacogenetic aspects of therapy with cholinesterase inhibitors: the role of CYP2D6 in Alzheimer's disease pharmacogenetics. *Curr Alzheimer Res.* 2007;4(4):479-500.

135. PI A. Aricept (donepezil hydrochloride) [package insert]. Woodcliff Lake, NJ: Eisai Inc.; 2012.

136. Gaedigk A, Ryder DL, Bradford LD, et al. CYP2D6 poor metabolizer status can be ruled out by a single genotyping assay for the -1584G promoter polymorphism. *Clin Chem.* 2003;49(6 Pt 1):1008-1011.

137. Pilotto A, Franceschi M, D'Onofrio G, et al. Effect of a CYP2D6 polymorphism on the efficacy of donepezil in patients with Alzheimer disease. *Neurology.* 2009;73(10):761-767.

138. Albani D, Martinelli Boneschi F, Biella G, et al. Replication study to confirm the role of CYP2D6 polymorphism rs1080985 on donepezil efficacy in Alzheimer's disease patients. *J Alzheimers Dis.* 2012;30(4):745-749.

139. Klimkowicz-Mrowiec A, Wolkow P, Sado M, et al. Influence of rs1080985 single nucleotide polymorphism of the CYP2D6 gene on response to treatment with donepezil in patients with alzheimer's disease. *Neuropsychiatr Dis Treat.* 2013;9:1029-1033.

140. Liu M, Zhang Y, Huo YR, et al. Influence of the rs1080985 single nucleotide polymorphism of the CYP2D6 gene and APOE polymorphism on the response to donepezil treatment in patients with Alzheimer's disease in China. *Dement Geriatr Cogn Dis Extra.* 2014;4(3):450-456.

141. Zhong Y, Zheng X, Miao Y, et al. Effect of CYP2D6*10 and APOE polymorphisms on the efficacy of donepezil in patients with Alzheimer's disease. *Am J Med Sci.* 2013;345(3):222-226.

142. Lu J, Fu J, Zhong Y, et al. The roles of apolipoprotein E3 and CYP2D6 (rs1065852) gene polymorphisms in the predictability of responses to individualized therapy with donepezil in Han Chinese patients with Alzheimer's disease. *Neurosci Lett.* 2016;614:43-48.

143. Yoon H, Myung W, Lim SW, et al. Association of the choline acetyltransferase gene with responsiveness to acetylcholinesterase inhibitors in Alzheimer's disease. *Pharmacopsychiatry.* 2015;48(3):111-117.

144. Ma SL, Tang NLS, Wat KHY, et al. Effect of CYP2D6 and CYP3A4 Genotypes on the Efficacy of Cholinesterase Inhibitors in Southern Chinese Patients With Alzheimer's Disease. *Am J Alzheimers Dis Other Demen.* 2019;34(5):302-307.

145. Yaowaluk T, Senanarong V, Limwongse C, et al. Influence of CYP2D6, CYP3A5, ABCB1, APOE polymorphisms and nongenetic factors on donepezil treatment in patients with Alzheimer's disease and vascular dementia. *Pharmgenomics Pers Med.* 2019;12:209-224.

146. Bradford LD. CYP2D6 allele frequency in European Caucasians, Asians, Africans and their descendants. *Pharmacogenomics.* 2002;3(2):229-243.

147. Campbell NL, Skaar TC, Perkins AJ, et al. Characterization of hepatic enzyme activity in older adults with dementia: potential impact on personalizing pharmacotherapy. *Clin Interv Aging.* 2015;10:269-275.

148. Farrer LA, Cupples LA, Haines JL, et al. Effects of age, sex, and ethnicity on the association between apolipoprotein E genotype and Alzheimer disease. A meta-analysis. APOE and Alzheimer Disease Meta Analysis Consortium. *JAMA.* 1997;278(16):1349-1356.

149. Michaelson DM. APOE ε4: the most prevalent yet understudied risk factor for Alzheimer's disease. *Alzheimers Dement.* 2014;10(6):861-868.

150. Deelen J, Evans DS, Arking DE, et al. A meta-analysis of genome-wide association studies identifies multiple longevity genes. *Nat Commun.* 2019;10(1):1-14.

151. Poirier J, Delisle MC, Quirion R, et al. Apolipoprotein E4 allele as a predictor of cholinergic deficits and treatment outcome in Alzheimer disease. *Proc Natl Acad Sci USA.* 1995;92(26):12260-12264.

152. Braga IL, Silva PN, Furuya TK, et al. Effect of APOE and CHRNA7 genotypes on the cognitive response to cholinesterase inhibitor treatment at different stages of Alzheimer's disease. *Am J Alzheimers Dis Other Demen.* 2015;30(2):139-144.

153. Miranda LF, Gomes KB, Tito PA, et al. Clinical response to donepezil in mild and moderate dementia: Relationship to drug plasma concentration and CYP2D6 and APOE genetic polymorphisms. *J Alzheimers Dis.* 2017;55(2):539-549.

154. Savitz J, Hodgkinson CA, Martin-Soelch C, et al. The functional DRD3 Ser9Gly polymorphism (rs6280) is pleiotropic, affecting reward as well as movement. *PloS One.* 2013;8(1):1-9.

155. Xu S, Liu J, Yang X, et al. Association of the DRD2 CA(n)-STR and DRD3 Ser9Gly polymorphisms with Parkinson's disease and response to dopamine agonists. *J Neurol Sci.* 2017;372:433-438.

156. Redenšek S, Flisar D, Kojović M, et al. Dopaminergic pathway genes influence adverse events related to dopaminergic treatment in Parkinson's disease. *Front Pharmacol.* 2019;10(8):1-10.

157. Rieck M, Schumacher-Schuh AF, Altmann V, et al. Association between DRD2 and DRD3 gene polymorphisms and gastrointestinal symptoms induced by levodopa therapy in Parkinson's disease. *Pharmacogenomics J.* 2018;18(1):196-200.

158. Hassan A, Heckman MG, Ahlskog JE, et al. Association of Parkinson disease age of onset with DRD2, DRD3 and GRIN2B polymorphisms. *Parkinsonism Relat Disord.* 2016;22:102-105.

159. Theken KN, Lee CR, Gong L, et al. Clinical Pharmacogenetics Implementation Consortium Guideline (CPIC) for CYP2C9 and Nonsteroidal Anti-Inflammatory Drugs. *Clin Pharmacol Ther.* 2020;108(2):191-200.

160. Macías Y, Gómez Tabales J, García-Martín E, et al. An update on the pharmacogenomics of NSAID metabolism and the risk of gastrointestinal bleeding. *Expert Opin Drug Metab Toxicol.* 2020;16(4):319-332.

161. Johnson BA, Ait-Daoud N, Bowden CL, et al. Oral topiramate for treatment of alcohol dependence: a randomised controlled trial. *Lancet (London, England).* 2003;361(9370):1677-1685.

162. Johnson BA, Rosenthal N, Capece JA, et al. Topiramate for treating alcohol dependence: a randomized controlled trial. *JAMA.* 2007;298(14):1641-1651.

163. Miranda R,Jr., MacKillop J, Monti PM, et al. Effects of topiramate on urge to drink and the subjective effects of alcohol: a preliminary laboratory study. *Alcohol Clin Exp Res.* 2008;32(3):489-497.

164. Kranzler HR, Covault J, Feinn R, et al. Topiramate treatment for heavy drinkers: moderation by a GRIK1 polymorphism. *Am J Psychiatry.* 2014;171(4):445-452.

165. Zhang Y, Wang D, Johnson AD, et al. Allelic expression imbalance of human mu opioid receptor (OPRM1) caused by variant A118G. *J Biol Chem.* 2005;280(38):32618-32624.

166. Ray LA, Hutchison KE. Effects of naltrexone on alcohol sensitivity and genetic moderators of medication response: a double-blind placebo-controlled study. *Arch Gen Psychiatry.* 2007;64(9):1069-1077.

167. Anton RF, Oroszi G, O'Malley S, et al. An evaluation of mu-opioid receptor (OPRM1) as a predictor of naltrexone response in the treatment of alcohol dependence: results from the Combined Pharmacotherapies and Behavioral Interventions for Alcohol Dependence (COMBINE) study. *Arch Gen Psychiatry.* 2008;65(2):135-144.

168. Oslin DW, Berrettini W, Kranzler HR, et al. A functional polymorphism of the mu-opioid receptor gene is associated with naltrexone response in alcohol-dependent patients. *Neuropsychopharmacology.* 2003;28(8):1546-1552.

169. Chamorro AJ, Marcos M, Mirón-Canelo JA, et al. Association of μ-opioid receptor (OPRM1) gene polymorphism with response to naltrexone in alcohol dependence: a systematic review and meta-analysis. *Addict Biol.* 2012;17(3):505-512.

170. Hartwell EE, Feinn R, Morris PE, et al. Systematic review and meta-analysis of the moderating effect of rs1799971 in OPRM1, the mu-opioid receptor gene, on response to naltrexone treatment of alcohol use disorder. *Addiction.* 2020;115(8):1426-1437.

171. Findlay JW, Jones EC, Butz RF, et al. Plasma codeine and morphine concentrations after therapeutic oral doses of codeine-containing analgesics. *Clin Pharmacol Ther.* 1978;24(1):60-68.

172. Persson K, Hammarlund-Udenaes M, Mortimer O, et al. The postoperative pharmacokinetics of codeine. *Eur J Clin Pharmacol.* 1992;42(6):663-666.

173. Volpe DA, McMahon Tobin GA, Mellon RD, et al. Uniform assessment and ranking of opioid μ receptor binding constants for selected opioid drugs. *Regul Toxicol Pharmacol.* 2011;59(3):385-390.

174. Eckhardt K, Li S, Ammon S, et al. Same incidence of adverse drug events after codeine administration irrespective of the genetically determined differences in morphine formation. *Pain.* 1998;76(1-2):27-33.

175. Kirchheiner J, Schmidt H, Tzvetkov M, et al. Pharmacokinetics of codeine and its metabolite morphine in ultra-rapid metabolizers due to CYP2D6 duplication. *Pharmacogenomics J.* 2007;7(4):257-265.

176. Gasche Y, Daali Y, Fathi M, et al. Codeine intoxication associated with ultrarapid CYP2D6 metabolism. *N Engl J Med.* 2004;351(27):2827-2831.

177. PI C. Codeine (codeine sulfate) [package insert]. Eatontown, NJ: West-Ward Pharmaceuticals; 2017.

178. Crews KR, Gaedigk A, Dunnenberger HM, et al. Clinical Pharmacogenetics Implementation Consortium guidelines for cytochrome P450 2D6 genotype and codeine therapy: 2014 update. *Clin Pharmacol Ther.* 2014;95(4):376-382.

179. Smith DM, Weitzel KW, Elsey AR, et al. CYP2D6-guided opioid therapy improves pain control in CYP2D6 intermediate and poor metabolizers: a pragmatic clinical trial. *Genet Med.* 2019;21(8):1842-1850.

180. Gillen C, Haurand M, Kobelt DJ, et al. Affinity, potency and efficacy of tramadol and its metabolites at the cloned human mu-opioid receptor. *Naunyn Schmiedebergs Arch Pharmacol.* 2000;362(2):116-121.

181. Grond S, Sablotzki A. Clinical pharmacology of tramadol. *Clin Pharmacokinet.* 2004;43(13):879-923.

182. Stamer UM, Lehnen K, Höthker F, et al. Impact of CYP2D6 genotype on postoperative tramadol analgesia. *Pain.* 2003; 105(1-2):231-238.

183. Kirchheiner J, Keulen JT, Bauer S, et al. Effects of the CYP2D6 gene duplication on the pharmacokinetics and pharmacodynamics of tramadol. *J Clin Psychopharmacol.* 2008;28(1):78-83.

184. Tobias JD, Green TP, Coté CJ. Codeine: Time to Say "No". *Pediatrics.* 2016;138(4):e1-e7.

185. Savill NC, Buitelaar JK, Anand E, et al. The efficacy of atomoxetine for the treatment of children and adolescents with attention-deficit/hyperactivity disorder: a comprehensive review of over a decade of clinical research. *CNS Drugs.* 2015;29(2):131-151.

186. Sauer JM, Ponsler GD, Mattiuz EL, et al. Disposition and metabolic fate of atomoxetine hydrochloride: the role of CYP2D6 in human disposition and metabolism. *Drug Metab Dispos.* 2003;31(1):98-107.

187. Brown JT, Abdel-Rahman SM, van Haandel L, et al. Single dose, CYP2D6 genotype-stratified pharmacokinetic study of atomoxetine in children with ADHD. *Clin Pharmacol Ther.* 2016;99(6):642-650.

188. Michelson D, Read HA, Ruff DD, et al. CYP2D6 and clinical response to atomoxetine in children and adolescents with ADHD. *J Am Acad Child Adolesc Psychiatry.* 2007;46(2):242-251.

189. Ring BJ, Gillespie JS, Eckstein JA, et al. Identification of the human cytochromes P450 responsible for atomoxetine metabolism. *Drug Metab Dispos.* 2002;30(3):319-323.

190. Trzepacz PT, Williams DW, Feldman PD, et al. CYP2D6 metabolizer status and atomoxetine dosing in children and adolescents with ADHD. *Eur Neuropsychopharmacol.* 2008;18(2):79-86.

191. Fijal BA, Guo Y, Li SG, et al. CYP2D6 predicted metabolizer status and safety in adult patients with attention-deficit hyperactivity disorder participating in a large placebo-controlled atomoxetine maintenance of response clinical trial. *J Clin Pharmacol.* 2015;55(10):1167-1174.

192. de Leon J. Translating pharmacogenetics to clinical practice: Do cytochrome P450 2D6 ultrarapid metabolizers need higher atomoxetine doses? *J Am Acad Child Adolesc Psychiatry.* 2015;54(7):532-534.

193. Brown JT, Bishop JR, Sangkuhl K, et al. Clinical Pharmacogenetics Implementation Consortium Guideline for Cytochrome P450 (CYP)2D6 Genotype and Atomoxetine Therapy. *Clin Pharmacol Ther.* 2019;106(1):94-102.

194. PI S. Strattera (atomoxetine) [package insert]. Indianapolis, IN: Eli Lilly and Company; 2020.

195. Lachman HM, Papolos DF, Saito T, et al. Human catechol-O-methyltransferase pharmacogenetics: description of a functional polymorphism and its potential application to neuropsychiatric disorders. *Pharmacogenetics.* 1996;6(3):243-250.

196. Mattay VS, Goldberg TE, Fera F, et al. Catechol O-methyltransferase val158-met genotype and individual variation in the brain response to amphetamine. *Proc Natl Acad Sci USA.* 2003;100(10):6186-6191.

197. Hart AB, de Wit H, Palmer AA. Candidate gene studies of a promising intermediate phenotype: failure to replicate. *Neuropsychopharmacology.* 2013;38(5):802-816.

198. Wardle MC, Hart AB, Palmer AA, et al. Does COMT genotype influence the effects of d-amphetamine on executive functioning? *Genes Brain Behav.* 2013;12(1):13-20.

199. Hamidovic A, Dlugos A, Palmer AA, et al. Catechol-O-methyltransferase val158met genotype modulates sustained attention in both the drug-free state and in response to amphetamine. *Psychiatr Genet.* 2010;20(3):85-92.

200. Ilieva I, Boland J, Farah MJ. Objective and subjective cognitive enhancing effects of mixed amphetamine salts in healthy people. *Neuropharmacology.* 2013;64:496-505.

201. Gruber R, Grizenko N, Schwartz G, et al. Sleep and COMT polymorphism in ADHD children: preliminary actigraphic data. *J Am Acad Child Adolesc Psychiatry.* 2006;45(8):982-989.

202. Sengupta S, Grizenko N, Schmitz N, et al. COMT Val108/158Met polymorphism and the modulation of task-oriented behavior in children with ADHD. *Neuropsychopharmacology.* 2008;33(13):3069-3077.

203. McGough JJ, McCracken JT, Loo SK, et al. A candidate gene analysis of methylphenidate response in attention-deficit/hyperactivity disorder. *J Am Acad Child Adolesc Psychiatry.* 2009;48(12):1155-1164.

204. Froehlich TE, Epstein JN, Nick TG, et al. Pharmacogenetic predictors of methylphenidate dose-response in attention-deficit/hyperactivity disorder. *J Am Acad Child Adolesc Psychiatry.* 2011;50(11):1129-1139.e2.

205. Contini V, Victor MM, Bertuzzi GP, et al. No significant association between genetic variants in 7 candidate genes and response to methylphenidate treatment in adult patients with ADHD. *J Clin Psychopharmacol.* 2012;32(6):820-823.

206. Pagerols M, Richarte V, Sánchez-Mora C, et al. Pharmacogenetics of methylphenidate response and tolerability in attention-deficit/hyperactivity disorder. *Pharmacogenomics J.* 2017;17(1):98-104.

207. Cheon KA, Jun JY, Cho DY. Association of the catechol-O-methyltransferase polymorphism with methylphenidate response in a classroom setting in children with attention-deficit hyperactivity disorder. *Int Clin Psychopharmacol.* 2008;23(5):291-298.

208. Kereszturi E, Tarnok Z, Bognar E, et al. Catechol-O-methyltransferase Val158Met polymorphism is associated with methylphenidate response in ADHD children. *Am J Med Genet B Neuropsychiatr Genet.* 2008;147B(8):1431-1435.

209. Park S, Kim JW, Kim BN, et al. Catechol-O-methyltransferase Val158-Met polymorphism and a response of hyperactive-impulsive symptoms to methylphenidate: A replication study from South Korea. *J Psychopharmacol.* 2014;28(7):671-676.

210. Myer NM, Boland JR, Faraone SV. Pharmacogenetics predictors of methylphenidate efficacy in childhood ADHD. *Mol Psychiatry.* 2018;23(9):1929-1936.

211. Salatino-Oliveira A, Genro JP, Zeni C, et al. Catechol-O-methyltransferase valine158methionine polymorphism moderates methylphenidate effects on oppositional symptoms in boys with attention-deficit/hyperactivity disorder. *Biol Psychiatry.* 2011;70(3):216-221.

212. McCracken JT, Badashova KK, Posey DJ, et al. Positive effects of methylphenidate on hyperactivity are moderated by monoaminergic gene variants in children with autism spectrum disorders. *Pharmacogenomics J.* 2014;14(3):295-302.

213. National Guideline C. National Institute for Health and Care Excellence: Clinical Guidelines. *Attention deficit hyperactivity disorder: diagnosis and management.* National Institute for Health and Care Excellence (UK) Copyright © NICE 2018.; 2018.

214. Naguy A. Clonidine Use in Psychiatry: Panacea or Panache. *Pharmacology.* 2016;98(1-2):87-92.

215. Deupree JD, Smith SD, Kratochvil CJ, et al. Possible involvement of alpha-2A adrenergic receptors in attention deficit hyperactivity disorder: radioligand binding and polymorphism studies. *Am J Med Genet B Neuropsychiatr Genet.* 2006;141B(8):877-884.

216. Polanczyk G, Zeni C, Genro JP, et al. Association of the adrenergic alpha2A receptor gene with methylphenidate improvement of inattentive symptoms in children and adolescents with attention-deficit/hyperactivity disorder. *Arch Gen Psychiatry.* 2007;64(2):218-224.

217. da Silva TL, Pianca TG, Roman T, et al. Adrenergic alpha2A receptor gene and response to methylphenidate in attention-deficit/hyperactivity disorder-predominantly inattentive type. *J Neural Transm (Vienna).* 2008;115(2):341-345.

218. Cheon KA, Cho DY, Koo MS, et al. Association between homozygosity of a G allele of the alpha-2a-adrenergic receptor gene and methylphenidate response in Korean children and adolescents with attention-deficit/hyperactivity disorder. *Biol Psychiatry.* 2009;65(7):564-570.

219. Kim BN, Kim JW, Cummins TD, et al. Norepinephrine genes predict response time variability and methylphenidate-induced changes in neuropsychological function in attention deficit hyperactivity disorder. *J Clin Psychopharmacol.* 2013;33(3):356-362.

220. Park S, Kim JW, Kim BN, et al. No significant association between the alpha-2A-adrenergic receptor gene and treatment response in combined or inattentive subtypes of attention-deficit hyperactivity disorder. *Pharmacopsychiatry.* 2013;46(5):169-174.

221. Huang HC, Wu LS, Yu SC, et al. The alpha-2A adrenergic receptor gene -1291C/G single nucleotide polymorphism is associated with the efficacy of methylphenidate in treating Taiwanese children and adolescents with attention-deficit hyperactivity disorder. *Psychiatry Investig.* 2018;15(3):306-312.

222. Contini V, Victor MM, Cerqueira CC, et al. Adrenergic α2A receptor gene is not associated with methylphenidate response in adults with ADHD. *Eur Arch Psychiatry Clin Neurosci.* 2011;261(3):205-211.

223. Hong SB, Kim JW, Cho SC, et al. Dopaminergic and noradrenergic gene polymorphisms and response to methylphenidate in Korean children with attention-deficit/hyperactivity disorder: is there an interaction? *J Child Adolesc Psychopharmacol.* 2012;22(5):343-352.

224. Gomez-Sanchez CI, Carballo JJ, Riveiro-Alvarez R, et al. Pharmacogenetics of methylphenidate in childhood attention-deficit/hyperactivity disorder: long-term effects. *Sci Rep.* 2017;7(1):10391-10398.

225. Unal D, Unal MF, Alikasifoglu M, et al. Genetic variations in attention deficit hyperactivity disorder subtypes and treatment resistant cases. *Psychiatry Investig.* 2016;13(4):427-433.

226. Hegvik TA, Jacobsen KK, Fredriksen M, et al. A candidate gene investigation of methylphenidate response in adult

attention-deficit/hyperactivity disorder patients: results from a naturalistic study. *J Neural Transm (Vienna).* 2016;123(8):859-865.

227. Camilleri M, Busciglio I, Carlson P, et al. Pharmacogenetics of low dose clonidine in irritable bowel syndrome. *Neurogastroenterol Motil.* 2009;21(4):399-410.

228. Yang YY, Lin HC, Lee WP, et al. Association of the G-protein and α2-adrenergic receptor gene and plasma norepinephrine level with clonidine improvement of the effects of diuretics in patients with cirrhosis with refractory ascites: a randomised clinical trial. *Gut.* 2010;59(11):1545-1553.

229. Yang L, Qian Q, Liu L, et al. Adrenergic neurotransmitter system transporter and receptor genes associated with atomoxetine response in attention-deficit hyperactivity disorder children. *J Neural Transm (Vienna).* 2013;120(7):1127-1133.

230. Zeni CP, Guimarães AP, Polanczyk GV, et al. No significant association between response to methylphenidate and genes of the dopaminergic and serotonergic systems in a sample of Brazilian children with attention-deficit/hyperactivity disorder. *Am J Med Genet B Neuropsychiatr Genet.* 2007;144B(3):391-394.

231. Tharoor H, Lobos EA, Todd RD, et al. Association of dopamine, serotonin, and nicotinic gene polymorphisms with methylphenidate response in ADHD. *Am J Med Genet B Neuropsychiatr Genet.* 2008;147B(4):527-530.

232. Winsberg BG, Comings DE. Association of the dopamine transporter gene (DAT1) with poor methylphenidate response. *J Am Acad Child Adolesc Psychiatry.* 1999;38(12):1474-1477.

233. Kooij JS, Boonstra AM, Vermeulen SH, et al. Response to methylphenidate in adults with ADHD is associated with a polymorphism in SLC6A3 (DAT1). *Am J Med Genet B Neuropsychiatr Genet.* 2008;147B(2):201-208.

234. Mc GJ, Mc CJ, Swanson J, et al. Pharmacogenetics of methylphenidate response in preschoolers with ADHD. *J Am Acad Child Adolesc Psychiatry.* 2006;45(11):1314-1322.

235. van der Meulen EM, Bakker SC, Pauls DL, et al. High sibling correlation on methylphenidate response but no association with DAT1-10R homozygosity in Dutch sibpairs with ADHD. *J Child Psychol Psychiatry.* 2005;46(10):1074-1080.

236. Seeger G, Schloss P, Schmidt MH. Marker gene polymorphisms in hyperkinetic disorder--predictors of clinical response to treatment with methylphenidate? *Neurosci Lett.* 2001;313(1-2):45-48.

237. Hamarman S, Fossella J, Ulger C, et al. Dopamine receptor 4 (DRD4) 7-repeat allele predicts methylphenidate dose response in children with attention deficit hyperactivity disorder: a pharmacogenetic study. *J Child Adolesc Psychopharmacol.* 2004;14(4):564-574.

238. Tahir E, Yazgan Y, Cirakoglu B, et al. Association and linkage of DRD4 and DRD5 with attention deficit hyperactivity disorder (ADHD) in a sample of Turkish children. *Mol Psychiatry.* 2000;5(4):396-404.

239. Cheon KA, Kim BN, Cho SC. Association of 4-repeat allele of the dopamine D4 receptor gene exon III polymorphism and response to methylphenidate treatment in Korean ADHD children. *Neuropsychopharmacology.* 2007;32(6):1377-1383.

240. Ji HS, Paik KC, Park WS, et al. No Association between the Response to Methylphenidate and DRD4 Gene Polymorphism in Korean Attention Deficit Hyperactivity Disorder: A Case Control Study. *Clin Psychopharmacol Neurosci.* 2013;11(1):13-17.

241. Orliaguet G, Hamza J, Couloigner V, et al. A case of respiratory depression in a child with ultrarapid CYP2D6 metabolism after tramadol. *Pediatrics.* 2015;135(3):e753-e755.

CHAPTER 9

TRANSPLANT PHARMACOGENOMICS

Christine L. Cadiz and David R. Ha

LEARNING OBJECTIVES

1. Discuss the clinical considerations of pharmacogenomics in solid organ and hematopoietic stem cell transplantation.

2. Describe general mechanisms of action, pharmacokinetics/pharmacodynamics, adverse drug reactions, and drug interactions of transplant immunosuppressant agents.

3. Identify gene targets that influence pharmacokinetic or pharmacodynamic phenotypes of transplant immunosuppressant agents.

4. Given a case with pharmacogenetic testing results, provide recommendations regarding selection, dosing, monitoring, and other considerations for transplant immunosuppressant agents.

INTRODUCTION

Immunosuppression is an essential component of therapy to prevent and treat allograft rejection in transplant patients.[1] Many commonly prescribed post-transplant immunosuppressive agents have narrow therapeutic indexes, requiring a balance to maintain efficacy and avoid toxicity. These agents carry a risk for transplant/allograft rejection if a patient does not have adequate immunosuppression. Additionally, there are risks for complications from immunosuppression such as opportunistic infections, as well as adverse effects associated with these agents. Given that these immunosuppressive agents are associated with significant adverse effects, drug interactions, and variation in drug metabolism, it makes sense to study pharmacogenetic variation in metabolism of and response to these agents. This chapter focuses primarily on pharmacogenomics of immunosuppressive agents.

Pharmacogenomics in the transplantation domain is complex. Genetic polymorphisms may lead to variation in both response to drugs and response to transplantation. Tissue antigenicity needs to be considered, and genetic differences in human leukocyte antigen (HLA) typing, cytokines, chemokines, and restrictive allograft syndrome (RAS) may be related to risk of rejection.[2] Organ failure syndromes and cancers leading to transplant and complications of infection are also of significant concern in this patient population and are covered in other chapters.

Transplant pharmacogenomics research is ongoing, and clinically actionable recommendations are still emerging for many drugs in the field. Published evidence-based clinical guidelines from the Clinical Pharmacogenetics Implementation Consortium (CPIC) are available for tacrolimus. Although genotype-based guidelines are not currently available for other immunosuppressive agents, there are published studies for drug–gene pairs in the transplantation literature that describe genetic polymorphisms associated with altered pharmacokinetics and pharmacodynamics for cyclosporine, mycophenolate, sirolimus, and everolimus.[1,3] Azathioprine, which is no longer a common component of maintenance immunosuppression regimens following solid organ transplantation, is discussed in Chapter 7.

CALCINEURIN INHIBITORS

Calcineurin inhibitors (CNIs) have become the mainstay in immunosuppression regimens given to patients following solid organ transplantation, usually administered in combination with an antiproliferative and a glucocorticoid. Two significant CNIs are cyclosporine and tacrolimus. Cyclosporine was approved by the Food and Drug Administration (FDA) in 1983. At that time, it offered the most effective therapy to prevent allograft rejection and represented a major advancement in improving survival prospects for transplant recipients. Tacrolimus was approved by the FDA in 1994 and is currently one of the most commonly prescribed immunosuppressive agents in the setting of solid organ transplantation. Both CNIs are used as antirejection medications in kidney, liver, heart, and lung transplant, as well as for treatment of graft-versus-host disease (GVHD) and other severe autoimmune diseases.[4–6]

Most of the literature describing effects of genetic variants on CNI response have focused on genes encoding for enzymes and efflux transporters primarily responsible for drug metabolism and transport: CYP3A4, CYP3A5, and ATP-binding cassette transporter B1 (ABCB1). Other studies have investigated the effect of variation in other genes on pharmacodynamics and pharmacokinetics. With the exception of tacrolimus and CYP3A5, evidence has not been consistent in demonstrating strong associations between known genetic polymorphisms and tacrolimus and cyclosporine response. Additional studies and meta-analyses are needed to help elucidate these associations and potentially develop recommendations for genotype-guided dosing.[7,8]

Tacrolimus

Background

Tacrolimus is a CNI that binds to a calcineurin-dependent intracellular protein, FKBP-12, and forms a complex that inhibits calcineurin activity. It exerts its immunosuppressive effects through inhibition of the production and liberation of interleukin-2 (IL-2) and other cytokines by T cells. IL-2 plays a central role in allograft rejection through activation and proliferation of cytotoxic T lymphocytes (Figure 9-1).[1,5] Clinically, tacrolimus is used as part of standard immunosuppressive regimens to prevent, not treat, acute allograft rejection after solid organ and hematopoietic stem cell transplantation.

Tacrolimus is available in both intravenous and oral formulations. The bioavailability of oral tacrolimus and cyclosporine, another CNI, is highly variable. Compared to cyclosporine, tacrolimus's absorption is more predictable, with time to peak concentration usually between one and three hours.[9] Immediate-release formulations (Prograf) are not interchangeable with once-daily extended-release products (Astagraf XL and Envarsus XR), and both

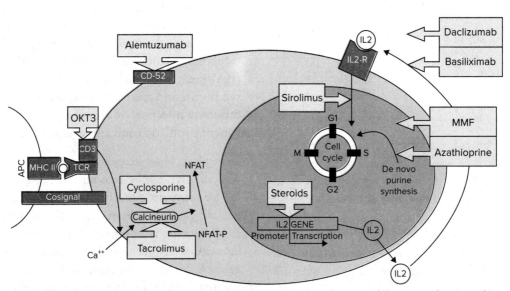

FIGURE 9-1 • Stages of CD4 T-cell activation and cytokine production with identification of the sites of action of immunosuppressive agents. (Reproduced, with permission, from Mueller XM. Drug immunosuppression therapy for adult heart transplantation. Part 1: immune response to allograft and mechanism of action of immunosuppressants. *Ann Thorac Surg.* 2004;77(1):354–362.)

extended-release products also cannot be substituted for each other due to signification variation in pharmacokinetics.[5] Tacrolimus is extensively hepatically metabolized by CYP3A, largely by CYP3A4 and CYP3A5, and is a substrate of P-glycoprotein. Studies have demonstrated that CYP3A5 is the principal enzyme responsible for tacrolimus metabolism and CYP3A4 is the primary enzyme for cyclosporine metabolism.[7,8,10] The importance of CYP3A5 in tacrolimus metabolism explains the relationship between genotype and dosing requirements, but CYP3A4 also plays a role in tacrolimus clearance.[11]

Goal blood levels of tacrolimus vary depending on the type of transplant, time since transplant, and other factors. Typical blood levels measured are trough levels drawn 30 minutes before the next dose.[5] Because tacrolimus is a substrate of CYP enzymes and the P-glycoprotein efflux transporter, drug interactions primarily occur with agents that inhibit or induce these proteins (Table 9-1).[7] Polymorphisms in genes involved in drug metabolism and drug transport are described here, along with associated predicted phenotypes. However, it is important to note that drug interactions and other clinical factors may be considerable enough to convert a patient from a predicted phenotype to a different phenotype.

Tacrolimus and CYP3A5

Mechanism of Drug–Gene Interaction

Tacrolimus is extensively hepatically metabolized by CYP3A5, the principal enzyme responsible for tacrolimus metabolism.[7,8,10] Numerous studies have shown that tacrolimus blood concentrations are affected by CYP3A5 genotype and predicted metabolism phenotype. Metabolism by CYP3A5 leads to inactivation of the drug, with poor metabolizers having a higher likelihood of achieving target drug trough concentrations in comparison to intermediate or normal metabolizers.[4]

To date, there are nine defined star allele designations based on genotype at particular single nucleotide polymorphisms (SNPs) of the CYP3A5 gene. CYP3A5 *3, *6, and *7 are associated with shortened messenger RNA (mRNA) and loss of function. Other allelic variants are considered rare variants with unknown significance related to effect on function. Wild-type, or homozygotes with a *1/*1 allele designation carrying two functional alleles, are expected to exhibit extensive metabolism. Heterozygotes with one functional allele and one loss-of-function allele are predicted to be intermediate metabolizers. Carriers with at least one functional allele are considered CYP3A5 expressers. Homozygotes with two

TABLE 9-1. Common Drug Interactions That Affect Calcineurin Inhibitor Concentrations

Drug	Impact on TAC Concentrations	Impact on CSA Concentrations
Anti-Infective Agents		
Azole antifungals (Fluconazole, Voriconazole, Itraconazole, Posaconazole)	↑	↑
Azithromycin	↑	↑
Clarithromycin	↑	↑
Erythromycin	↑	↑
Levofloxacin	↑	↑
Lopinavir/Ritonavir	↑	↑
Saquinavir	↑	↑
Glecaprevir/ Pibrentasvir	↑	—
Nafcillin	↓	↓
Rifampin	↓	↓
Efavirenz	↓	↓
Diltiazem	↑	↑
Verapamil	↑	↑
Central Nervous System Agents		
Nefazodone	↑	↑
Carbamazepine	↓	↓
Phenytoin	↓	↓
Phenobarbital	↓	↓
Phosphate Binders		
Sevelamer	↓	↓
Food		
Grapefruit juice	↑	↑
Herbal Supplements		
St. John's wort	↓	↓

TAC = tacrolimus, CSA = cyclosporine
Data from references 5, 6, 59, and 60.

loss-of-function alleles are predicted to be poor metabolizers and are considered CYP3A5 nonexpressers.[4]

Consequence of Drug–Gene Interaction

Individuals carrying two functional alleles (CYP3A5*1/*1), CYP3A5 expressers, are likely to exhibit extensive metabolism, resulting in lower dose-adjusted tacrolimus trough concentrations. Similarly, CYP3A5 expressers carrying one functional allele are projected to have lower dose-adjusted trough concentrations compared to nonexpressers due to predicted intermediate metabolizer phenotype. CYP3A5 expressers have a decreased chance of achieving target tacrolimus concentrations with standard recommended initiation doses.[4,8] Delay in achieving target tacrolimus concentrations potentially exposes patients to risks of inadequate immunosuppression, namely rejection. Thus, transplant recipients carrying at least one functional CYP3A5 allele may require starting doses higher than standard recommended initiation doses of tacrolimus.[8]

CYP3A5 nonexpressers, individuals carrying two nonfunctional alleles, are anticipated to have higher dose-adjusted tacrolimus trough concentrations closer to expected values after administration of standard recommended initiation doses. These individuals would have a higher likelihood of achieving target tacrolimus trough concentrations.[4,8]

Treatment Recommendation

Clinical guidelines that provide recommendations for tacrolimus CYP3A5 genotype-guided dosing have been published by both CPIC and the Dutch Pharmacogenetics Working Group (DPWG). It is recommended to start with increased tacrolimus doses for normal and intermediate metabolizers and with standard doses for poor metabolizers.[4] The most recent CPIC guidelines for tacrolimus recommend initiating therapy with doses 1.5 to 2 times the standard recommended starting dose for CYP3A5 intermediate or extensive metabolizers, with a maximum recommended starting dose of 0.3 mg/kg/day.[4] See Table 9-2 for a summary of genotypes, predicted phenotypes, implications for tacrolimus trough concentrations, and therapeutic dosing recommendations from the PharmGKB annotation of CPIC guidelines for tacrolimus and CYP3A5.[8] After initiation, adjustments to maintenance therapy should be based on therapeutic drug monitoring, and patients need to be evaluated for other clinical factors, including drug interactions, that can affect drug metabolism and dosing requirements.

In summary, therapeutic drug monitoring is necessary to ensure that patients achieve therapeutic tacrolimus trough concentrations to decrease risk of rejection and avoid overexposure that increases risk of toxicity, including nephrotoxicity, hypertension, hyperglycemia, and neurotoxicity. Due to the ability to monitor drug concentrations, pharmacogenetic tests would be most beneficial prior to starting therapy. CYP3A5 pharmacogenetic testing can play an important role in determining an appropriate initial dose that may prevent delays in achieving therapeutic trough concentrations. However, the body of evidence regarding CYP3A5 variability is linked primarily to pharmacokinetic

differences, and we currently do not have sufficient evidence on effects related to clinical outcomes. Thus, CPIC guidelines do not specifically recommend whether or not to test, but do recommend adjusting initial tacrolimus doses accordingly if CYP3A5 genotype is known.[4]

Tacrolimus and CYP3A4

Although there are currently no published CPIC guidelines with CYP3A4 genotype-based recommendations, many studies have demonstrated an association between genotype and pharmacokinetic phenotype. One reason for the lack of published CPIC guidelines may be due to a stronger body of evidence linking CYP3A5 genotype variability with pharmacokinetic differences, partly attributed to high frequency of CYP3A5 poor metabolizer phenotypes in many patient populations (80% to 85% frequency in Caucasians), compared to CYP3A4, for which variants leading to poor metabolism are rare.[4] Additionally, conclusions from studies have not been consistent, with some studies reporting association with CYP3A4 genotypes and tacrolimus exposure and other studies reporting no association.

Mechanism of Drug–Gene Interaction

While studies have demonstrated that CYP3A5 is the primary enzyme responsible for tacrolimus metabolism, CYP3A4 also plays a role in tacrolimus clearance.[11] CYP3A4*22 is a variant associated with decreased CYP3A4 activity. In a study of 99 stable kidney transplant recipients to assess influence of the CYP3A4*22 allele on tacrolimus concentrations, this variant was found to be associated with reduced tacrolimus metabolism. Furthermore, the effect was more pronounced for patients who were carriers of loss-of-function alleles for both CYP3A4 and CYP3A5.[12] Multiple additional studies have confirmed the influence of combined consideration of nonfunctional alleles of CYP3A5 (most notably *3/*3) and nonfunctional alleles of CYP3A4 (CYP3A4*22). CYP3A4*1B is a genetic polymorphism associated with enhanced CYP3A4 activity and increased tacrolimus metabolism.[13,14] Although published data have not been consistent, additional studies have concluded that other CYP3A4 determinants have a marked effect on dose-adjusted tacrolimus concentrations, including a newly described allelic variant, CYP3A4*20, which has been associated with decreased tacrolimus metabolism.[15]

Consequence of Drug–Gene Interaction

One study evaluated a cohort of 272 renal transplant patients for associations between CYP3A4*22 and CYP3A5*3

TABLE 9-2. Tacrolimus Genotype-Guided Therapeutic Recommendations

Likely Phenotype[a]	Genotypes	Examples Of Diplotypes[b]	Implications For Tacrolimus Pharmacologic Measures	Therapeutic Recommendations[c]	Classification Of Recommendations[e]
Extensive metabolizer (CYP3A5 expresser)	An individual carrying two functional alleles	*1/*1	Lower dose-adjusted trough concentrations of tacrolimus and decreased chance of achieving target tacrolimus concentrations	Increase starting dose 1.5 to 2 times recommended starting dose.[d] Total starting dose should not exceed 0.3 mg/kg/day. Use therapeutic drug monitoring to guide dose adjustments.	Strong
Intermediate metabolizer (CYP3A5 expresser)	An individual carrying one functional allele and one nonfunctional allele	*1/*3, *1/*6, *1/*7	Lower dose-adjusted trough concentrations of tacrolimus and decreased chance of achieving target tacrolimus concentrations	Increase starting dose 1.5 to 2 times recommended starting dose.[d] Total starting dose should not exceed 0.3 mg/kg/day. Use therapeutic drug monitoring to guide dose adjustments.	Strong
Poor metabolizer (CYP3A5 non-expresser)	An individual carrying two nonfunctional alleles	*3/*3, *6/*6, *7/*7, *3/*6, *3/*7, *6/*7	Higher ("normal") dose-adjusted trough concentrations of tacrolimus and increased chance of achieving target tacrolimus concentrations	Initiate therapy with standard recommended dose. Use therapeutic drug monitoring to guide dose adjustments.	Strong

[a]*Typically with other CYP enzymes, an extensive metabolizer would be classified as a "normal" metabolizer, and therefore, the drug dose would not change based on the patient's genotype. However, in the case of CYP3A5 and tacrolimus, a CYP3A5 expresser (i.e., CYP3A5 extensive metabolizer or intermediate metabolizer) would require a higher recommended starting dose and the CYP3A5 nonexpresser (i.e., poor metabolizer) would require the standard recommended starting dose.*

[b]*Additional rare variants such as CYP3A5*2, *8, and *9 may be found that are of unknown functional significance. However, if a copy of *1 is present, the expected phenotype would be intermediate metabolizer.*

[c]*This recommendation includes the use of tacrolimus in kidney, heart, lung, and hematopoietic stem cell transplant patients and liver transplant patients where the donor and recipient genotypes are identical.*

[d]*Further dose adjustments or selection of alternative therapy may be necessary due to other clinical factors (e.g., medication interactions or hepatic function).*

[e]*Rating scheme is described in 2015 Supplement of the CPIC Guideline for tacrolimus and CYP3A5.*

Source: Reproduced, with permission, from Whirl-Carrillo M, McDonagh EM, Hebert JM, et al. Pharmacogenomics knowledge for personalized medicine. Clin Pharmacol Ther. 2012;92(4):414–417.

and dose-adjusted tacrolimus trough concentrations. Patients were genotyped and assigned phenotypic designations as follows: extensive metabolizers (CYP3A4*1/*1 and CYP3A5*1 carriers), intermediate metabolizers (CYP3A4*1/*1 with CYP3A5*3/*3 or CYP3A4*22 carriers with CYP3A5*1 carriers), or poor metabolizers (CYP3A4*22 carriers with CYP3A5*3/*3).[16] Based on combined consideration of CYP3A4*22 and CYP3A5*3 loss-of-function alleles, poor metabolizers were significantly more likely to have overexposure associated with supratherapeutic dose-adjusted tacrolimus concentrations, while extensive metabolizers were significantly more likely to have subtherapeutic concentrations five to seven days after transplantation.[16]

TABLE 9-3. Proposed Consideration of CYP3A4 and CYP3A5 Combined Genotype-Guided Dosing

Dosing Guideline	CYP3A5*3/*3 + CYP3A4*22	CYP3A5*3/*3 + CYP3A4*1/*1	CYP3A5*1/*3 + CYP3A4*1/*1	CYP3A5*1/*1 + CYP3A4*1/*1
Universal dose	Standard recommended dose (0.20 mg/kg/day)	Standard recommended dose (0.20 mg/kg/day)	Standard recommended dose (0.20 mg/kg/day)	Standard recommended dose (0.20 mg/kg/day)
Current CPIC recommendation	Standard recommended dose (0.20 mg/kg/day)	Standard recommended dose (0.20 mg/kg/day)	1.5–2 times the standard dose but do not exceed 0.3 mg/kg/day	1.5–2 times the standard dose but do not exceed 0.3 mg/kg/day
Proposed revisions based on Elens et al.	0.14 mg/kg/day	0.2–0.25 mg/kg/day	0.3–0.4 mg/kg/day	0.3–0.4 mg/kg/day

Note: Standard recommended doses may vary according to transplantation type and immunosuppressive regimen. Genotype-guided dosing recommendations should be adjusted accordingly, and other clinical factors should be taken into consideration.

Source: Reproduced, with permission, from Whirl-Carrillo M, McDonagh EM, Hebert JM, et al. Pharmacogenomics knowledge for personalized medicine. Clin Pharmacol Ther. 2012;92(4):414–417.

A meta-analysis evaluating seven studies involving renal transplant recipients reported that carriers of the CYP3A4*1B SNP had lower dose-adjusted tacrolimus concentrations compared to CYP3A4*1/*1 homozygotes. The authors concluded that the CYP3A4*1B polymorphism affects tacrolimus dose requirements.[14] Patients with the CYP3A4*1B/*1B or CYP3A4*1B/*1 genotype may require increased tacrolimus doses compared to transplant recipients with the *1/*1 genotype.[8]

Treatment Recommendation

Based on a discriminant analysis comparing the relevance of CYP3A4/CYP3A5 combined and CYP3A5*3, Elens and Haufroid[17] recommend incorporating CYP3A4*22 genotype–based initial dosing recommendations for Caucasian patients into existing CPIC guidelines for tacrolimus, which currently only consider CYP3A5 genotype. They further provide drug dosing recommendations based on combined genotype (Table 9-3).[8]

Carriers of the CYP3A4*1B variant may require increased tacrolimus dose requirements. Because there are currently no published guidelines with CYP3A4 genotype–based recommendations, consideration of CYP3A4 variants should be coupled with evaluation of other genetic factors such as CYP3A5 genotype, as well as relevant clinical information.

Tacrolimus and ABCB1

Mechanism and Consequence of Drug–Gene Interaction

A number of studies have found no significant association between dose-adjusted tacrolimus levels and various polymorphisms of ABCB1, which encodes for the efflux transporter P-glycoprotein. However, one study suggests a potential pharmacodynamic effect with ABCB1 3435C>T SNP associated with a decrease in mRNA stability and effects on IL-2 production.[18] Another recently published study identified an ABCB1 donor polymorphism (ABCB1 c.1199GA/AA) that results in altered efflux of CNIs and may be associated with increased risk of rejection in patients receiving a tacrolimus-based immunosuppressive regimen, although the variant identified is rare.[19] A different study investigating ABCB1 as a determinant of tacrolimus levels identified ABCB1 61A>G as a novel variant that can affect dose-adjusted tacrolimus levels in kidney transplant recipients.[20] While various studies so far suggest associations, they have not demonstrated a substantial effect on tacrolimus pharmacokinetics and pharmacodynamics. ABCB1 genotyping is not currently recommended to guide tacrolimus dosing.[21,22]

Tacrolimus and NR1I2 and NR1I3

Mechanism and Consequence of Drug–Gene Interaction

NR1I2 and NR1I3 are genes that encode for nuclear receptors that function to regulate transcription of drug-metabolizing enzymes and drug transporters.[23] Although studies have reported significant differences in tacrolimus concentrations associated with the NR1I2 rs3814055 SNP, other studies did not report any significant associations with NR1I2.[23,24] Due to the lack of consistent associations, there are no current recommendations to address genotyping NR1I2 and NR1I3 in the standard of care for transplant patients.

Cyclosporine

Background

Cyclosporine is a CNI that, like tacrolimus, exerts its immunosuppressive effects through inhibition of the production and liberation of IL-2.[1,6] IL-2 plays a central role in allograft rejection through activation and proliferation of cytotoxic T lymphocytes. Clinically, cyclosporine is used to prevent, not treat, acute allograft rejection.[1]

Multiple cyclosporine formulations exist.[1,6] The original formulation, cyclosporine nonmodified (Sandimmune), is formulated in olive oil, which leads to variable and potentially erratic absorption, especially in the case of biliary dysfunction or diarrhea. Newer formulations, cyclosporine modified (Neoral and Gengraf), are microemulsions, which affords greater bioavailability and more rapid, more extensive, and less variable absorption compared with cyclosporine nonmodified.[1] For these reasons, cyclosporine nonmodified and cyclosporine modified are not bioequivalent and cannot be used interchangeably. Cyclosporine distributes widely with a volume of distribution between 4 and 6 liters per kilogram. Cyclosporine is extensively hepatically metabolized via CYP3A, is a substrate of P-glycoprotein, and has significant first-pass metabolism with oral administration. As with tacrolimus, drug interactions primarily occur with agents that inhibit or induce these proteins (Table 9-1). Goal blood levels of cyclosporine vary depending on the type of transplant, time since transplant, and other factors. Typical blood levels assessed are trough levels and at two hours post-oral administration.[6]

Cyclosporine and ABCB1

Mechanism of Drug–Gene Interaction

ABCB1 variants may influence P-glycoprotein expression and result in modifications to drug efflux. In a study of 64 stable renal, liver, and lung transplant patients, ABCB1 1199A carriers presented a 1.8-fold decreased cyclosporine intracellular concentration, whereas the 3435C>T carriers presented a 1.7-fold increased intracellular, as well as a 1.2-fold increased blood concentration. In contrast, ABCB1 61A>G, 1236C>T, and 2677G>T polymorphisms did not influence cyclosporine intracellular and blood concentrations.[25]

Consequence of Drug–Gene Interaction

In an investigation of 4471 white, CNI-treated kidney transplant patients in the United Kingdom, kidney donor CC genotype at C3435T (rs1045642) within ABCB1, a variant known to alter the expression of P-glycoprotein, was associated with an increased risk for long-term graft failure compared with non-CC genotype.[26] In a case-control study, 18 of 97 patients developed cyclosporine-associated nephrotoxicity and showed complete recovery of renal function in all cases when switched to a CNI-free regimen. Both recipients and donors were genotyped for ABCB1 polymorphisms at the positions 3435C-->T and 2677G-->T/A. Donor ABCB1 3435TT genotype was strongly associated with cyclosporine-associated nephrotoxicity.[27]

Treatment Recommendation

In summary, ABCB1 3435C>T has been associated with altered intracellular and blood cyclosporine concentrations, increased risk of long-term renal allograft failure, and increased risk of cyclosporine-associated nephrotoxicity. However, no currently published clinical guidelines address genotyping ABCB1 in the standard of care for transplant patients.

Cyclosporine and CYP3A4/CYP3A5

Mechanism of Drug–Gene Interaction

In a study of 103 Chinese renal transplant patients, those with CYP3A4*18B alleles were found to have lower dose-adjusted concentrations of cyclosporine compared with CYP3A4*1/*1 in the first month post-transplant. No association was found with multidrug-resistant 1 (MDR1) and CYP3A5*3 polymorphisms.[28] In a study of 151 kidney and heart transplant patients, those carrying the CYP3A4*1B variant allele had a significantly higher oral cyclosporine clearance compared with patients homozygous for CYP3A4*1.[29]

Consequence of Drug–Gene Interaction

CYP3A4*18B association with lower dose-adjusted cyclosporine concentrations suggest that higher doses of cyclosporine may be needed in patients with CYP3A4*18B alleles.[28] Although patients carrying the CYP3A4*1B variant allele had higher oral cyclosporine clearance, the effect was small and determined by the investigators to be unlikely to affect cyclosporine dosing practically.[29]

A number of studies have found no association between dose-adjusted cyclosporine levels and various polymorphisms. No significant dose-adjusted cyclosporine trough level associations were found in a study of 110 kidney transplant patients who were genotyped for CYP3A4*1B and *3, CYP3A5*3 and *6, and MDR-1 C3435T polymorphisms.[30] In a separate study of 171 patients genotyped for CYP3A5*3; CYP3A4*1B;

and the ABCB1 1236 C>T, 2677 G>T/A, and 3435 C>T SNPs, no significant dose-adjusted cyclosporine trough or two-hour post-dose-level associations were found.[31] Similar findings were seen in a study of 137 kidney transplant patients, in which no associations were found between CYP3A5*3 and *6 genotypes and dose-adjusted cyclosporine trough levels.[32] Finally, in a study of renal transplant patients, no significant association was found between CYP3A5*3/*3, CYP3A5*1/*3, and CYP3A5*1/*1 polymorphisms, with cyclosporine and metabolite levels suggesting minimal effect of these polymorphisms on cyclosporine metabolism.[33]

Treatment Recommendation

Results from small-scale studies suggest that transplant recipients who are carriers of CYP3A4*18B may need higher doses of cyclosporine. For other genetic variants, small effect sizes and lack of association with altered drug metabolism do not support genotype-based dosing. Currently, there are no clinically actionable pharmacogenomic relationships for cyclosporine and CYP3A4 or CYP3A5, and no published clinical guidelines address genotyping prior to cyclosporine initiation.

OTHER IMMUNOSUPPRESSIVE AGENTS

Mycophenolate

Background

Mycophenolate was approved by the FDA in 1995.[34] It was originally developed to treat autoimmune diseases and is used for conditions such as lupus, psoriasis, scleroderma, and autoimmune hepatitis. The most common use of mycophenolate in transplantation is after solid organ transplantation, and it has become the first-line antimetabolite in immunosuppressive regimens. It is administered concomitantly with other immunosuppressants, most often with a CNI.[34] Mycophenolate has also been used as adjunct therapy for prevention and treatment of GVHD in bone marrow transplant recipients.[34,35] Although not recommended to be used as monotherapy to prevent rejection due to increased risk of graft failure, it has become a key component of CNI-sparing regimens used to reduce CNI exposure and toxicity.[36] A meta-analysis of 56 randomized clinical trials for renal transplant patients suggested that decreasing exposure to CNI after kidney transplant may improve graft function without evidence for increased risk of rejection.[36]

Mycophenolic acid (MPA) is the active metabolite and has a cytostatic effect on T and B lymphocytes by suppressing proliferation. It is an inhibitor of inosine-5'-monophosphate dehydrogenase (IMPDH), an important enzyme for nucleotide synthesis that is essential for the T- and B-lymphocyte proliferation pathway. It is available in intravenous and oral formulations as a prodrug, mycophenolate mofetil (MMF, Cellcept), and as the active moiety in a delayed-release oral sodium salt formulation as mycophenolic acid (Myfortic). MMF is hydrolyzed by plasma and tissue esterases to MPA.[34] MPA is further glucuronidated to an inactive metabolite in the liver by uridine diphosphate–glucuronosyl transferase (UGT) enzymes.[35] Inactive metabolites conjugated with glucuronic acid can undergo enterohepatic recycling via organic anion transporter proteins (OATPs) coded for by solute carrier organic anion (SLCO) transporter genes and are reactivated to MPA, often resulting in a secondary peak after administration.[34] Glucuronidated metabolites are also transported by efflux transporters, such as ATP-binding cassette transporter C2 and MDR-related protein 2 (ABCC2/MRP2) for renal excretion.[22] Variation in genes responsible for MPA metabolism, enterohepatic recycling, transport, and pharmacologic targets may contribute to variability in pharmacokinetics or drug response and have been described in the literature.[34] The most common adverse effects are gastrointestinal effects and hematologic effects such as anemia, leukopenia, neutropenia, pancytopenia, and thrombocytopenia.[37] Some studies have investigated the effects of gene variants on adverse effects such as gastrointestinal intolerance and leukopenia.[8]

Mycophenolate and IMPDH

Mechanism of Drug–Gene Interaction

Because MPA is an inhibitor of IMPDH, gene variants of this drug target have the potential to affect T- and B-lymphocyte proliferation and degree of immunosuppression. Multiple studies have examined the potential effects of gene variants of the mycophenolic acid target IMPDH on efficacy in preventing acute rejection and on risk of adverse effects.[8]

Consequence of Drug–Gene Interaction

A study published in 2008 genotyped 191 renal transplant recipients and concluded that the IMPDH1 rs2278293 and rs2278294 variants were significantly associated with the incidence of acute rejection within one year following renal transplantation.[38] Gensburger et al.[39] evaluated multiple IMPDH1 and IMPDH2 polymorphisms in 456 patients and reported an association with IMPDH1 rs277294 and lower risk of biopsy-proven acute rejection, as well as a higher risk for leukopenia within the first year after transplantation. They concluded that there was no significant association with clinical outcomes for any of the other polymorphisms studied, including IMPDH1 rs2778293.[39] A separate study of 82 renal transplant patients suggested a potential influence of IMPDH1 rs2278293 polymorphism on risk of subclinical acute rejection within one month following transplantation.[40] However, a larger-scale study conducted later genotyped 1040 random samples of renal transplant recipients for IMPDH1 rs2278293 and rs2278294 and IMPDH2 rs11706052 variants. No association was found between these variants and MMF tolerated dose, and evidence did not support that presence of these IMPDH variants was associated with risk for rejection and graft survival.[41]

A study investigating the influence of IMPDH1 haplotypes on gastrointestinal intolerance was conducted in 59 pediatric heart transplant patients who were also taking either cyclosporine or tacrolimus.[42] Investigators identified ten haplotypes in this patient population and found one that was significantly associated with gastrointestinal intolerance, with 59.1% experiencing gastrointestinal intolerance among carriers and 21.6% experiencing gastrointestinal intolerance among non-carriers ($p = 0.005$).[42]

Treatment Recommendation

While polymorphisms within genes encoding drug targets IMPDH have been reported to affect pharmacokinetics, risk for adverse effects and, to a small degree, clinical outcomes, evidence has not been conclusive enough to make strong genotype-based recommendations.[1,22,34] Currently, there are no clinically actionable pharmacogenomic relationships for mycophenolate and IMPDH, and no published clinical guidelines address genotyping prior to drug initiation.

Mycophenolate and UGT, ABCC1, ABCC2, SLCO1B1, and SLCO1B3

Mechanism of Drug–Gene Interaction

UGT1A9, UGT1A8, and UGT2B7 are enzymes involved in glucuronidation of MPA to its inactive metabolite, and variants have been reported to influence MPA response or pharmacokinetics, but evidence is not consistent for any strong associations.[43]

Consequence of Drug–Gene Interaction

Various UGT1A9 alleles have been associated with potential increased risk of allograft rejection or decreased graft function in renal transplant patients, as was seen with the UGT1A9 98C allele and reduced kidney function following renal transplantation.[43] A pharmacokinetic study evaluating several SNPs of UGT1A9, UGT1A8, UGT2B7, and ABCC2 found statistically significant increased MPA exposure resulting from more extensive enterohepatic circulation for patients with the UGT1A9-118(dT)(10) allele. The study also found increased exposure to a pharmacologically active metabolite associated with one ABCC2 polymorphism (1249G>A), but no other significant pharmacokinetic differences for any of the other SNPs studied.[44]

Additional studies have found UGT polymorphisms associated with increased risk of adverse events, including anemia and leukopenia, while others have identified potential SLCO1B1 (SLCO1B1*5) variants associated with decreased risk for MPA-related adverse effects.[45,46]

Treatment Recommendation

While polymorphisms within genes encoding UGT enzymes responsible for drug metabolism, transporters involved in enterohepatic recycling (SLCO), and MRP2 transporters (ABCC2) have been reported to affect pharmacokinetics, risk for adverse effects, and, to a small degree, clinical outcomes, evidence has not been conclusive enough to make strong genotype-based recommendations for mycophenolate.[1,22,34]

Mycophenolate and Hypoxanthine–Guanine Phosphoribosyltransferase (HGPRT) Deficiency

HGPRT is not a gene directly involved in MPA pharmacokinetics or pharmacodynamics. Regardless, it is worth mentioning that because MPA is an inhibitor of IMPDH, MMF and MPA use should be avoided in patients with hereditary HGPRT deficiency such as Lesch-Nyan and Kelley-Seegmiller syndromes.[38,39] Administration of MPA can exacerbate symptoms of the disease related to gout and elevated uric acids levels, including renal failure.[47,48]

MECHANISTIC TARGET OF RAPAMYCIN (mTOR) INHIBITORS

Inhibitors of the kinase mTOR have become increasingly used in transplantation. Inhibition of mTOR suppresses

T-cell proliferation, thereby preventing acute allograft rejection. Two mTOR inhibitors, sirolimus and everolimus, will be discussed in this chapter.[49,50]

Sirolimus

Background

Sirolimus was approved by the FDA in 1999 and is available in tablets and oral solution.[49] Bioavailability of the tablet and oral solution formulations is 27% and 14%, respectively. Thus, these two formulations are not considered interchangeable. Sirolimus distributes extensively and has a volume of distribution of 4 to 20 liters per kilogram. Sirolimus is metabolized extensively in the intestinal wall and liver by CYP3A4 and is a substrate of P-glycoprotein.[51] The therapeutic range of sirolimus is 5 to 15 mcg/L in blood. Concentrations lower than 5 mcg/L are associated with rejection, while concentrations higher than 15 mcg/L are associated with adverse effects.[1]

Sirolimus and CYP3A5

Mechanism and Consequence of Drug–Gene Interaction

In a study of 47 renal transplant patients, the CYP3A5*3 polymorphism was associated with decreases in sirolimus metabolic activity and oral clearance.[52] In a later study of 105 healthy volunteers and 50 renal transplant patients, those with the CYP3A5*3 polymorphism had significantly higher sirolimus concentration-to-dose ratios compared with those with the *1 allele, which required significantly less sirolimus to achieve adequate blood trough concentrations.[53] Although patients with the CYP3A5*3 polymorphism may require lower sirolimus doses, there are currently no published guidelines with recommendations for genotype-based dosing. Consideration of genetic polymorphisms should be coupled with evaluation of other clinical factors.

Sirolimus and ABCB1 and IL-10

Mechanism and Consequence of Drug–Gene Interaction

In a study of 86 renal transplant patients, ABCB1 3435C>T and IL-10 -1082G>A were significantly associated with long-term sirolimus dose requirements. Mean sirolimus weight-normalized trough concentrations were 48% higher in patients with the ABCB1 3435CT/

TT genotype than those with the 3435CC genotype and was 24% higher in IL-10-1082GG compared with -1082AG/AA.[54] As with CYP3A5, there are currently no published guidelines with recommendations for genotype-based sirolimus dosing for ABCB1 or IL-10.

Sirolimus and Subclinical or Negligible Pharmacogenetic Associations

In an in vitro study of microsomes from 113 stable kidney transplant recipients, no significant association was found between CYP3A4, CYP3A5, or peroxisome proliferator–activated receptor alpha (PPARα) genotypes and sirolimus dose, blood concentration, or concentration-to-dose ratio. The CYP3A4*22 allele resulted in approximately 20% lower metabolic rates of sirolimus.[55]

Everolimus

Background

Everolimus was approved by the FDA in 2009 and is available in a tablet formulation. Absorption is rapid, and bioavailability is approximately 30%. Everolimus distributes widely with an apparent volume of distribution of 128 to 589 liters.[50] Everolimus is extensively metabolized in the liver and is a substrate of CYP3A4 and P-glycoprotein.[56] The therapeutic range of everolimus is 5 to 15 mcg/L in blood.[50]

Everolimus and Clinically Significant Pharmacogenetic Associations

No studies have thus far shown clinically significant pharmacogenetic associations related to everolimus exposure or clinical outcomes in solid organ transplant recipients, and there are currently no recommendations for genotype-guided dosing.

Everolimus and Subclinical or Negligible Pharmacogenetic Associations

In a study of 53 renal transplant patients, ABCB1, CYP3A5, CYP2C8, and PXR polymorphisms had no clinically relevant effect on everolimus pharmacokinetics.[57] In another study of 65 lung transplant patients, ABCB1 c.1236C>T, ABCB1 c.2677G>T/A, and ABCB1 c.3435C>T; CYP3A4*1B, CYP3A5*3, and CYP2C8*2/*3/*4; and pregnane X receptor (NR1I2) c.44477T>C, c.63396C>T, and c.69789A>G polymorphisms did not significantly affect everolimus dose-adjusted levels (Table 9-4).[58]

TABLE 9-4. Genes and Alleles with Clinical and Subclinical Pharmacogenetic Associations

Drug	Gene	Polymorphism	rs Number	Effect	Clinical Significance	CPIC Recommendations Available?
Tacrolimus	CYP3A5	Homozygous *3 *6 *7	rs776746 rs10264272 rs41303343	Poor drug metabolism (CYP3A5 nonexpresser)	Higher likelihood of achieving target trough concentrations with standard dosing.	Yes
		*1/*3, *1/*6, *1/*7	—	Intermediate drug metabolism (CYP3A5 expresser)	Lower likelihood of achieving target trough concentrations with standard dosing. Initiating therapy with 1.5–2 times starting dose recommended.	
		Wildtype or *1/*1	—	Extensive drug metabolism (CYP3A5 expresser)		
	CYP3A4	*22	rs35599367	Decreased drug metabolism	Potential for increased likelihood of achieving target trough concentrations, especially when combined with CYP3A5 variants. May require lower initiation doses.	No
		*1B	rs2740574	Enhanced drug metabolism	Potential for decreased likelihood of achieving target trough concentrations. May require higher tacrolimus doses.	
	ABCB1	3435C>T	rs1045642	Potential for altered clearance and IL-2 production	None demonstrated; theoretical effect on risk of rejection.	No
		1199G>A	rs2229109	Modified drug efflux and altered drug levels		
		61A>G	rs9282564	Altered drug levels		
	NR1I2	T/T	rs3814055	Altered drug levels		No
Cyclosporine	ABCB1	3435C>T	rs1045642	Altered intracellular and blood levels	Increased risk of long-term renal allograft failure and increased risk of cyclosporine-associated nephrotoxicity.	No
	CYP3A4	*18B (8266G>A)	Not assigned	Increased drug clearance	None demonstrated.	No

(Continued)

TABLE 9-4. Genes and Alleles with Clinical and Subclinical Pharmacogenetic Associations (*Continued*)

Drug	Gene	Polymorphism	rs Number	Effect	Clinical Significance	CPIC Recommendations Available?
Mycophenolate	IMPDH1	IVS7+125G>A	rs2278293	Acute rejection	Conflicting evidence for risk of rejection, but potential for decreased risk of biopsy-proven acute rejection and increased risk for leukopenia.	No
		IVS8-106G>A	rs2278294	Acute rejection and higher risk for leukopenia		
		1572C>T	rs2228075	Gastrointestinal intolerance	Increased risk of gastrointestinal intolerance.	
	UGT1A9	98T>C	rs17868320	Reduced kidney function	Potential for reduced kidney function following renal transplantation, but studies report contradictory findings.	No
		118(dT)(10)	rs3832043	More extensive enterohepatic circulation	Increased drug exposure.	
	ABCC2	1249G>A	rs2273697	Altered expression of drug-efflux protein	Increased exposure to pharmacologically active metabolite.	No
	SLCO1B1	*5	rs4149056	Altered hepatic uptake	Decreased risk of adverse effects.	No
Sirolimus	CYP3A5	*3	rs776746	Decreased drug metabolism and oral clearance	Increased drug concentrations	No
	ABCB1	3435C>T	rs1045642	Altered ABCB1 function		No
	IL-10	1082G>A	rs1800896	Altered CYP3A activity and P-gp expression		No

CASE SCENARIO

Patient Case

A 57-year-old, 80-kg African American male with end-stage renal disease secondary to diabetes and hypertension has been undergoing hemodialysis three times a week for the past two years. Other significant medical problems include anemia, hyperlipidemia, seizures, depression, and right foot amputation two years ago. The patient is admitted to the hospital for a deceased kidney transplant. Home medications include insulin glargine 30 units injected subcutaneously twice a day, insulin lispro 20 units injected subcutaneously three times a day before meals, amlodipine 10 mg taken orally once daily, epoetin alfa 10,000 units administered intravenously three times a week, ferrous sulfate 325 mg taken orally once daily, carbamazepine extended-release 200 mg taken orally twice daily, and pravastatin 20 mg taken orally once daily.

The transplant center protocol includes induction immunosuppressive therapy with rabbit antithymocyte globulin, followed by a maintenance immunosuppressive regimen containing oral tacrolimus, oral mycophenolate mofetil, and a glucocorticoid (intravenous methylprednisolone for the first three days, followed by oral prednisone).

Question 1. Which statement regarding pharmacogenetic testing for immunosuppressive agents is true?

a. Due to safety concerns, CYP3A5 genotyping is required before tacrolimus can be administered to this patient.
b. Evidence-based clinical guidelines recommend avoiding mycophenolate in patients with specific IMPDH genotypes.
c. Evidence-based clinical guidelines recommend genotype-based adjustments to initial tacrolimus dose if CYP3A5 genotype is known.
d. If CYP3A5 genotype is not known, the patient should be placed on cyclosporine instead of tacrolimus.

Question 2. Planned maintenance immunosuppression includes oral tacrolimus 0.1 mg/kg/day, with a tacrolimus target trough of 7 to 10 ng/mL for the first month after transplantation. The patient previously completed a comprehensive pharmacogenomics test panel that included testing for CYP3A5 variants. His CYP3A5 diplotype is *1/*3.

Which statement is consistent with information from published CPIC guidelines for tacrolimus?

a. The predicted phenotype is intermediate metabolizer (CYP3A5 expresser), with a decreased likelihood of achieving goal tacrolimus concentrations.
b. The predicted phenotype is intermediate metabolizer (CYP3A5 expresser), with an increased likelihood of achieving goal tacrolimus concentrations.
c. The predicted phenotype is CYP3A5 nonexpresser, with a decreased likelihood of achieving goal tacrolimus concentrations.
d. The predicted phenotype is extensive metabolizer (CYP3A5 expresser), with a decreased likelihood of achieving goal tacrolimus concentrations.

Question 3. Which recommendation is consistent with information from published CPIC guidelines for tacrolimus?

a. Decrease initial tacrolimus dose to 0.05 mg/kg/day.
b. Increase initial tacrolimus dose to 0.15 mg/kg/day.
c. Initiate therapy with standard recommended tacrolimus dose of 0.1 mg/kg/day.
d. Increase initial tacrolimus dose to 0.4 mg/kg/day.

Question 4. Considering CYP3A5 genotype-based recommendations, the team initiates immediate-release tacrolimus 0.15 mg/kg/day (6 mg orally twice daily). A whole-blood tacrolimus trough concentration, drawn two days later, comes back at 5 ng/mL. Which recommendation is appropriate?

a. Use the CYP3A5 genotype to determine if it is necessary to adjust the current tacrolimus dose.
b. Increase the patient's tacrolimus dosage and monitor to re-evaluate whole-blood trough concentration.
c. Decrease the patient's tacrolimus dosage and monitor to re-evaluate whole-blood trough concentration.
d. Continue the current tacrolimus regimen, as the dose was based on CYP3A5 genotype and drug-level monitoring is not indicated.

Answers:

Question 1. *c.* There are no requirements for tacrolimus pharmacogenetic testing described in evidence-based clinical guidelines or FDA drug labels. However, the CPIC guideline for tacrolimus and CYP3A5 does recommend adjustments to initial tacrolimus doses for CYP3A5 expressers. There are currently no evidence-based clinical guidelines for drug-gene pairs for mycophenolate.

Question 2. *a.* The predicted phenotype for *1/*3 is an intermediate metabolizer (CYP3A5 expresser). Patients with this diplotype have lower dose-adjusted tacrolimus trough concentrations and a decreased likelihood of achieving target drug trough concentrations. Therefore, they will likely require higher initial doses to achieve target drug concentrations.

Question 3. *b.* The CPIC guidelines for tacrolimus and CYP3A5 recommend an initial starting dose 1.5 to 2 times the standard recommended dose for CYP3A5 expressers, with a starting dose not to exceed 0.3 mg/kg/day.

Question 4. *b.* Current CPIC guidelines recommend adjustments to initial tacrolimus doses based on CYP3A5 genotype. However, with its narrow therapeutic index, therapeutic drug monitoring is vital in achieving target levels to prevent rejection and avoid toxicity. The patient's current tacrolimus concentration is low, which can represent inadequate immunosuppression. Therefore, it would be appropriate to increase the tacrolimus dosage and assess the trough concentration to assess the effect of the dosage increase. It is important to consider additional clinical factors to determine further tacrolimus dose adjustments, or even continuation of the drug itself. The patient is on carbamazepine, a known CYP3A4 inducer, which can lead to decreased tacrolimus blood concentrations. Additional clinical factors that should be monitored and considered include hepatic function, adverse effects, and allograft function.

PHARMACOGENOMICS CLINICAL PEARLS

Pharmacogenomics in the transplantation domain remain complex. Currently, for the drugs discussed in this chapter, the only published evidence-based clinical guideline from CPIC is for tacrolimus and CYP3A5. However, transplant pharmacogenomics research is ongoing, and discovery of additional genotype variants may contribute to the emergence of clinically actionable recommendations for other immunosuppressant drugs commonly used for patients in this setting.

ABBREVIATIONS AND ACRONYMS

ABCB1 = ATP-binding cassette transporter B1

ABCC2 = ATP-binding cassette transporter C2

CNI = calcineurin inhibitor

CPIC = Clinical Pharmacogenetics Implementation Consortium

CYP = cytochrome P450 enzymes

DPWG = Dutch Pharmacogenetics Working Group

GVHD = graft-versus-host disease

HGPRT = Hypoxanthine-guanine phosphoribosyl-transferase

IL = interleukin-2 (IL-2)

IMPDH = inhibitor of inosine-5'-monophosphate dehydrogenase

MDR = multidrug resistant

MMF = mycophenolate mofetil

MPA = mycophenolic acid

MRP 2 = multidrug resistance-related protein 2

mTOR = mechanistic target of rapamycin

OATPs = organic anion transporter proteins

PPARα = peroxisome proliferator-activated receptor alpha

SNP = single nucleotide polymorphism

REFERENCES

1. Kiang TK, Ensom MH. Immunosuppresants: Cyclosporine, tacrolimus, sirolimus, and mycophenolic acid. In: Beringer PM, ed. *Winter's Basic Clinical Pharmacokinetics.* 6th ed. Philadelphia, PA: Wolters Kluwer Health; 2018:320–347.

2. Hayney MS. Chapter 15. Immunology, transplantation, and vaccines. In: Bertino JS Jr, DeVane C, Fuhr U, Kashuba AD, Ma JD, eds. *Pharmacogenomics: An Introduction and Clinical Perspective.* New York, NY: McGraw-Hill. 2013:197–204.

3. van Gelder T, van Schaik RH., Hesselink DA. Pharmacogenetics and immunosuppressive drugs in solid organ transplantation. *Nat Rev Nephrol.* 2014;10:725–731.

4. Birdwell KA, Decker B, Barbarino JM, et al. Clinical Pharmacogenetics Implementation Consortium (CPIC) guidelines for CYP3A5 genotype and tacrolimus dosing. *Clin Pharmacol Ther.* 2015;98(1):19–24.

5. Tacrolimus. Lexi-Drugs. Lexicomp Online. Hudson, OH: Lexicomp; 2019. Available at https://online-lexi-com.ccl.idm.oclc.org/lco/action/doc/retrieve/docid/patch_f/1801799?cesid=3ZvFk86TC-cJ&searchUrl=%2Flco%2Faction%2Fsearch%3Fq%3Dtacrolimus%26t%3Dname%26va%3Dtacrolimus. Accessed September 20, 2019.

6. Cyclosporine. Lexi-Drugs. Lexicomp Online. Hudson, OH: Lexicomp; 2019. Available at https://online-lexi-com.ccl.idm.oclc.org/lco/action/doc/retrieve/docid/patch_f/1772084?cesid=35zGMMiMX-mR&searchUrl=%2Flco%2Faction%2Fsearch%3Fq%3Dcyclosporine%26t%3Dname%26va%3Dcyclosporine. Accessed September 20, 2019.

7. Barbarino JM, Staatz CE, Venkataramanan R, et al. PharmGKB summary: Cyclosporine and tacrolimus pathways. *Pharmacogenet Genomics.* 2013;23(10):563–585.

8. Whirl-Carrillo M, McDonagh EM, Hebert JM, et al. Pharmacogenomics knowledge for personalized medicine. *Clin Pharmacol Ther.* 2012;92(4):414–417.

9. Johnson HJ, Schonder KS. Solid-organ transplantation. In: DiPiro JT, TalbertL RL, Yee GC, Matzke GR, Wells BG, Posey L, eds. *Pharmacotherapy: A Pathophysiologic Approach.* 10th ed. New York, NY: McGraw-Hill; 2017:1395–1418.

10. Dai Y, Hebert MF, Isoherranen N, et al. Effect of CYP3A5 polymorphism on tacrolimus metabolic clearance in vitro. *Drug Metab Dispos.* 2006;34(5):836–847.

11. Kamdem LK, Streit F, Zanger UM, et al. Contribution of CYP3A5 to the in vitro hepatic clearance of tacrolimus. *Clin Chem.* 2005;51(8):1374–1381.

12. Elens L, van Schaik RH, Panin N, et al. Effect of a new functional CYP3A4 polymorphism on calcineurin inhibitors' dose requirements and trough blood levels in stable renal transplant patients. *Pharmacogenomics*. 2011;12(10):1383–1396.

13. Tavira B, Coto E, Diaz-Corte C, et al. A search for new CYP3A4 variants as determinants of tacrolimus dose requirements in renal-transplanted patients. *Phamacogenet Genomics*. 2013;23(8):445–448.

14. Shi WL, Tang HL, Zhai SD. Effects of the CYP3A4*1B genetic polymorphism on the pharmacokinetics of tacrolimus in adult renal transplant recipients: a meta-analysis. *PLoS One*. 2015;10(6):e0127995.

15. Gomez-Bravo MN, Apellaniz-Ruiz M, Salcedo M, et al. Influence of donor liver CYP3A4*20 loss-of function genotype on tacrolimus pharmacokinetics in transplanted patients. *Phamacogenet Genomics*. 2018;28(2):41–48.

16. Lloberas N, Elens L, Llaudó I, et al. The combination of CYP3A4*22 and CYP3A5*3 single-nucleotide polymorphisms determines tacrolimus dose requirement after kidney transplantation. *Pharmacogenet Genomics*. 2017;27(9):313–322.

17. Elens L, Haufroid V. Genotype-based tacrolimus dosing guidelines: With or without CYP3A4*22? *Pharmacogenomics*. 2017;18(16):1473–1480.

18. Vafadari R, Bouamar R, Hesselink DA, et al. Genetic polymorphisms in ABCB1 influence the pharmacodynamics of tacrolimus. *Ther Drug Monit*. 2013;35(4):459–465.

19. Woillard JB, Gatault P, Nicolas P, et al. A donor and recipient candidate gene association study of allograft loss in renal transplant recipients receiving a tacrolimus-based regimen. *Am J Transplant*. 2018;18(12):2905–2913.

20. Hu R, Barratt DT, Coller JK, et al. CYP3A5*3 and ABCB1 61A>G significantly influence dose-adjusted trough blood tacrolimus concentrations in the first three months post-kidney transplantation. *Basic Clin Pharmacol Toxicol*. 2018;123(3):320–326.

21. Crowley LE, Mekki M, Chand S. Biomarkers and pharmacogenomics in kidney transplantation. *Mol Diagn Ther*. 2018;22(5):537–550.

22. Cascorbi I. The pharmacogenetics of immune-modulating therapy. *Adv Pharmacol*. 2018;83:275–296.

23. Kurzawski M, Malinowski D, Dziewanowski K, Drozdik M. Analysis of common polymorphisms within NR1I2 and NR1I3 genes and tacrolimus dose-adjusted concentration in stable kidney transplant recipients. *Pharmacogenet Genomics*. 2017;27(10):372–377.

24. Birdwell K, Grady B, Choi L, et al. The use of a DNA biobank linked to electronic medical records to characterize pharmacogenomic predictors of tacrolimus dose requirement in kidney transplant recipients. *Pharmacogenet Genomics*. 2012;22(1):32–42.

25. Crettol S, Venetz JP, Fontana M, et al. Influence of ABCB1 genetic polymorphisms on cyclosporine intracellular concentration in transplant recipients. *Pharmacogenet Genomics*. 2008;18(4):307–315.

26. Moore J, McKnight AJ, Dohler B, et al. Donor ABCB1 variant associates with increased risk for kidney allograft failure. *J Am Soc Nephrol*. 2012;23(11):1891–1899.

27. Hauser IA, Schaeffeler E, Gauer S, et al. ABCB1 genotype of the donor but not of the recipient is a major risk factor for cyclosporine-related nephrotoxicity after renal transplantation. *J Am Soc Nephrol*. 2005;16:1501–1511.

28. Qiu XY, Jiao Z, Zhang M, et al. Association of MDR1, CYP3A4*18B, and CYP3A5*3 polymorphisms with cyclosporine pharmacokinetics in Chinese renal transplant recipients. *Eur J Clin Pharmacol*. 2008;64:1069–1084.

29. Hesselink D, van Gelder T, van Schaik RH, et al. Population pharmacokinetics of cyclosporine in kidney and heart transplant recipients and the influence of ethnicity and genetic polymorphisms in the MDR-1, CYP3A4, and CYP3A4 genes. *Clin Pharmacol Ther*. 2004;76:545–556.

30. Hesselink D, van Schaik RH, van der Heiden IP, et al. Genetic polymorphisms of the CYP3A4, CYP3A4, and MDR-1 genes and pharmacokinetic of the calcineurin inhibitors cyclosporine and tacrolimus. *Clin Pharmcol Ther*. 2003;74:245–254.

31. Bouamar R, Hesselink DA, van Schaik RH, et al. Polymorphisms in CYP3A4, CYP3A4, and ABCB1 are not associated with cyclosporine pharmacokinetics nor with cyclosporine clinical end points after renal transplantation. *Ther Drug Monit*. 2011;33:178–184.

32. Zhao Y, Song M, Guan D, et al. Genetic polymorphisms of CYP3A4 genes and concentration of the cyclosporine and tacrolimus. *Transplant Proc*. 2005;37:178–181.

33. Chu XM, Hao HP, Wang GJ, et al. Influence of CYP3A5 genetic polymorphism on cyclosporine A metabolism and elimination in Chinese renal transplant recipients. *Acta Pharmacol Sin*. 2006;27:1504–1508.

34. Staatz CE, Tett SE. Pharmacology and toxicology of mycophenolate in organ transplant recipients: an update. *Arch Toxicol*. 2014;88(7):1351–1389.

35. Mycophenolate. Lexi-Drugs. Lexicomp Online. Hudson, OH: Lexicomp; 2019. Available at https://online-lexi-com.ccl.idm.oclc.org/lco/action/doc/retrieve/docid/patch_f/7327?cesid=a2Y-ThkHiVh9&searchUrl=%2Flco%2Faction%2Fsearch%3Fq%3Dmycophenolate%26t%3Dname%26va%3Dmycophenolate. Accessed September 20, 2019.

36. Sharif A, Shabir S, Chand S, et al. Meta-analysis of calcineurin-inhibitor-sparing regimens in kidney transplantation. *J Am Soc Nephrol*. 2011;22(11):2107–2118.

37. Mycophenolic Acid. In-Depth Answers. Micromedex Healthcare Series [database online]. Greenwood Village, CO: Truven Health Analytics; 2019. Available at https://www-micromedexsolutions-com.ccl.idm.oclc.org/micromedex2/librarian/CS/71424D/ND_PR/evidencexpert/ND_P/evidencexpert/DUPLICATIONSHIELDSYNC/3E37C2/ND_PG/evidencexpert/ND_B/evidencexpert/ND_AppProduct/evidencexpert/ND_T/evidencexpert/PFActionId/evidencexpert.DoIntegratedSearch?SearchTerm=Mycophenolate+Mofetil&fromInterSaltBase=true&false=null&false=null&=null#. Accessed October 27, 2019.

38. Wang J, Yang JW, Zeevi A, et al. IMPDH1 gene polymorphisms and association with acute rejection in renal transplant patients. *Clin Pharmacol Ther*. 2008;83(5):711–717.

39. Gensburger O, Van Schaik RH, Picard N, et. al. Polymorphisms in type I and II inosine monophosphate dehydrogenase genes and association with clinical outcome in patients on mycophenolate mofetil. *Pharmacogenet Genomics*. 2010; 20(9):537–543.

40. Kagaya H, Miura M, Saito M, et al. Correlation of IMPDH1 gene polymorphisms with subclinical acute rejection and mycophenolic acid exposure parameters on day 28 after renal transplantation. *Basic Clin Pharmacol Toxicol*. 2010;107(2):631–636.

41. Shah S, Harwood SM, Döhler B, et al. Inosine monophosphate dehydrogenase polymorphisms and renal allograft outcome. *Transplantation*. 2012;94(5):486–491.

42. Ohmann EL, Burckart GJ, Chen Y, et al. Inosine 5′ monophosphate dehydrogenase 1 haplotypes and association with mycophenolate mofetil gastrointestinal intolerance in pediatric heart transplant patients. *Pediatr Transplant*. 2010;14(7):891–895.

43. Pazik J, Ołdak M, Dąbrowski M, et al. Association of UDP-glucuronosyltransferase 1A9 (UGT1A9) gene polymorphism with kidney allograft function. *Ann Transplant*. 2011;16(4):69–73.

44. Zhang WX, Chen B, Jin Z, et al. Influence of uridine diphosphate (UDP)-glucuronosyltransferases and ABCC2 genetic polymorphisms on the pharmacokinetics of mycophenolic acid and its metabolites in Chinese renal transplant recipients. *Xenobiotica*. 2008;38(11):1422–1436.

45. Woillard JB, Picard N, Thierry A, Touchard G, Marquet P; DOMINOS study group. Associations between polymorphisms in target, metabolism, or transport proteins of mycophenolate sodium and therapeutic or adverse effects in kidney transplant patients. *Pharmacogenet Genomics*. 2014;24(5):256–262.

46. Michelon H, König J, Durrbach A, et al. SLCO1B1 genetic polymorphism influences mycophenolic acid tolerance in renal transplant recipients. *Pharmacogenomics*. 2010;11(12):1703–1713.

47. Cellcept (mycophenolate mofetil) [package insert]. South San Francisco, CA: Genentech USA, Inc.; 2019.

48. Myfortic (mycophenolic acid) [package insert]. East Hanover, NJ: Novartis Pharmaceuticals Corporation; 2016.

49. Sirolimus. Lexi-Drugs. Lexicomp Online. Hudson, OH: Lexicomp; 2019. Available at https://online-lexi-com.ccl.idm.oclc.org/lco/action/doc/retrieve/docid/patch_f/7670?cesid=24RDoJhJ-clP&searchUrl=%2Flco%2Faction%2Fsearch%3Fq%3Dsirolim-us%26t%3Dname%26va%3Dsirolimus. Accessed October 13, 2019.

50. Everolimus. Lexi-Drugs. Lexicomp Online. Hudson, OH: Lexicomp; 2019. Available at https://online-lexi-com.ccl.idm.oclc.org/lco/action/doc/retrieve/docid/patch_f/1700399?cesid=1NvhUFvlP-FO&searchUrl=%2Flco%2Faction%2Fsearch%3Fq%3Deverolim-us%26t%3Dname%26va%3Deverolimus. Accessed October 13, 2019.

51. Rapamune (sirolimus) [package insert]. Philadelphia, PA: Wyeth Pharmaceuticals, Inc.; 2017.

52. Le Meur Y, Djebli N, Szelag JC, et al. CYP3A5*3 influences sirolimus oral clearance in de novo and stable renal transplant recipients. *Clin Pharmacol Ther*. 2006;80(1):51–60.

53. Miao LY, Huang CR, Hou JQ, Qian MY. Association study of ABCB1 and CYP3A5 gene polymorphisms with sirolimus trough concentration and dose requirements in Chinese renal transplant recipients. *Biopharm Drug Dispos*. 2008;29(1):1–5.

54. Sam WJ, Chamberlain CE, Lee SJ, et al. Associations of ABCB1 3435C>T and IL-10-1082G>A polymorphisms with long-term sirolimus dose requirements in renal transplant patients. *Transplantation*. 2011;92(12):1342–1347.

55. Woillard JB, Kamar N, Coste S, et al. Effect of CYP3A4*22, POR*28, and PPARα rs4253728 on sirolimus in vitro metabolism and trough concentrations in kidney transplant recipients. *Clin Chem*. 2013;59(12):1761–1969.

56. Afinitor (everolimus) [package insert]. East Hanover, NJ: Novartis Pharmaceuticals Corporation; 2010.

57. Moes DJ, Press RR, den Hartigh J, et al. Population pharmacokinetics and pharmacogenetics of everolimus in renal transplant patients. *Clin Pharmacokinet*. 2012;51(7):467–480.

58. Schoeppler KE, Aquilante CL, Kiser TH, et al. The impact of genetic polymorphisms, diltiazem, and demographic variables on everolimus trough concentrations in lung transplant recipients. *Clin Transplant*. 2014;28(5):590–597.

59. Kuypers DR. Immunotherapy in elderly transplant recipients: A guide to clinically significant drug interactions. *Drugs Aging*. 2009;26(9):715–737.

60. Jennings DL, Johnson HJ. Solid-organ transplantation. In: DiPiro JT, Yee GC, Posey LM, Haines ST, Nolin TD, Ellingrod V, eds. *Pharmacotherapy: A Pathophysiologic Approach*. 11th ed. New York, NY: McGraw-Hill; 2019:1473–1496.

INDEX

Page numbers followed by "f" denote figures; those followed by "t" denote tables